YOGALIGN

PAIN-FREE YOGA FROM YOUR INNER CORE

by Michaelle Edwards, LMT, ERYT

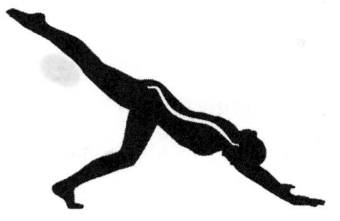

Hihimanu Press

Hanalei, Kauai, Hawaii

2011

Written by Michaelle Edwards
Developmental Edit by Erin Wascher
Edited by Jennifer Regan
Layout by Daria Lacy
Illustrations and book design by Julia O'Reilly
Cartoons by MItch McPeek and Kirstie Beneke
Cover photo by Joel Guy
Cover design by Daria Lacy and Michaelle Edwards
Book photos by Sarah Wall and Zak Gilbert
Photo of Gabrielle Reece by Amber Crago

Printed in the US

The YogAlign Method is a trademarked process.

Hihimanu Press
PO Box 681, Hanalei, Hawaii 96714
Phone   808-826-9230
E-mail   manayoga@yahoo.com
www.yogalign.com • www.yogainjuries.com

First Edition
SBN 9780615544755
Library of Congress Control Number: 2011917334

The publisher/author of this material make no medical claims for its use.
This material is not intended to treat, diagnose, or cure and illness.
If you are in serious pain, please consult with your medical practitioner.

PRAISE FOR YOGALIGN

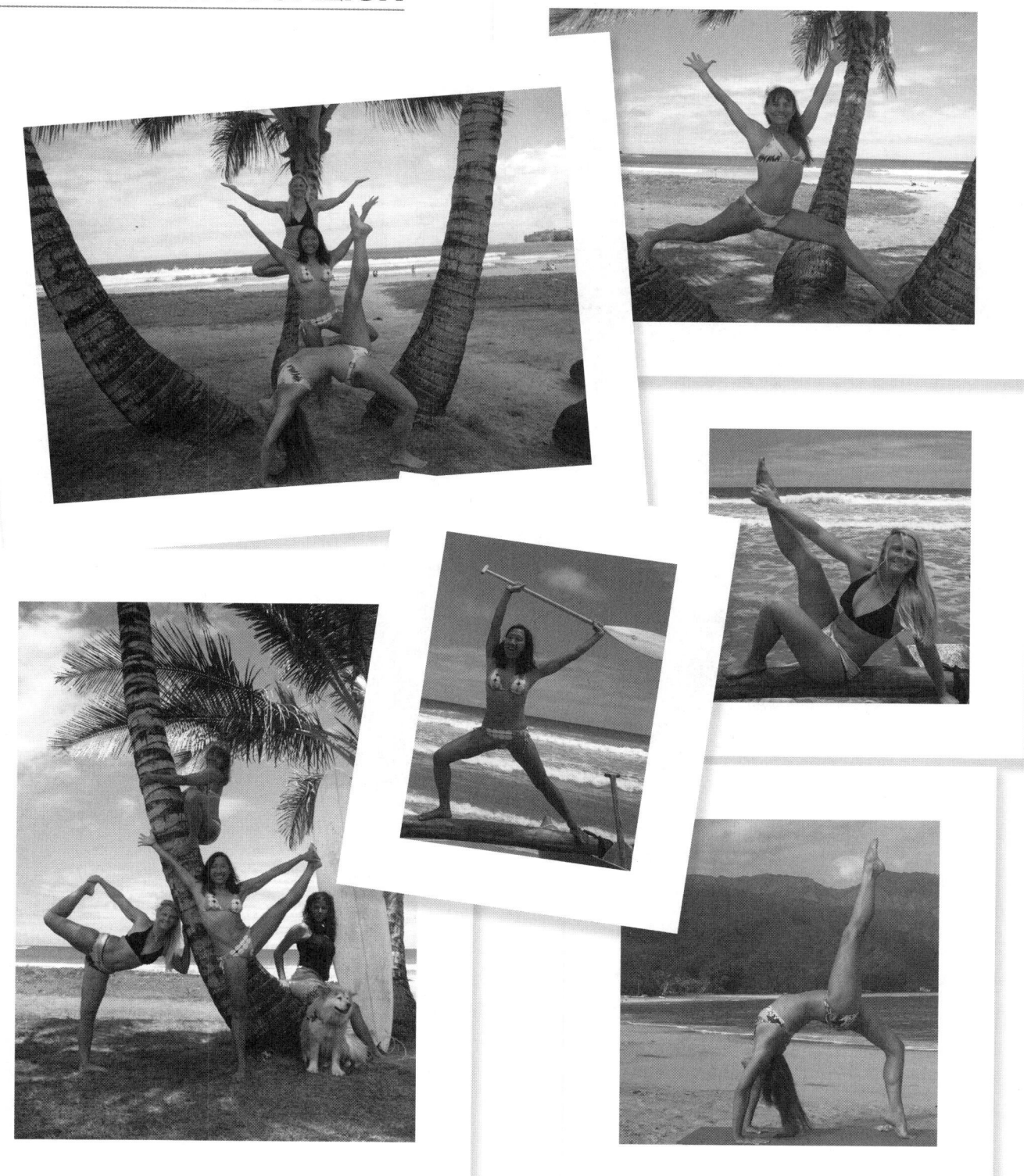

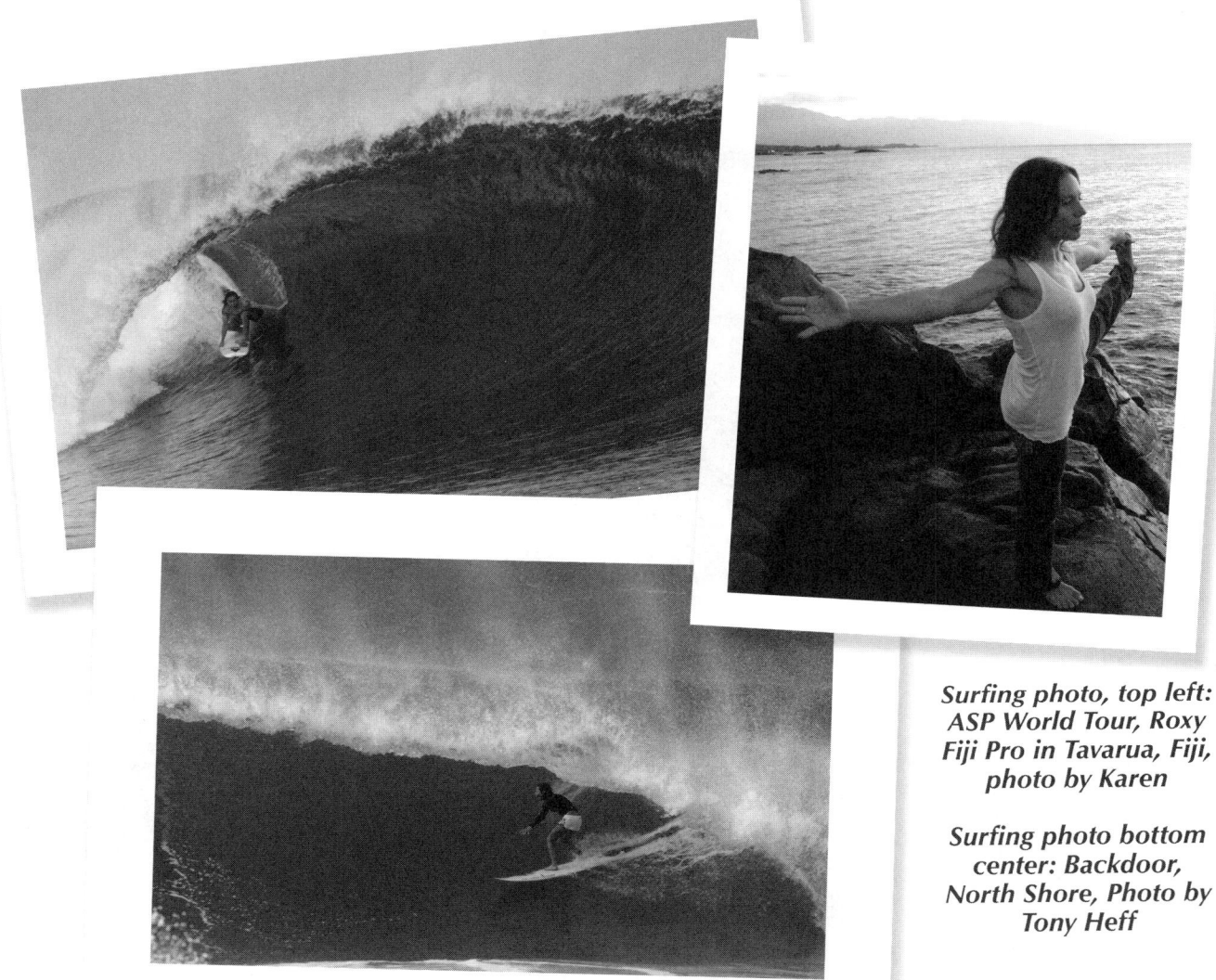

Surfing photo, top left: ASP World Tour, Roxy Fiji Pro in Tavarua, Fiji, photo by Karen

Surfing photo bottom center: Backdoor, North Shore, Photo by Tony Heff

""I have been a surfing professional for over 20 years. Working with Michaelle and learning the Yogalign method of moving the body with structural alignment, and practicing breath work has been the most effective yoga and training I have ever practiced. I no longer have the chronic pain in my shoulders and the sciatica that had plagued me for years. I feel lighter, stronger, and aligned. My shoulders used to be chronically rotated forward and I suffered pain and frequent injuries. With YogAlign, I learned to shift my paddling techniques when surfing and my shoulders are now aligned in all my activities. I know how to keep my body aligned whether surfing, practicing bodywork, or hiking the trails on Kauai. I am now teaching YogAlign and my clients are all experiencing the same effects.

Rochelle Ballard, Professional Surfer, YogAlign Instructor, and Bodyworker.

YOGALIGN **Pain-Free Yoga From Your Inner Core**

"What I experienced with YogAlign was the creation of more space in the fascia, and more muscle control with an increased ability to "turn muscles on and off." YogAlign addresses both chronically tight and shortened anterior flexors, and overstretched and weak shoulder girdle muscles, while also opening up the respiratory system and strengthening intercostal muscles and the diaphragm. It is easy to understand that if the fascia is constricted the muscles alone cannot sustain a change of posture and the ability to breathe fully. I believe the fascia is remodeled by the relief of unhealthy stresses to new more functional stresses applied through the YogAlign method; at the same time muscles are strengthened, stretched, and reprogrammed to sustain a more healthy, energy efficient, alignment. Healthy not only because it helps to decrease wear and tear on a misaligned skeletal structure and joints, but also by allowing more space for the vital organs to function, thereby improving blood supply and respiration. I feel YogAlign promotes awareness and experience of the benefit of unlearning old habits and neurological patterning, which are restrictive and ultimately destructive to one's wellbeing. This awareness and first-hand experience leads to a new feeling of comfort and freedom in our bodies. With YogAlign you have created a safe and accessible path to health, wellness, and longevity that will benefit many. Mahalo (Thank you) Michaelle!"

David Kahle, Physical Therapist, Orcas Island Washington

"After my first group YogAlign class, I feel like I just had the benefits of 10 sessions of rolfing, without the pain."

Bob Shambron, Retired Natural Foods Restauranteur

"I have been practicing YogAlign with Michaelle for 16 months now, and have had huge improvements in my range of motion, breathing function and overall wellbeing. I feel great, with no pain or stiffness even after playing a tough game of volleyball. My body feels fluid and it makes me laugh because I feel as though I am actually doing less now in terms of muscle effort when I exercise. When I went for my physical recently and they measured my height, the nurse did it twice thinking she had made a mistake. The nurse announced with surprise to me that I am now an inch and a quarter taller than the records show at my physical last year. At 61 years old I feel like I am growing younger and my volleyball and surfing are getting better."

Greg Close, National Senior Men's Division Volleyball Player and Stand Up Paddler.

"I am fast approaching my sixth decade. My profession as a pharmacist requires me to stand 8 – 10 hours a day. I would wake up stiff and go to bed exhausted. I booked a YogAlign session with Michaelle and asked my husband of 34 years to join me. He has had scoliosis and back and neck problems his entire life. He is a bigger skeptic than I am but he agreed to try it. Well, two weeks later, after four private sessions with Michaelle, we are feeling and looking better than we have in years. We take with us a Yoga program that we can use in the office, at home, on vacation, walking the dogs, driving the car, or watching TV. I am amazed at how easy the exercises are and how profound the results. YogAlign is designed to create comfort and natural spine alignment while avoiding positions that could cause pain or injury. My husband and I are pleased beyond belief with our results."

William Nations, Satellite Design Engineer and VP, Lynn Nations, Doctor of Pharmacy

❀ ✿

"Recently I spent seven days practicing YogAlign on Oahu at a retreat with pro-surfer Rochelle Ballard, who is a certified YogAlign teacher. We were at her beautiful studio on the north shore of Oahu in April of 2010. I found YogAlign at the right time. It was nice having the adjustments and I was amazed at how much my body changed in such a short amount of time. I don't think my body has opened up that much in the 4 1/2 years of Power Yoga I had practiced previously. I work at a yoga studio that offers a lot of yoga, but YogAlign is what I practice. It has really helped me with my injuries."

Lonnie Butler, Santa Monica, CA.

❀ ✿

"Sheer amazement was how I felt at the end of the first Yogalign class with Michaelle Edwards! Having pain from scoliosis, I could hardly believe how not just my back, but the whole body opened up, became aligned and was completely relaxed! Even my legs felt relaxed and energetically expanded! And yes, the pain was gone and stayed gone for three days after the first class. Now I am going to focus on doing the breathing and poses so I can program the movements into the body by doing them daily. Having done many forms of movement, including ballet and alternative therapeutic movement, I was deeply impressed at how simple, yet extremely useful, the routine Michaelle has created truly is. This would be great for everyone including those who are aging. So five stars and high praise to Michaelle for her discovery and work, which makes it possible for people to learn a new and revolutionary way to help the body. Now people just need to discover it."

Michele Turetzky

"While doing the reclining rest position after a wonderful Yogalign class, I was aware of this bright light expanding inside of me. The masks and armor that I have carried most of my life for survival are being released. As the breathing strengthens my psoas and diaphragm connection, my body's fascial lines are being reprogrammed to hold me balanced in a web. What a gift it is to access this inner light and to have the core strength to walk through life in the truth of who I am. I am deeply grateful to Michaelle for this revolutionary form of yoga and for the changes I am experiencing in all levels of my being: physical, emotional, mental and spiritual."

Juliette LaFleur, Princeville, Kauai

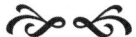

"Michaelle has discovered something innovatively beneficial in the yoga world that many teachers over look: spine alignment. This is a crucial part of one's being, allowing us to grow spiritually and maintain correct body posture for balance, happiness, and energy. What I discovered from studying with Michaelle is that her method—YogAlign— is applicable to all. It not only benefits yoga practitioners, but it can also correct anybody's body posture. Once I started to apply her method to my own asana (yoga) practice, not only have I noticed my own practice deepen, but I also found myself carrying out this method in my everyday routine, which helped to correct my standing and sitting posture. I now experience more happy states of mind and less body aches and pains."

Anthony P. Biduck, Rolfer and Founder of Anahata Healing

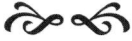

"For years I suffered from low back pain and neck tension especially after a paddling session. In just one session with Michaelle and the YOGALIGN METHOD, I understood natural spine alignment and how to engage it by using my psoas muscles. Learning how to let go of unconscious tension through the PNF (proprioceptive) techniques gave me a huge awakening about how to experience yoga from within. I felt a freedom and comfort in body that I had not felt in years. I discovered how to feel more economical in my body and experience effortless effort. Michaelle has a deep understanding of alignment and breath and yet the teaching was simple and precise. I can apply the principles to all my activities and other yoga classes and I am no longer in pain or misalignment."

Margo Turner, Mother, Triathlete, Hawaiian Canoe Paddler, and Marketing Professional.

"For the last 5 years, I have received frequent sessions of bodywork with very skilled practitioners. I suffered from migraine headaches and lower back pain. I tried many forms of therapy including deep tissue sports massage, chiropractic, osteopathic, cranial sacral, and an orthopedic physician. I would feel some relief for a few weeks and then the pain would return. After just a few weeks of working with Michaelle to align my spine with the YOGALIGN method, the sciatic pain that plagued me for years was gone! It has now been about six months since I began practicing the YOGALIGN method and my sciatic pain and headaches have completely disappeared. I have attained a level of health and fitness that I have not felt since I was a child. The natural blueprint for alignment has become intrinsic in my body, and I feel alive and vibrant. I am even doing hand stands and deep back bends with no pain. As I learned to stretch with resistance and protect my joints, I was never at any time sore from the deep work. After each session I would feel highly energized and yet deeply relaxed. Michaelle is a very gifted teacher and healer and I feel grateful to her for the amazing YOGALIGN system. The system is very easy to learn and I feel I have been given the tools to be my own healer."

John Steinmann, Avocado rancher, Entrepreneur, Surfer, Cyclist, Father.

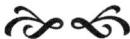

"I have studied YogAlign with Michaelle for over five years and I have attained a high level of fitness and alignment. My hammer toes have disappeared and in my 50's I developed a waist! One of the most profound aspects of her work was the clear instruction on breathing. I was able to discover how to breathe more fully with my ribs and diaphragm. I experienced a release of buried emotions and belief patterns as well. We always have fun and her sense of humor and boundless energy made learning pure joy. Thank you Michaelle!"

Barbi Clements, Mother, Body Boarder, Hiker, Traveler, Artist.

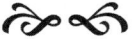

"After five weeks of YOGALIGN, I cancelled my surgery. Due to a bone spur in my shoulder, I could no longer do many of the things I loved to do (swimming, gardening, putting my arm around my sweetie) without pain. I had tried intensive physical therapy, ice, ibuprofen, even cortisone injections. I was a motivated and compliant patient. But re-aligning my shoulders and the rest of my body through Michaelle's Yogalign techniques corrected the cause of the pain and has brought relief. I am well on my way to recovery. Thank you Michaelle! I'm a believer!"

Linda Pizzatola, Graphic Artist, Gardener, Swimmer, Counselor.

"When I began YOGALIGN classes with Michaelle, I suffered from plantar fasciitis, forward head carriage, and migraine headaches. My posture was stooped and my neck and shoulders were always sore from overworked muscles that were not designed to hold the weight of my head. I was starting to feel trapped in my body and it was exhausting just to be in it. In just a few classes with Michaelle, my pain and misalignment disappeared as if by magic. I had been developing core strength from my pilates classes but Michaelle helped me learn to access my core in a way I had never been shown. My tennis game is getting better all the time and I feel relaxed and comfortable in my body. The natural blueprint for alignment I learned in the YogAlign method is intrinsic in my body now and I don't have to work at doing it. I have let go of my old posture and feel youthful and energized. I highly recommend her training to anyone with a spine!"

Sherry Latif, Pharmacist, Artist, Pilates Practitioner, Tennis Player, and Mother of three.

"I have been waiting all my life for this. I got tremendous relief from my C7 cervical injury in just one class."

Andrea St. Clair

"My butt has always looked flat and I have never had a lumbar curve even after I did 10 sessions of Rolfing. In my spine, my first lumbar vertebrae has been protruding as long as I can remember and I am now in my forties. To my amazement, doing YogAlign realigned my spinal curves in one group class and the vertebrae protrusion disappeared. I love having a lumbar spinal curve and I can feel my gluteus muscles strong and activated. This is the biggest shift I have felt happen in my body since I went through puberty."

Anne Paquin, Nia instructor, CPA

"I am an osteopathic physician and student of many types of energy healing and bodywork. The muscular and energetic releases I felt in my first YogAlign class were the fastest and most beneficial of all healing modalities I have every experienced."

Jessica Bacon, DO

"After an acute trauma from jumping off of a cliff into the ocean, I was in severe back pain. Standard methods of treatments like rest, ice and ibuprofen were not touching it. Although I had never even done yoga and was nervous about trying it with an injury, Michaelle explained to me how YogAlign is safe, comfortable and would give me relief from back pain."

"I took a group YogAlign class with Michaelle and experienced immediate relief both during the class and for several days after the yoga class. Her attention to detail and in particular how the movement of breath affects posture and spine alignment were informing and comfortable. She helped me understand both cerebrally and experientially that pain results from posture imbalances that get mapped into our brain, similar to the software programs in our computers. By rewiring the signals the brain sends out to the muscles, bad patterning can be erased and new body map "software" can be uploaded quickly and safely. My experience with YogAlign has inspired me to incorporate it into my work as an acupuncturist and I look forward to learning more."

Mike Osborn MS, Licensed Acupuncturist and Herbalist

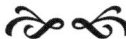

"Over the past 16 years, I have watched Michaelle's practice of yoga evolve into the most beneficial yoga I have ever seen or done. I had been practicing traditional yoga postures in a way that created an injury and left me with severe neck and back pain. Since I started learning YogAlign with Michaelle, my general posture is so much better and I breathe with ease. I had a flat thoracic spine and very tense shoulder blade muscles that were causing a lot of internal tension. By practicing the breathing and imagery work in YogAlign, I learned how to be in my body without the effort of trying to pull my shoulders back to stand up straight. I had suffered for a long time with chronic neck and back pain but since doing YogAlign, my neck and back pain are virtually gone. I have realized that I need only do yoga poses that simulate how I use my body in real life. I now have posture that keeps my spine and sacral joint healthy. YogAlign is by far the best yoga out there for a healthy spine and a pain-free existence!"

Lee Thompson, Yoga Teacher, Medical Assistant

"Three years ago I had three serious, consecutive accidents that crippled my passions as an athletic young woman and put me in so much pain that at times I could not walk. This escalated over the course of three years. I tried Pilates, chiropractors, doctors, and massage, but nothing seemed to work long term. Being a licensed massage therapist, I always emphasized to my clients the connective importance of breathing, the diaphragm, and the psoas muscle. However, in my own self-care practice, a piece of the puzzle was missing. Michaelle's YogAlign method was that missing piece, as it combines the science of breathing with posture conscious Yoga poses that unwind tension in the body while building strength with flexibility. Her emphasis on "self-care health care" puts the tools for healing back into the hands of people. Through her teachings the pain in my body melted away, freeing a part of my spirit that had been locked down for years. My experience and studies in body work allow me to understand the scientific mechanics behind YogAlign's long term effectiveness—how you can literally reprogram your brain to create new patterns of movement, quickly creating an aligned and pain-free body."

"YogAlign is the missing link in health and wellness that has the potential to change the world—inside and out."

Amber Crago: LMT, YogAlign Teacher, Photographer, Chef, Musician, and Japanese Translator

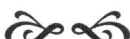

"In 2008 I moved to Kauai in search of increased healing after suffering the ravages of breast cancer treatment in 2006 which included a mastectomy, TRAM flap reconstructive surgery and severe radiation scarring. The benefits I gained from Michaelle's YogAlign weekly classes led me to take the six-week teacher training course. During the training course I was astounded to regain full range of motion and strength in my shoulder and arm, as well asto find that painwhich had plagued me since the surgeries was now drastically diminished. I feel great about myself! My desire is to teach these powerful techniques to other women recovering from breast cancer treatments and lead them along the path to increased healing ,radiant health, and a full range of motion."

Linda McSwain, RN

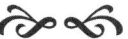

"I am confident this book will be a useful manual for yogis—both beginners and more seasoned practitioners recovering from injuries. Michaelle is performing a really useful and courageous service by bringing attention to this information. I am amazed to see how much yoga has become a "sacred cow", not to be questioned."

Kathleen Porter, Ageless Spine, Lasting Vitality

*We do not have a health
care crisis. We have a
self care crisis.*

CONTENTS

FOREWORD
BY ALISON SCOLA

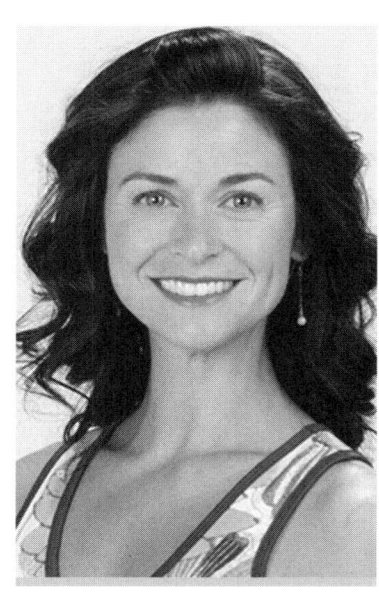

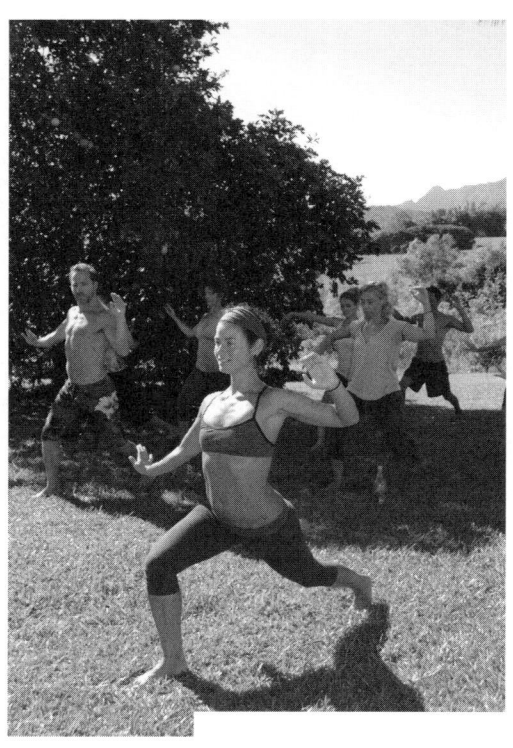

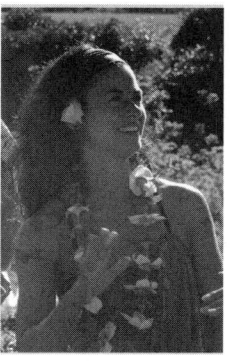

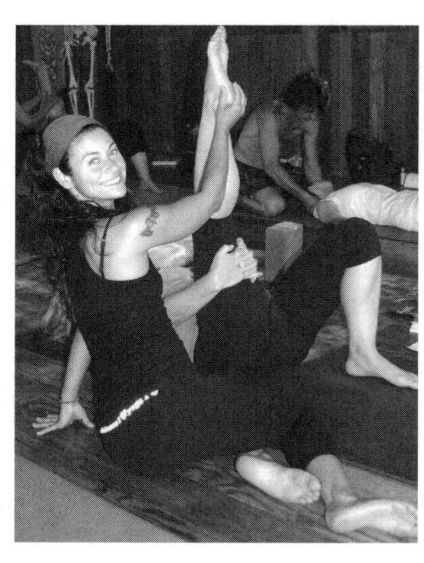

My quest to find relief from pain and a sense of freedom and joy in my physical body began over 25 years ago. This quest ended this year when I found Michaelle Edwards and discovered the powerful self-healing yoga method she developed called YogAlign.

Without knowing what to expect of YogAlign, I booked a session with Michaelle. During our first session, I was amazed by the deep release that I experienced in areas of my body that had for years been locked in chronic tension. She began to explain the unique experience I was having: that YogAlign was an evolution, a hybrid, a complete healing modality that integrated everything human beings need to heal—breath work, massage, fascial restructuring, neuromuscular repatterning, anatomical road maps, and the use of functional postures based on natural alignment of the spine and healthy biomechanics.

I was absolutely amazed that the combination of these methods allowed my body to open in ways that I thought were impossible, in just one session and without pain! I knew I had found something profound. I knew I had met my next teacher. I wanted to learn everything I could from Michaelle.

For the following five months I practiced YogAlign daily and experienced release in the locked areas of my body for the first time ever. My chronic neck pain disappeared. As I began to feel freedom in my body my depression started to lift, my energy returned, fears that dictated my choices vanished. I was healing a deep emotional wound and emerging as a woman of confidence, vitality and joy.

Before YogAlign I had pain so severe that it interfered with my quality of life; this began as early as 11 years of age. I experienced headaches, neck pain, anxiety and fatigue. I had suffered a series of minor car accidents and had symptoms of whiplash but was never treated for it. There was an assumption that my body would heal without any therapy. By the time I was in my early twenties, I was crippled by low back pain, lived a sedentary existence, and struggled with anxiety, depression and addiction.

In the hope of a solution, I sought out regular chiropractic care and deep tissue massage. These were temporary fixes and the results lasted only for a few hours or for a couple of days at best. I was constantly trying to figure out why my body would not hold the chiropractic adjustment or stay relaxed after a massage. I spent most of my time seated or lying down because I thought activity aggravated my symptoms. I had to quit my job and could not tolerate school because sitting in class or reading in any position exacerbated my neck pain and gave me a headache. It was at this time that someone suggested I try yoga.

I felt intimidated by going to yoga class because my body was very inflexible and out of shape. I thought to myself, "I can't even touch my toes and now someone is going to teach me to put my legs behind my head?" Despite my fears and doubts, I was desperate enough to even try yoga.

This was the beginning of my journey. Practicing yoga helped me understand how my posture was playing a role in my low back pain, and I began to learn about the powerful relationship between my physical body, my mind and my emotions. My emotions and past traumas were "trapped" inside my structure and affecting how I was unconsciously wired to move. My yoga practice revealed that it was all interconnected and brought immediate awareness to the fact that I had spent most of my life taking shallow breaths. I found that just deepening my breath with a focused awareness had a tremendous effect on how I felt emotionally and physically. This experience begged the questions: Was my anxiety, depression and physical pain informing my posture and breath? Or was my posture and breath causing my anxiety, depression and physical pain? The answer? All of the above.

I began to understand and experience the mind-body connection as I unraveled the mystery of my pain. I had found in yoga a milestone in my quest for wellbeing, but I had to practice diligently twice a day to manage my pain level. The headaches and neck pain always returned which sent me, baffled and frustrated, in search of more therapeutic options.

It was suggested to me that I give Rolfing a try. This technique massages and reorganizes fascia, the connective tissue running throughout our entire body. It was explained to me that my car accidents had left "scars" in my fascial tissues that would always pull the muscles into tension, which would then pull the bones of my spine out of alignment. This made good sense and explained to me why the pain always came back. What I did not know then was that the Rolfing could only access the superficial layer of my fascia and my issues ran deeper than any Rolfer could access and palpate. The fascial restrictions I had were not just scar tissue, because my body had been absorbed in poor postural habits for years before the accidents. My fascia had organized itself to support my bad posture and misalignment, and was clearly keeping me in a cycle of pain. I needed to change the programming for how I moved in my body.

I sometimes felt pain during and after my yoga sessions, too. It was all very confusing and at times I felt despair, no longer wanting to inhabit a bodily structure that was so full of pain. I needed solutions. One day, my amazing chiropractor suggested that my yoga practice was actually harming me. I was creating hyper-mobility in my ligaments from overstretching. So while I was still locked in tension in certain areas of my body, I was now too loose in others. The solution was to begin to exercise to strengthen my joint functions and build muscle. After about a year of regular exercise—at times painful due to trial and error based on suggestions from others—I started to notice that if I missed a workout, I was in a lot of pain. I needed to use my muscles because the increased circulation relieved my pain, boosted my energy level and made me feel happy.

As a result of my extensive therapeutic regime, over the following ten years I was able to pursue an active lifestyle and discovered one of my greatest joys to be dance. I became a professional swing dancer and instructor, and toured the world teaching and performing. I witnessed the number of injuries to which dancers' bodies were subjected. I also realized that, even while they were running the risk of injury, people were coming to dance in search of release from discomfort in their bodies and their lives.

Paradoxically, the lifestyle of travel and the physical demands of being a professional dancer and teacher were challenging and ultimately unhealthy for me. As a result of my own journey, I felt a deeper sense of purpose and a desire to teach others a holistic approach to healing. I decided to shift my focus to the original reason that I was able to dance—yoga therapy. In the six years that I have been teaching yoga and yoga therapy, I have been grateful and honored to be a guide and a witness to people's transformations.

It is the most rewarding work I have ever done.

While doing this beautiful work I was going through a divorce that caused an intense transformation of my own, and which sent me spiraling into old patterns of pain in my body. I was completely depleted and struggling with all of the stress that intense life changes can bring about. I then decided to take a trip to the beautiful Mana Yoga Center in Kauai. There I met Michaelle Edwards and was introduced to YogAlign.

When I arrived, it was her loving, playful nature that immediately struck me. She was so welcoming, and she radiated zest for life and joyfulness in her body. She was active and invited me to run, swim, surf, kayak, hike, and dance. She was beautiful and open and very passionate about sharing YogAlign with me. I was intrigued by her nature, lifestyle, and method. It seemed like a miracle, but with just a few sessions of YogAlign, I was joyful and pain-free.

When I left Kauai, I began to teach YogAlign to my clients and in my therapeutic group classes. The change I have witnessed in people, in a short period of time, is profound and has impacted me deeply. I have seen people surprised by how flexible they actually are once they learn that flexibility happens in their brain, and is acquired without painful stretching or body positions. Clients acquire grace and ease quickly, using the unique breathing techniques of YogAlign and the functionally-based exercises that rewire the brain and direct the body to move in graceful, centered alignment. I saw firsthand in my students the shift I myself went through from, "I am not flexible and yoga is going to hurt" to "I am flexible, free from pain, relaxed yet energized, and yoga feels good!"

I had one particular client who was not able to take a full breath because of kyphosis (a rounded upper back and forward head position), scarring from surgery, and multiple traumas. Her postural habits affected her ability to breathe well, which had led to symptoms of anxiety, depression and chronic fatigue. I also wondered if over the years her poor alignment and shallow breathing would lead to more serious conditions such as a diagnosis of congestive heart failure, resulting from the compression of her heart and lungs.

Practicing YogAlign breathing exercises has given this client the ability to breathe deeply for the first time in 10 years. With this seemingly simple change, she was able to start walking for exercise, has begun to eliminate medications, and can now enjoy the simple things that she couldn't before such as going out to dinner with her children or taking her daughter shopping. She has relief from anxiety attacks and constant exhaustion. Her emotional state now includes a sense of serenity and hope regarding her future quality of life. With her alignment now functional, she is using the movements of breathing in her daily life to support her in good posture.

I feel hopeful and excited when I think about the capacity for healing and living well that YogAlign offers people of all ages and fitness levels. It is the only method of therapy I have experienced that affects change on all levels of the mind/body/emotional being. It heals the root of almost all chronic pain in the human body, which is postural misalignment. YogAlign reorganizes the superficial and deep lines of fascia, restoring ease and functionality of movement. It combines self-massage and natural human body postures that align the spine while fostering an awareness of loving kindness and self-care over performance routines. YogAlign uses a special core breath technique developed by Michaelle that re-educates the nervous system until great posture becomes innate and effortless.

I have learned how to rewire my brain in order to direct my body to use less effort. YogAlign has created a balanced tone of my muscles and fascia, and I feel a sense of joy which seems to radiate from inside of me. Core stabilizations are orchestrated with the movements of breathing and are unique from any other form of abdominal exercise I have ever experienced. Externalized actions such as exercises for a tight six-pack actually lead to an inhibition of feeling, movement, and breathing. As I practiced with Michaelle, my core shifted from being rigid and firm to feeling fluid and dynamic. In YogAlign, the tone in the core is created from the inside out, lengthening and trimming the waist without any external effort to hold and tighten the abdomen. I discovered how wonderful it feels to let my belly go and release chronic holding patterns in my solar plexus area that were negatively affecting not only my mind and emotions, but also my digestion, metabolism, and elimination. We are never directed to hold our tummy in or tuck our tail bone under; in fact, Michaelle reminds us constantly that we do not get comfortable by being uncomfortable.

One learns quickly to let go of excess tension and align from the center, replacing old patterns that cause us to originate movements from our periphery. YogAlign re-examines the benefits of classical yoga postures and transforms them into functional movements that work within our natural alignment and biomechanics. Michaelle's work with stabilizing the sacral area and protecting the sacral ligaments from over-stretching provides clients with the tools that empower the body to release chronic lower back pain and sciatica, while providing people with the knowledge to practice yoga without harming the delicate sacral platform.

Many clients are surprised to learn that the chronic pain they suffer is oftentimes caused by yoga routines and fitness exercises that they erroneously believed were helping them. YogAlign allows the body to get back to a place of balance, back to the perfect design that nature intended. One of the greatest benefits of YogAlign is the internal feeling of freedom, lightness, energy, joy, and bliss that happens so quickly and effortlessly. We call that feeling the kid body, and it is a feeling of floating that allows the spirit to soar and the feet to fly, just as we experienced long ago in childhood.

For me, YogAlign represents the completion of my quest—a journey of healing to find happiness in my body. YogAlign has given me a quality of life that I never dreamed possible. I am so grateful to Michaelle Edwards for her years of exploration, study, passion, writing, and teaching. She has tremendous courage to come forward and share these revolutionary ideas with us all.

YogAlign is accessible. Anyone can do it, and its effect can be felt immediately. To the reader, I simply say, if you have found this book you have been given a gift. It is an opportunity to experience a new body and perhaps a chance to experience a form of yoga that is based on self-love, and the movement of the human body according to its natural design.

Alison Scola, January 2011

Every human being carries within him his own doctor. People come to us without knowing this fact. We will be most successful if we provide this doctor who resides inside everyone the chance to go to work.

Albert Schweitzer
Theologian, organist, philosopher, physician, and medical missionary.

YOGALIGN™

Pain-free Yoga from Your Inner Core

PREFACE

Over the past 40 years, I have worked with thousands of people of all ages and fitness levels, hailing from all over the globe. What I've noticed throughout this experience is an epidemic loss of self-reliance when it comes to our own health. Most of us feel pain in our body and we put ourselves at the mercy of others, looking to others to find the cure for what ails us. We have become overly-dependent upon prescription drugs, doctor visits, and surgeries—all of which depend upon someone else to "fix" what seems to be broken. Yoga, when practiced with awareness of what you are doing and why, is a powerful tool leading to inner healing and self-reliance. In writing this book, it is my true hope that the YogAlign system will help you develop the tools and self-reliance that exists within you, allowing your body to heal itself by supporting it with proper alignment, breathing, nutrition, self-awareness and self-love.

YogAlign grew out of my own commitment to trust that my body would heal itself, and a belief that there was an innate source of wisdom and intelligence guiding the whole experience. Many times we ignore our bodies until they scream in pain, and we wonder that our injuries and ills come on so suddenly. In truth, if we were listening to our bodies everyday, as we ought to, we would find that the body gives ample warning when things are going awry. The techniques I have developed in YogAlign allow you to hear the subtle language of your body when it whispers and nudges you to pay attention, telling you to tread lightly and release the unnecessary tensions that go along with modern life.

Our human body is intelligently organized to heal itself if we support it in that process, and we muster that support by listening and paying attention to what the body tells us.

For thousands of years, man lived a natural life, moving about to hunt, gather, and grow food while living with the natural changes of the seasons. As civilization advanced and machines were invented to do the hard work, man began to sit for most of the day—away from the natural world and stuck in a building or chair, focused on mental tasks that don't involve movement of the body. Amazingly, this state of affairs has only come about in the last 150 years. Now many of us are sitting in chairs, engaging in poor posture with poor breathing habits that have become innate and are sabotaging our health and strength.

Oddly enough, many yoga and exercise positions put the body in the same right-angled position that is the baneful result of sitting in a chair. We are so used to the discomfort of a chair-sitting lifestyle (and the resultant feelings of stiffness and age) that we are oblivious to the pain and may not notice that some yoga poses create the very same tension issues as chair sitting does. YogAlign banishes the chair-sitting position, instead focusing upon pain-free natural poses that allow the body to be in a position simulating real life movement, instead of static positioning.

I have spent years studying anatomy and working with clients using techniques that support a reconnection to the language of the inner body. In the process of listening, feeling, and paying attention, one begins to gain the tools of awareness that promote the body to heal itself. In a short time, through poses, breathing exercises, self-massage, and a developed self-awareness, you will begin to feel how you are using your body. Without thinking, your body will begin to move with more efficiency and fluidity, and your posture will be comfortable—no pain, no strain, and no extraneous effort.

Among those who have learned YogAlign and become pain-free and aligned are highly-skilled athletes, folks with desk jobs, teens and seniors. All of them had some type of alignment and breathing dysfunction causing them to suffer pain and injuries in their back, hips, shoulders, knee, and neck. Many also suffered from chronic conditions such as vertigo, TMJ, plantar fasciitis, sciatica, chronic fatigue, headaches and countless other "issues in the tissues." Instead of realizing the root of the problem (their postural alignment and poor breathing techniques), many of these clients simply labeled their knees as bad, their body as inflexible, or their painful feet as "just like mom's." This external blame game of pain focused their troubles on genetics, or an idea of a flawed body that was destined to fail. YogAlign taught them that strength, flexibility and fluidity were always within them... they just had to make some simple changes that would release that potential.

Many of us feel dense, solid, constricted, and trapped in a cycle of pain and postural problems. The good news is that we do have the power to change our bodily reality, because posture is a code dictated by our very own movement software and belief systems. None of us wakes up in the morning and makes a conscious decision to have poor postural patterning. We don't tell our shoulders to round, our knees to bow or our back to tighten. The body simply does what it has been programmed to do via unique "movement software" encoded automatically by our nervous system from the moment of our birth. Our habits and lifestyles and even our emotions have all contributed to a set programming that determines how we breathe, how we sit, how we stand and how we move and how we sense the feeling of our body.

Changing these movement codes is at the heart of the YogAlign method, which uses special techniques and life-imitating poses to change the wiring in the brain, and revitalize one's ability to live and move in connection with their own body.

Our physical body is truly only a dense representation of our thoughts, emotions, memories and experiences, and we are not "solid" as we have believed ourselves to be. Science tells us that the body is about 65–72 percent water, and our atoms are composed of more space than actual solid matter. If our body at this cellular level is mostly space, how can this space be dense, solid, or misaligned? What I have found is that because our bodies are mostly space and water, we can easily and fluidly reshape our bodies out of the cycle of chronic pain and misalignment by changing the neural codes that direct our movement. It can happen fast, and without painful exercises. The process is amazingly simple, fun, and educational.

You may be surprised at what you read in this book because it often seems the antithesis of what we have all come to believe is true. Many of the techniques that I have developed are the opposite of what I was originally taught to do in yoga and stretching classes—and for good reason. People are getting seriously hurt doing yoga poses, but because yoga is not regulated by the government, exact data on these injuries is hard to come by. Almost every person I know who seriously practices hatha (posture-based) yoga on a regular basis has been injured. Many have torn the hamstring from the sit bone, ripped knee and sacral ligaments, herniated discs, and become so overly-flexible that they are in constant joint pain due to a lack of structural support. The overstretching of the ligaments and nerves caused by some yoga poses has led some of my friends to receive hip and knee replacements. The numbers of the affected just keep growing.

I, myself, had a serious knee ligament injury from doing a yoga pose. Because of the injury, I could no longer do extreme poses, but even in the course of a basic practice I could notice a pain in my right SI joint that worsened each time I reached for my big toe in Triangle. I also noticed that my neck would "go out" on a regular basis, particularly after doing a plow or shoulder stand pose. I turned to a chiropractor for regular adjustments, and needed more and more regular massages, too. I had a serious daily practice but sometimes, after missing a day or two in a row, I noticed that I didn't feel soreness in my neck or instability in my hip. As soon as I practiced again, back would come the increasingly-familiar aches and pains. Yoga teachers would tell me that the hip pain was a sign that my hips were opening; one yoga teacher even told me it would take five years of intense practice before my hips would fully "open." Since being injured, I was not so quick to believe everything that yoga teachers told me and I had to face the truth. When I did not practice, my body felt more stable. I began to question what I was gaining from my practice. As I listened to friends talk about how sore they were from yoga and how much their body parts hurt. I started to take a step back and re-evaluate my yoga practice. What was I doing this for, and why?

Anxious to understand my body's messages, I started to think about how the body works as a whole, and I began to consider the elements of each pose that may be causing pains and injury in different parts of my body. As a body worker and a yogi, I knew that yoga was supposed to be about healing and the connection among body, mind, and spirit. What if the problem was not my body, but rather the yoga and fitness techniques that I had learned and followed as a student, teacher and practitioner?

I went into my studio and began to dissect and analyze every single pose and movement, including the way I had been told to breathe and hold bandhas. As I did each pose and movement, I tuned into the feeling of my body and the movement of the breath. Some poses simply did not feel good. I questioned the reasoning and the biomechanics behind it all.

Yogic knowledge teaches that the spine is part of the brain and you are as young as your spine. Yet it was unclear how my spine was benefiting from many of the poses I was doing. Even among my clients, many had poor posture; as I watched them do a seated forward bend, all I could see was a rounded spine and hunched shoulders. So I wondered: how do these poses—which seem to reinforce slouching by strengthening muscles engaged in improper alignment—assist people to open up and let go? How can these poses assist me or my clients in real life? What is the reason for each pose? Who made this position up and why?

That last question led me to the book *Yoga Body* where I found out that yoga poses are not the ancient practice that many believe. Rather, it is the ancient Yoga philosophy teachings that have survived the centuries and that provide us with the wisdom to understand our true nature. This ancient philosophy that has been passed down for thousands of years was not based on a physical practice and certainly the focus was not doing difficult body positions with a room full of people. What many think of when they think of yoga is composed of poses that are only 50-100 years old, and that were devised by men from India who melded ancient yoga philosophy with physical disciplines that were European in origin. Influenced by British military drills, calisthenics, contortionism, body building and women's gymnastics, these yogis were combining religion and philosophy with exercise, as part of a global backlash against the sedentary influences of the Industrial Revolution. Because of high injury rates and the fact that these poses are not ancient and time-tested, I came to the conclusion that we all must take a look at yoga asana (positions) and assess their biomechanical value. After all, it is great that millions of people are doing yoga, but it is vitally important that the essence of yoga—know yourself—is not lost in a physically-based practice that makes no biomechanical sense. One of the basic tenets of yoga philosophy is to practice non-violence or ahimsa towards the self and others and yet the physical yoga many do today is not following that most basic principle based on self-care and self-love.

For twenty years, I have spent countless hours working on my own practice and creating yoga poses that are based on moving from the center with the least amount of effort. Being a massage therapist led me to combine self-massage techniques in each and every session, and I feel YogAlign has evolved into a practice of self-love, as well as a whole new way of doing yoga that is based upon the spiral design of the human body. Many of my clients came to me suffering from pain and misalignment. Yet after practicing YogAlign (even for short amounts of time) they looked and (reportedly) felt fabulous. Nobody was getting sore or injured during or after class and yet flexibility levels were increased along with strength and balance. My clients were taller, happier, better-aligned and felt in amazement as their aches and pains disappeared.

The YogAlign method works at the nervous system level, creating almost immediate transformation to a pain-free state of being in the body without effort. Practitioners of YogAlign say the transformation feels like "floating" or being freed. Having a youthful spine, functional fascia lines, and a powerful diaphragm and rib cage are key to longevity and a pain-free body, and YogAlign effects these elements through a unique breathing process that inspires the strength and power of a functionally-stable core. As you start to practice the YogAlign system, you will begin to move and breathe with a feeling of power and lightness, in which movement requires very little effort. This is what I call "getting the kid body back."

As you continue on, you will find that much of my method centers on eliminating unnecessary muscle tension and establishing ease, synergy and balance. As muscles become more efficient, this enables a physical restructuring which restores health in the connective tissue web that defines, surrounds, supports, and directs our structure, movements, and physio-emotional being. Contrary to the collective belief that getting fit requires pain to gain, being fit and in balanced alignment takes effort that effectively feels effortless. In YogAlign, one is comfortable at all times with no strain or tension affecting the body and breathing function. Your body relaxes and you begin to feel more fluid and free in movement, just as you did when you were a kid.

My desire is to help people heal themselves of chronic pain or injury quickly and painlessly. When my clients adopt the proper tools to achieve their healing, they relearn their natural alignment patterning, resulting in more energy and less tension in their daily lives. They learn to let go of stress and muscle patterning that depletes and inhibits their life force, giving them instead a body that is actively and sustainably free.

Join me in becoming sustainable in your own body with the YogAlign™ Method.

To use this book, I suggest you begin by reading chapters One through Eight. Through those chapters, you will gain an anatomical overview of your body, facilitated by experiential exercises that allow you to actively sense and experience the anatomy about which you're reading. This anatomical road map will be vital once you begin to practice YogAlign's poses and exercises.

The second half of the book details the YogAlign Method, explaining each of the poses and providing photos for guidance. You can use this section to teach yourself YogAlign, safely and effectively. The included DVD will set you on your way toward becoming fit and pain-free as your own teacher and healer. I have also provided websites in the back of the book that will allow you to connect with a YogAlign teacher or become a YogAlign teacher through the Kauai Yoga School.

Mahalo (thank you) for joining me in YogAlign, the yoga with aloha. Aloha nui loa, Namaste,

~Michaelle Edwards
Hanalei, Kauai, July 2011

ACKNOWLEDGEMENTS

I would like to express gratitude for the many students and clients who have practiced and worked with me over the last 20 years during my development of YogAlign. The trust that they placed in me—and their willingness to actively participate in the process while thinking and feeling outside of the box—is what greatly lead to the formation of this method and to the creation of this book and my DVDs. It has been a group effort of many and I feel blessed to have known you all.

I want to thank Thomas Myers for his work in mapping out our fascia lines and explaining their importance to bodyworkers, yoga teachers, and movement therapists all over the world. His theory of the fascia trains educated me on the idea of tensegrity as the major determinant of our structural patterning. Because of him I remember to always think globally when addressing structural issues in the body.

Thanks also to Rosemary Feitis and the now-deceased Louis Schultz, who wrote a brilliant book called The Endless Web that has helped me understand how our fascia is the major determinant of our posture, movement, structure, and even our moods. Their kindness and generosity in loaning me illustrations from their book is a true gift of aloha, and I am greatly indebted to Rosemary and the artist Diana Salles.

I would like to acknowledge Judith Lasater, PT, for her important books on yoga asana, ethics, anatomy and non-violent communication. I have for many years respected and referred to her superior knowledge of the human body, and I feel greatly indebted to her for her brilliant teaching, and her books. I also thank her for her dedication in teaching the importance of anatomical guidelines to the safe and effective instruction of yoga. Her book What We Say Matters is a guiding light both for myself and for my students in regards to communication with ahimsa.

I will always have gratitude for my first yoga teacher, Swami Satchidananda who has now passed away. I began my practice of yoga with him at the age of 18 at Pomfret Center in Conneticut, when I went to meet him and stay at the ashram. He introduced me to the 8 limbs of yoga and illuminated me with his wisdom, wit, and deep compassion. He was a true yoga master who introduced me to the study of meditation, yoga philosophy, and pranayama at a very young age, encouraging me to go out into the world to practice my yoga.

Yoga teacher and author, Erich Schiffman, encouraged me to listen to the wisdom from within and teach from my heart. His humor, openness and huge generosity of spirit inspired me to be my own teacher and follow my own path, which evolved into my creation of YogAlign.

Eric Franklin is making huge contributions to the world of somatic education, guided imagery,and dance movement and I appreciate his books and workshops.

Special thanks to Joel Guy, filmmaker, artist, and water man, who was able to capture the beautiful cover shot. Thank you Susie Ayers for teaching me to dance and being my true friend and adventure partner. Thanks to Carl Wetzler for your many years of friendship, advice and trips into the Sawtooths to connect with nature.

Special mahalos (thanks in Hawaiian) to my son Zachary Gilbert, who took on the tasks of photographer, film editor and model for this book. You are a true blessing in my life.

Mahalo to waterman Laird Hamilton and athlete "Gabby" Gabrielle Reece for their support and enthusiasm for YogAlign and FitAlign. Surfer Rochelle Ballard, thank you for your generous spirit and energy as an icon of women's surfing, a YogAlign teacher, a fitness educator, and a massage therapist.

Thank you Mitch McPeek for the fabulous cartoons depicting the "abnormally normal" slouches of both teens and older folks. Kirstie Beneke, a YogAlign teacher training graduate also contributed some cartoons used throughout the book.

Alison Scola was a huge force in helping me align with my inner feminine goddess energy and dancing spirit. Gretchen Seaver gave me wonderful massages and soothed away my worries when the tasks seem insurmountable. Suzanne Dupree has been my friend throughout all my projects and I appreciate your love and support.

My brother, Jody Edwards, has closely advised and consulted me with regards to the technicalities of publishing and marketing. He cheered me on when tasks seem insurmountable to finish the book regardless of the hour and time involved. My sisters Geralene, Patrice, Eileen, Tara, and Tawn, as well as my brother Ken have all been there with a helping hand or an open heart. Thank you Julie, my step-mother, for supporting me in my work.

My father, Gerald (Jerry) Edwards has encouraged me all along to develop the genes I inherited from "Michael Monahan", my great grand-father. Monahan was a well known Irish author and philosopher, iconoclast, and an original thinker of his day. According to the Argonaut, "Monahan has a felicitous literary style, a chivalrous instinct, and a sincerity that never shrinks from the unpopular cause".

To my friend, neighbor, and client, Charlie Bass, thank you for your support and friendship in helping me to see this project through to the end. You came through for me when I needed help the most.

Mahalos to Helen and George Gilbert for their love and support through the years and thank you Mark for building the yoga barn and inspiring me to do my best.

Laura Christine of Kauai has been an immense help to the many (and huge) tasks involved in writing this book and keeping my websites tuned up. Her talents in computers, web design, writing, editing, bass playing, and advising greatly contributed to my success in writing about, and evolving, the YogAlign method. She is herself a brilliant YogAlign teacher and I look forward to many years of collaboration and friendship with her.

Jennifer Regan has been an editor extraordinaire. and cheered me on when things seemed insurmountable. Daria Lacy was able to do the final layout, cover design, and send the files to press in between running her ranch and chasing after loose dogs and horses. Special thanks to Julia O'Reilly for your masterful artwork and illustrations for the book. Your expertise and talent have been a huge contribution to my book.

Thank you Sarah Wall for your excellent photography and down to earth wit and wisdom.

Mahalos to Abigail Harris for helping me with the cyberworld and securing my domains.

Endless thanks to Erin Wascher of Kauai, my personal assistant, who spent a whole summer helping me edit my work and encouraging me to get it done. She kept me on track and organized my life and tasks when the tasks seem insurmountable Our early morning YogAlign practice, beach runs and surfing sessions helped to keep my body and spirit shining bright.

My other personal assistant Amber Crago kept me alive with her amazing cooking during the spring teacher training of 2011 when the book was in the birth canal.

To Lee Witmer, my friend from high school who has stood by my side through life's ups and downs and showed me what real friendship is: I am so blessed to have you in my life.

Cris Evatt, my neighbor and my writing mentor, inspired me to write and stay on task. Her wonderful books have filled me with insights on the human mind, relationships and keeping life simple. She passed away from cancer before I could give her a copy of this book, but she spent many hours encouraging me to finish it and get it out to the world. I owe a special thanks to her husband Dave Williams for keeping me powered up with fresh Kauai apple bananas and advice on love, money, and chickens.

Jean Kagan helped me edit my writings when I first began the project, and her faith in YogAlign encouraged me to get it out there from the very beginning.

Yoga teacher and musician, Denise Kaufman challenged me to wake up to my inner guide. Her dedication to the path of yoga philosophy and the human spirit along with her love of music, nature and the arts have truly inspired me.

Bob Smith of the Hatha Yoga center of Seattle was the first yoga teacher who gave me awareness of the psoas muscles at the core of our body. Liz Coch wrote a book about the psoas that contributed greatly to my understanding of doing exercises that contribute to a healthy functional psoas group: the core of your core.

Tamara Stryker, Mike Sposito, Dan and Lisa Ostermiller, Darlene Viggiano, Bill Hamilton, Betty Roi, Jan Peterson, Russell Wright, Janis Lyon, CC Waeschle, Greg and Linda Closegrazier, Shirley Shibao and family, Claire Woolger, Dennis Kain, James Larocco, Suzanne Dupree, Shelley Hack, Debbie Street, Sue and Bill Carpenter, Kathy Valier, Sherri Latif, Illeana Carrenos, Kirk Smart, Taj Jure, Dyna Kuehnle, Nameeta Lai, Terri Tico, Peter and Steph Sprague, Kevyn Lettau, the Knights, Robin Allen, Jerry and Barbie Wayne, Margaret Huang, Steve and Jan Drammer, Lael and Darryl Gray, Joy Morrell, Kirk, Dawn, and Jesse Peterson, Simon Potts, and many other friends and clients who have truly inspired me to do and be my best—I thank you.

ACKNOWLEDGEMENTS FOR THE DVD:

I am in great appreciation of Spence Palermo who is a film maker extraordinaire and a long time friend. Our friendship goes way back to our early 20's, when we both made our livings as professional musicians traveling across the great state of Montana. Our friendship continued on with his filming of my first DVD, Yoga from Kauai, and now the accompanying DVD in this book. Although he travels the globe working on documentaries for National Geographic, the Discovery Channel and more, he has always found time to work with me and help me bring these projects to fruition. His talent, professionalism, humor and patience in the filming and editing of the accompanying DVD are above and beyond both duty and friendship. Aloha to you, my dear friend.

Raymond Long of Bandha Yoga was extraordinarily generous in allowing me to reproduce his computer-generated imagery of the breathing muscles and the psoas muscle group; his computer graphics expert, Chris MacIvor, did a brilliant job in creating these. I am so thankful to Raymond for his kindness and his willingness to both share his own work and encourage mine.

Elizabeth Freeman lovingly lent us her beautiful gardens and estate overlooking Kahili Beach on Kauai for the setting of much of the DVD.

Thank you Jeff Peterson of Honolulu, for the gift of your beautiful slack key guitar music for the DVD. Your aloha and mana have enhanced and inspired me.

Finally, I want to acknowledge the power of source and the innate natural wisdom of the human body; the greatest teacher of all and a universe in itself. I have received much of the information for the development of YogAlign simply by paying attention to the subtle language of the body; a gift from our creator.

CHAPTER 1: INTRODUCTION TO THE YOGALIGN METHOD

ॐ **Recreating Your Innate Kid Body**

ॐ **The World Is Round—and So Is Your Body**

ॐ **There Is an Epidemic of Poor Posture in Our Modern Civilization**

ॐ **You Are Mostly Water and Space**

ॐ **Our Fascia Web Holds Us Up**

ॐ **The Six-Pack Is Overrated**

ॐ **Know Your Core Anatomy**

ॐ **Alignment Begins with Freeing the Breathing Process**

ॐ **Flexibility Is Wired in Your Brain**

ॐ **Why Are We Doing These Poses?**

ॐ **Natural Alignment for Life**

ॐ **Getting That "Kid Body" Back**

The world is round—
and so is your body.

❝In essence, our quality of life has more to do with how we feel, rather than with how much we own.**❞**

Michaelle Edwards, creator of YogAlign

RECREATING YOUR INNATE KID BODY

If you watch very young children at play, you will see the joyful balance in how they move. Kids are

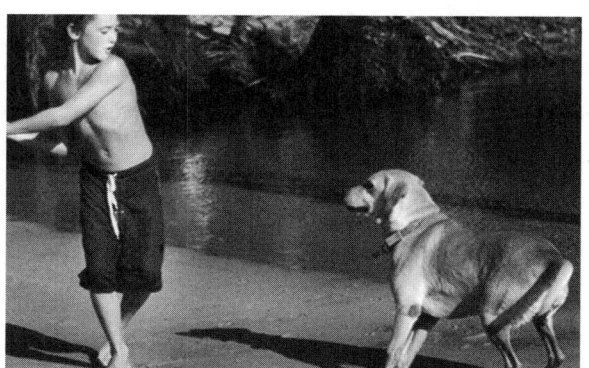

not inhibited in their body or in their beliefs about themselves; the absence of physical and emotional inhibitions gives children the fluidity and balance that we lose as we grow into adults. We spend hours driving in cars, and sitting at desks engaging in poor body positions that compress the spine and weaken the breathing muscles. Our bodily awareness seems limited to our latest aches and pains.

Being sedentary is a fact of our modern lifestyle. If we are to keep the kid body alive and well in us, it makes sense to adapt functional ways of sitting and exercising. In YogAlign, all poses are similar to how we use our body in real life. YogAlign allows you to create a new template for natural alignment that keeps you in perfect posture whether you are doing yoga, cycling, gardening, sitting at your desk or walking the dog. You begin to truly feel your body in its entirety, with all parts connected into a cohesive whole. You feel light, powerful and strong, and a deep sense of joy arises from inside you, harkening back to the simplicity of your childhood days.

So what is the "kid body"? Take a moment to observe the way children and animals move, and you will notice that they naturally have good postural alignment, without force or effort. Cats never look clumsy and birds are always graceful in flight, while dogs sit in perfect alignment. When children pick up something from the ground, they don't bend over with straight legs and a flexed spine—instead, kids will bend their knees and use the strength of their legs and butt muscles, with their feet grounded and hip-distance apart.

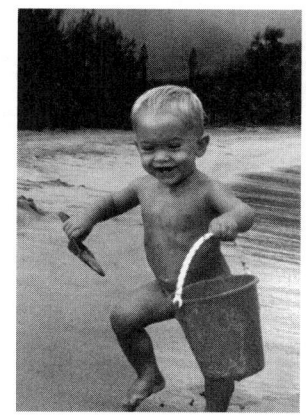

Kids instinctually know how to move, using inner support from their center while maintaining the natural curves of their spine.

YogAlign focuses on keeping this kid-like fluidity by using poses and breathing that encourage natural spine alignment and functional movements. For instance, in YogAlign, we do not try to keep our legs straight in a seated or standing forward bend, even when there is the flexibility to do so. Our bodies are designed to move, and our knees are designed to bend to create movement. Trying to make our bodies flexible by limiting natural motion is counter-intuitive, and only impedes our functional movement abilities.

When practicing YogAlign, our body is kept safe, stable, and free of injury by using positions that simulate real-life movement. By repeatedly using natural body positions in the practice of YogAlign, we learn to move intrinsically from our core, without an excess of muscle actions from our extremities. Practicing breathing, posture, and core movements that maintain a kid-like flexibility in our daily lives helps us reach a level of true sustainability.

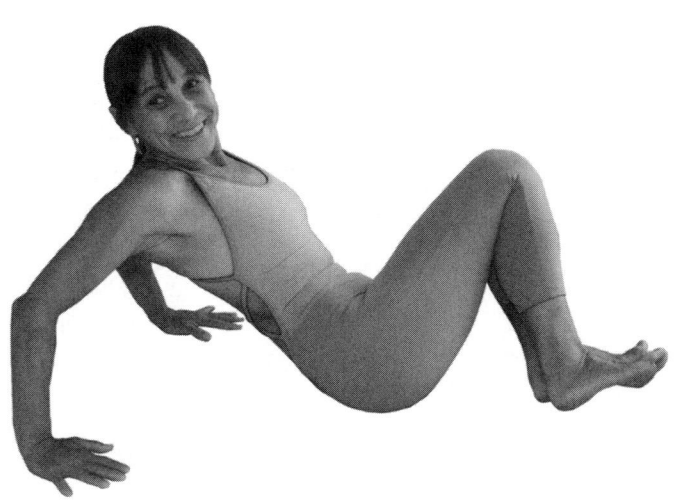

Fig. 1.1 – Rotator Rolls

By bringing our movements back to our true center, we establish beneficial innate patterning that happens without thinking, and is directed by the movements of breathing.

YogAlign practice also includes self-massage techniques that bring blood flow and oxygen to chronically strained areas of the body. As you roll and massage, you keep your body aligned from your core, using deep-breathing and trunk-synergy exercises that tone your body.

For YogAlign's "Rotator Rolls" (**Fig. 1.1**), circular movements use the weight of the body to massage the hips and butt (or gluteal) muscles.

THE WORLD IS ROUND—AND SO IS YOUR BODY

There are no straight lines in nature. Creation celebrates roundness, starting with the beautiful double helix of our very DNA. All of life in the natural world is designed in spirals and curves that foster graceful, fluid movements. Think of the shape of a flower, an orange, a shell, a tree, or the moon. The human body is no different in its form. From early on we are educated with ideas that are linear, and go from point "A" to point "B"; in reality we live in a continuity of roundness and spirals, where all parts of the body and the world connect in a seamless whole.

We are round—eyes, head, mouth, neck, trunk, breasts, arms and legs. Our spine, limbs and trunk are cylinders, and even our inner body is composed of tubes running liquid from head to toe. Because our body is *round* in nature, sitting in chairs in a right-angle bracket position (or stretching in this same position) goes against nature's design for the spine, and for the human body in general.

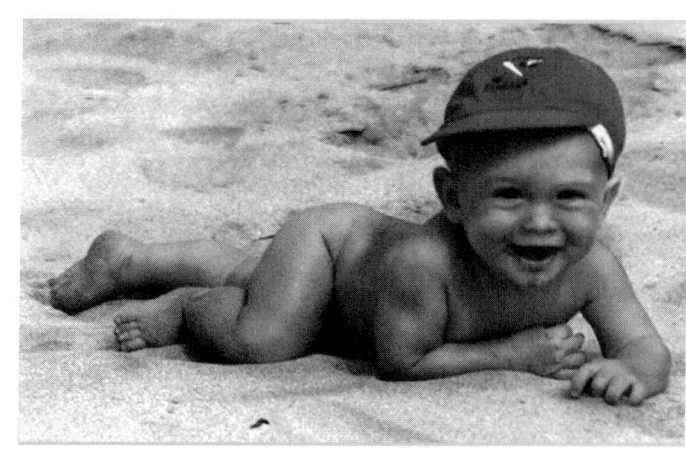

The spine itself is designed to hold four complimentary curves that support and cushion our movements. From birth, we begin to establish our own unique movement patterns, which affect these spinal curves and how they function. At birth, we have one C-shaped curve in our spine, established as we developed in the fetal position. As babies, we learn to move in a new world of gravity; as we lie on our belly and lift our heads to look about our new world, we develop strong, deep muscles in our back that help to establish the complimentary cervical (neck) and lumbar (lower back) curves. These curves serve as shock absorbers, protecting our spinal nerves and vertebrae from compression when we walk or move about. Sitting in chairs and rounding over our desks reverses these protective curves, leading to pain, poor posture and premature aging of the spine.

THERE IS AN EPIDEMIC OF POOR POSTURE IN OUR MODERN CIVILIZATION

Poor posture, chronic pain and tension are seen everywhere in the Western world, and sitting in chairs is the biggest reason why. Many people suffer exhaustion and pain on a daily basis, and many encounter tension and tightness throughout their lives. There is a general—yet erroneous—belief in our culture that it is normal to shrink with age, and that chronic aches and pain are inevitable. On the contrary, your body is miraculously and exquisitely engineered to be pain-free and flexible, well into old age.

Yet in the Western world, most people over the age of fifty have little suppleness to their spine, and lack freedom in their movement and breathing processes. This is because our lifestyle is built around sitting in positions that put our hips in a constant right angle to our legs. The L-shaped position taken during sitting causes compression of the spine and damages the spine's functional and supportive natural curves. After years of being in these static, unnatural positions, our bodies develop bad posture, toughened connective tissue, compressed vertebrae and nerves, chronic pain, and arthritis. These right-angled positions also affect our breathing process—the expansion of our lungs, the contraction of our diaphragm, etc. The diaphragm weakens and the breath becomes shallow as we lose the connection to our deep core breathing and spinal muscles. Poor alignment also invites us to rely on our extremities for support, forcing muscles to perform unnatural functions. We begin to overengage our neck and upper back muscles, leading to ingrained (and unconscious) bad postural habits.

Sitting in chairs is unnatural, often uncomfortable, and is counter to our natural design. Yet we live in a chair-sitting culture. Over time, we begin to adapt patterns of movement and alignment that are not functional, sabotaging the ability to move and breathe from our center. Our nervous system becomes imprinted with movement patterns and positions that waste precious energy, impeding our ability to be at ease in our body. Unless you know how to reboot the brain's signals that direct the intricate posture and movements of your body, you are stuck with a less-than-optimal wiring. YogAlign works to re-pattern this neuromuscular wiring, enabling you to acquire optimal alignment on an innate and intrinsic level.

You Are Mostly Water and Space

Many of us frequently feel tight and stiff and believe that it would be nearly impossible for us to be flexible, or achieve good posture. Yet enclosed within our skin, we are mostly composed of water and space. Muscles themselves are estimated to be 65—75 percent water, while our blood is 95 percent water. If all of this space could be removed from the cells in our entire body, the average human body would be a three-inch ball of matter. Denseness, stiffness and inflexibility are illusions when you realize that there is not much to us!

Flexibility is usually determined by the resting length of a muscle. If a muscle feels tight, that's because the nervous system is keeping it contracted when it does not need to be. A great athlete appears to move without any effort because he has so fine-tuned his body that only what is needed is engaged; there's no unnecessary contraction, so his body moves fluidly. Contraction occurs when we have adopted habits or alignments that use muscles in ways in which they were not intended. To eliminate these habits, we must wake up parts of the body that are not doing their jobs and turn off muscles that contribute to poor posture habits. In YogAlign we focus on becoming aligned by teaching our bodies to do "less."

The process of yoga is about removing obstacles like excess muscle tension, or excessive worry. YogAlign is about creating a "sustainable body", the most energy-efficient body possible. The same way that we are seeking to live on our planet using efficient, natural sources of energy that don't waste or pollute, we must seek out ways to conserve energy in our bodies. Those who are out of alignment and have chronically bad posture waste the lion's share of their energy because poor posture uses muscles inefficiently. When we are misaligned, we waste our precious energy stores, sap our strength, compress our joints, compromise our organ function, and—in the long run—develop a life of chronic aches and pains.

YogAlign focuses on: 1) understanding how the body is supported and controlled, and 2) teaching techniques to eliminate unnecessary tension and recover natural flexibility, tone and ease. Our bodies are permeated by systems of connective tissue that align our body through a balanced, tensile force. By practicing safe and easy breathing exercises and positions, we can learn to work with this connective tissue to regain our fluidity, moving more like the water and space that we truly are.

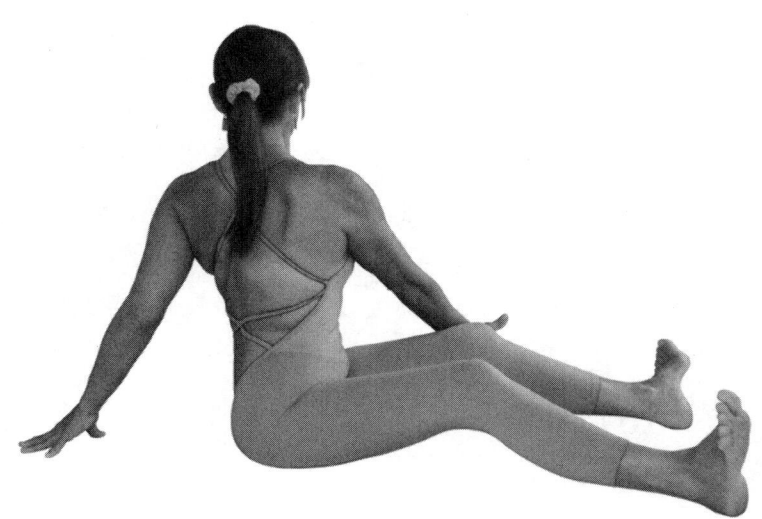

Fig. 1.2 – The Spine Aligner Twist

The YogAlign "Spine Aligner Twist" (**Fig. 1.2**) is an example of an exercise that simulates how we engage our body in real life. Special posture recalibrating techniques free the movement of the rib cage while slow, deep breathing creates fluidity and power.

Our Fascia Web Holds Us Up

Linear ideas about our shape and anatomy confuse us as to what really supports us. In truth we are supported by a web of connective tissue, or *fascia*, that permeates our entire body. This fascia connects bone to bone, supports our organs, and connects our muscles together in distinct pathways running from head to toe. Connective tissue is everywhere within us, making up 20 percent of our body weight and lining every cell, organ, and tissue. Many people think that our bones support us, envisioning the classroom skeleton. However, notice that the classroom skeleton has been artificially wired together to hold the bones in place. Similarly, the bones of the body would not stand freely without the attachments of connective tissue to support the skeleton. Peel an orange or grapefruit and you will see this same web of connective tissue; it's a structural support found throughout nature. The white cellulose holds the round shape of the grapefruit, even with the peel removed. Down to the tiniest juice sack, there is connective tissue that supports the fruit's structure. Like the structural walls of the grapefruit, fascia is everywhere in our body—down to the cell wall itself—determining our shape, structure and movement patterning.

EXPERIENTIAL EXERCISE #1

Our Fascia Web Connects the Body

Sit on the floor with your legs straight and your feet together. Do not do this exercise if you have disc problems or chronic back pain. Extend your toes back towards your shins, and sit up very straight. You may feel tightening in the lower back, or you might feel pain in the neck or upper shoulders. Even those who are very flexible will notice a slight pulling in the sacrum area. Now try to take a deep breath; you will notice that it is very difficult. This is because contracting our toes also contracts or tightens our belly and rib cage area, inhibiting the muscle actions needed for inhalation.

Because this is not a pose we recommend in YogAlign, don't stay in this position for more than a few moments, and do not use force to maintain it. To release tension, lie on your back on the floor and stretch your arms over head. Point your toes and extend your spine, relieving any compression along the vertebrae.

This exercise has allowed you to experience how our body position can affect our breath, and how our connective tissue spans the entirety of our body, binding it into a cohesive whole.

To balance movement in the body, you must balance the tensile forces of these connective tissues or "fascia lines." Our bodily structure can be compared to a tent, with our spine as the center pole. All of the tent lines are adjusted to hold the tent in a balanced, upright position. If the center pole is out of alignment, or the lines are shorter on one side and longer on the other, then the fabric of the tent is shifted in an uneven fashion. Like the tent, we need equal pull in the tensile structures of our body to be able to move freely, and stay aligned.

THE SIX-PACK IS OVERRATED

When the tensile forces of our fascia lines are balanced, the body can begin to move effortlessly. Many people teach or practice exercises that are based on pulling the belly *in* when doing sit-ups or other abdominal exercises. Our culture places a heavy focus on toning our outer belly—our "six-pack"—but toning just the outer belly makes the abdominals short and tight, over-training them to contract and compressing the natural curves in the spine. This causes the spine to be flexed, instead of extended, which can lead to long-term spine misalignments and chronic back pain. The tighter we make the lines of our front, the more tension we put on the lines of our back. When we train the core by tightening the front of our body, we unknowingly engage our superficial structures, like the outer belly and upper throat muscles, to support us. It is more useful to use exercises that create balance and stability from our core breathing center.

As they age many people appear to be much older because of a shortening in the front of the body, which draws the head forward and rounds the upper back. Many abdominal exercises and forward-bending yoga poses accelerate this forward-aging posture by repeatedly shortening the front of the body in order to "stretch the back." In addition, many people are doing exercises that further encourage the muscles of the front body to become short and "tight." It is important for long-term health and fitness to eliminate such exercises, as well as any body position that exacerbates dysfunctional posture patterns.

With YogAlign we learn to tone the belly in a way that allows ease in our movements, but we don't focus on keeping the navel area pulled in. The holding in of our belly is an aberration of natural function that sabotages our abdominal health. One simply does not need to pull in the navel to gain strength or create upright alignment. In YogAlign, the belly is toned through stabilization exercises. Through deep breathing and functional movements, you can encode your nervous system to enlist your core muscles as stabilizers, providing you with a built-in, internalized ring of support. YogAlign poses create an equalized balance of tensile forces between the front, back, lateral, spiral, and deep center regions of our body. In Chapter 7, you will learn how to stabilize and synergize the actions of the muscles and connective tissue in your core trunk region.

Because all parts of the body affect the whole, shortening and contraction in the front can put a tremendous strain, or pull, on the back line of our body. The body is interconnected; you cannot move one part of it without affecting another. For instance, abdominal muscles located in the front of the body naturally contract along with your feet when you pull your toes back towards your shins. The front of your body shortens because fascial forces connect the top of your feet to your ribs and belly, and even up to your jaw. Your abdominal muscles are also connected to your ribs, and when they shorten and contract, they prevent full expansion in the breathing process.

With YogAlign, we call these foot positions "driving with the parking brake on," and that is certainly what it feels like. If a pose is beneficial, you will always feel able to move and breathe while radiating out from the center of the body. YogAlign poses are designed to engage and balance the body, enabling free movement patterns of natural alignment. Even the smallest misalignment can cause restriction, so we need to focus on engaging the body in its entirety, with conscious awareness of the whole. With the YogAlign method, the emphasis and intention of each pose is to facilitate a deep breathing process that creates ideal body alignment. Deep breathing empowers the inner core, extends the spine, and creates more space in the body. Stabilization of the core muscles and equalized tensile factors in the connective tissue are the keys to pain-free biomechanics.

KNOW YOUR CORE ANATOMY

YogAlign seeks to activate the multi-tasking *psoas* (pronounced "so–az") muscles, which are the bridge between our emotional and our physical bodies. The psoas work in synergy with other important muscles of our trunk, including the superficial *rectus abdominus*, or the "six-pack"; the deeper *transverse abdominus* that acts as an inner ring of support; the *obliques*; and the *quadratus lumborum*, or deepest abdominal muscles. The psoas attach directly to the diaphragm, affecting breath, movement, and organ function. The psoas are also the link between the upper and lower body, connecting the spine to the legs and the trunk.

Sometimes called the fight-or-flight muscles, the psoas can contract when we feel stress or negative emotions. This is because the psoas muscles are part skeletal muscle and part smooth muscle. Skeletal muscles can be consciously contracted, such as when we flex the bicep to bend our elbow. But smooth muscles, like the heart, are controlled by the autonomic or automatic nervous system. Since the psoas are comprised of both kinds of muscle tissue, they can contract unconsciously when the nervous system is stressed. The body/mind connection becomes evident as worries, stresses and unexpressed tensions lead to contraction of the psoas, constricting movement throughout the body. Without functional psoas, the rest of the body can develop compensatory movement patterning, which lacks fluidness and efficiency. In YogAlign, we learn to engage the psoas functionally, elongating our posture and assisting with deeper breathing.

In Chapter 3, you will be fascinated to learn more about this relatively ignored muscle group, and the chapter will serve as your anatomical road map to the muscles of your inner core.

ALIGNMENT BEGINS WITH FREEING THE BREATHING PROCESS

Alignment is important in yoga and the poses we do should be consistent with good posture and good alignment. Good alignment should be practiced in all of our daily movements—both in our yoga practice and beyond the yoga mat. Becoming aware of how we use our body from moment to moment is the key to being well-aligned and pain-free. The ideal yoga practice enables one to create a state of presence in all actions of every moment.

Alignment, to a great degree, is dictated by how we are breathing. Shallow breathing creates poor posture. Deep-centered breathing aligns us in a natural position. In YogAlign, we emphasize that it's not what we're doing, but how we are breathing when we're doing it, that determines postural balance and quality of movement. YogAlign teaches us to have truly functional breathing skills, not just in our yoga practice or exercise positions, but in every way we use our body all day long. Using the movements of deep breathing, we can align ourselves from the inside out. The emphasis and intention of each pose in the YogAlign method is to practice functional body positions that empower our ability to move efficiently and breathe deeply. This supports our body's natural alignment and fosters function, ease, and comfort in our daily life. In Chapter 4, you will learn how to breathe your way to optimal health.

EXPERIENTIAL EXERCISE #2

Simple Movements Can Restrict Breathing

For this exercise put a drinking straw in your mouth. Stand with your feet in a natural hip-width stance, keeping your knees slightly bent. To align your trunk with the lower part of your body, press your feet into the floor. With your elbows bent, bring your hands out to the sides with your fingers widely spread. Pretend that you are pressing against a wall to engage the muscles that extend your spine and stabilize your shoulder blades.

Hold the feeling created by this position and then let your arms drop to your sides naturally.

Inhale by sipping on the straw, noticing how well you can breathe and how much your ribs can move. Notice how the movement of breathing lengthens your waist and stretches open the front of the body.

Now bring your feet close together and squeeze your inner thighs. Again try to sip on the straw and notice how the breathing muscles are now restricted. Because your feet are now close together, your body has responded by contracting muscles—through your connective tissue lines—all the way from your feet up to your belly and ribs, inhibiting inhalation.

FLEXIBILITY IS WIRED IN YOUR BRAIN

How well your muscles move is influenced by fascia quality, and your fascia quality is impacted by how much habituated muscle tension you have. How we control this tension, as well as how we control movement, is determined by our brain's messages to the muscles. Effective exercising for functional movement must happen at the brain level. Poor movement patterns can be changed when we learn to rewire what the brain is telling the muscles to do.

YogAlign uses techniques that train your brain to move your body differently. Think about it this way: you don't wake up in the morning and say, "I think I will have bad posture today" or "I think I will adopt the posture habit of tilting my head sideways when I walk." Yet over time, these unconscious messages become hard-wired and are part of what makes us unique. It takes thousands of intricate muscle signals just to walk across the room and we don't have the ability to direct each individual muscle to tell our body how to do it. The body knows what to do because the movement centers in our brain have encoded complex neuromuscular patterning, allowing us to move without thinking too much about it. The key to changing how we move is changing the codes in our nervous system to enable better posture, and encourage functional movement from our core.

The secrets to flexibility are in this book, along with the simple—but paradoxical—truth that to get flexible, one needs to practice tightening what already feels tight. Muscles need to be tightened in order to become flexible, and to stay safe we need to tighten them when we stretch; we also need to keep the body comfortable so that we do not invoke a *stretch reflex*. Stretch reflexes are the body's coping response to muscles being stretched beyond a certain point, which the body interprets as a danger. The reflex contracts the muscle out of self-protection, since a tightly contracted muscle is less likely to tear. Oftentimes when we stretch, there is a feeling of discomfort because we feel tight, and no matter how much we stretch, the body does not seem to want to let go. This is the stretch reflex in action, and it is there to protect the body against muscle strain and injury.

This stretch reflex can be outwitted, so that we can move beyond our normal tightness and gain flexibility and strength at the same time. We do this by tightening muscles beyond their normal range of tension, and by tightening what already feels tight. This is "resistance stretching," and it helps us to become strong and flexible, and is a foundation for much of the YogAlign system. In resistance stretching, we hold stretches while tightening muscles beyond the normal contraction rate. We release the "extra tightening" while staying in the stretching position, and our brain releases our muscles to a longer resting length. In doing so, we enable ourselves to become toned, extended, and flexible in each pose, and hardwire the new flexibility into the innate patterning that is coded in our brain.

While doing this resistance stretching, we make sure that we position the body in natural alignment, protecting our spinal curves and joint integrity, so that we are using the whole body functionally, rather than trying to compartmentalize movement. Many professional athletes are discovering that resistance stretching is the key to achieving elongated, toned muscles that allow a wide range of flexibility, foster strength and speed, and protect joints and ligaments from injury.

In this book, you will also learn a fascinating self-applied method to do "proprioceptive neuromuscular facilitation" (or PNF) which will help to rewire the brain's codes that control how you move. Chapter 5 shares the essentials of changing your brain to re-invent your movement. In your own home, you can use these techniques with resistance stretching and watch your body change shape, becoming flexible and aligned, and growing taller and toned after just the first session. It is fun and fascinating to discover that getting flexible is easy, if you follow the anatomical wiring of your body.

WHY ARE WE DOING THESE POSES?

Foremost among the reasons people practice yoga is a sincere desire to take care of their body, mind, and emotions. We practice conscious breathing, poses, and meditation to build strength and flexibility, to release stress, and to find calmness and inner peace. No one expects to be injured in a yoga practice, yet yoga-related injuries are happening to far too many people. YogAlign teaches the fine art of listening to your body. It is easy to hear the body when it is screaming in pain, yet few hear the body as it whispers and gives clues about subtle alignment and being at ease. In Chapter 8, you will learn that yoga does not have to hurt, and that you can protect yourself from the epidemic of yoga- and stretching-related injuries.

When you do a pose, listen to your body. Think about what you are doing and why. Ask your body if it *wants* to be in this position. Can you take a full, deep breath here? Does this pose have anything to do with how your body wants to move naturally? These are the questions we ask our bodies in YogAlign, and this inner dialogue empowers the practitioner with discernment and the ability to feel the body, and hear what it says at all times.

Many of the traditional poses taught by the majority of yoga schools are not practiced in YogAlign, because our body is just not designed for these positions. Many yoga students have heard "the pose begins when you want to come out of it" or "breathe through the pain," but in YogAlign, a pose feels effortless when done right, and we do not stay in positions that make us feel uncomfortable. We don't breathe through pain in the hopes that it will disappear, or imagine that staying in a pose that feels uncomfortable will somehow benefit us. In YogAlign we follow what feels good to our body and we know that one does not become *comfortable* by being *uncomfortable*. YogAlign teaches us to be our own teacher, and to trust our inner voice and discernment. People get hurt when they ignore their own body and try to follow the dictates of others.

So, in YogAlign we ask questions. What is beneficial about putting our body in a position where we cannot breathe deeply and which has nothing to do with how we naturally move throughout our day? Do we ever walk with both knees straightened at the same time? The body is designed to move by bending our knees, so we need to let go of the old, outdated idea that "straightening your knees and trying to bend forward" will make us flexible. or that it shows how flexible we are.

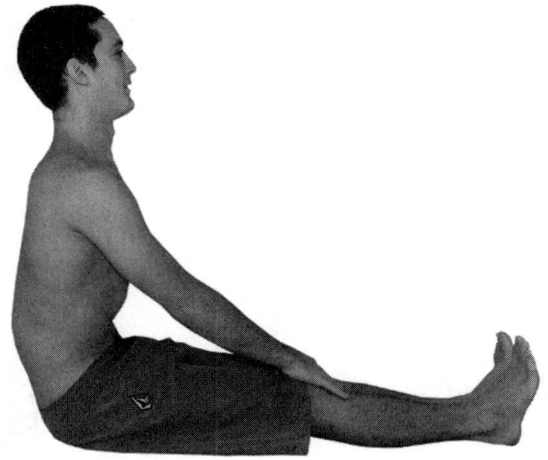

Fig. 1.3A – Shortening the front to stretch the back makes no anatomical sense.

In primitive villages you would never see people sitting like Zack (**Fig. 1.3A**). Many yoga students admit that they dislike the straight-leg seated positions, but feel that perhaps this is only because their bodies aren't flexible enough. The good news is that you are communicating well with your body if you know that certain poses simply do not feel good, and are unnatural to you. Many poses feel bad to us because they compress the lower back discs and flatten the natural tilt of our lumbar spine and sacrum. Our body is saying "This hurts!" and it is letting us know it is time to stop. Continuing to do harm to the body, even after it has sent a clear message to us to stop, is a violation of a fundamental yoga principle of *ahimsa*, or non-violence. This practice of non-violence must be applied to ourselves as well as to others.

People practice painful poses believing they will eventually become flexible. I did this for years until I realized that we will never get comfortable and flexible by being uncomfortable and trying to put the body in a position that has nothing to do with how we are designed to move in real life. Sitting poorly will not make you flexible; this makes no anatomical sense. There is a very good chance such positions will not improve your flexibility and, done over an extended period, could cause harm. Yoga injuries are on the rise and some physical therapists have estimated that 30–40 percent of people doing yoga get some type of injury[1]. According to the Consumer Product Safety Commission, 13,000 people who went to the emergency room between 2004 and 2007 reported being injured from practicing yoga[2]. YogAlign was developed in part to combat the rise in yoga injuries and encourage people to use the practice of yoga to develop better functionality in their bodies without causing harm.

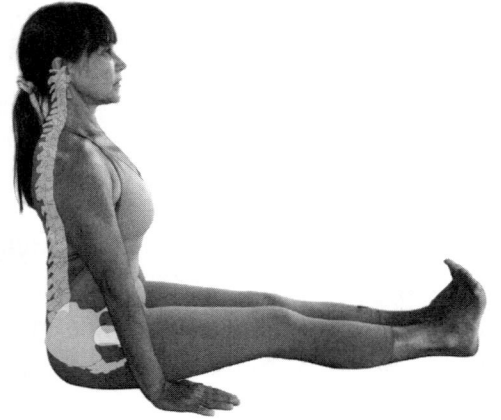

Fig. 1.3B– Flattened or convex sacrum creates tension in the lower back.

Life happens in the here and now and if you are not comfortable in a pose now, you never will be. People who are very flexible in the hips and hamstrings do certain exercises with ease, not seeing the inherent danger of flattening the curve of the lumbar spine (**Fig. 1.3B**). In these exercises, ligaments in the sacrum become overstretched, contributing to a straight, flat spinal line at the junction of the pelvis. This "saggy sacrum" leads to hip compression, knee pain, and a lack of shock absorption for the entire structure of the body.

In YogAlign, at least one knee is always bent, to maintain and support natural postural alignment of the body (**Fig. 1.3C**). If you're not convinced, just try walking across the room without bending your knees. You will immediately see that the human body is not designed for movement without bending the knees, and trying to keep your knees straight goes against our body's design. Foot positions in which one extends through the heel with the toes pulled towards the shin do not serve natural

[1] *The Perils of Posing,* by Susan Underwood, *Newsweek,* January 9, 2007

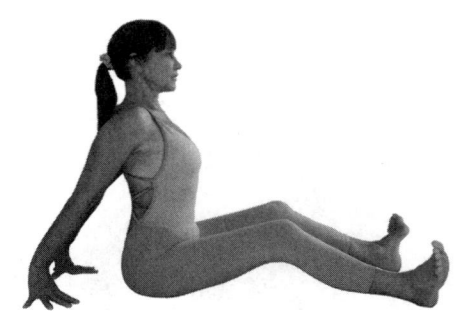

Fig. 1.3C – The Spine Aligner. Bent knees support the four natural curves of the spine.

alignment either. Next time you go for a swim, pull your toes in towards your shin, and you'll see that one cannot propel through the water unless the toes are pointed. Why have we been taught in most yoga poses to pull the toes back towards the shin as we press out through the heel? It makes no anatomical sense when one learns that the position of the foot affects the body's ability to move and breathe.

YogAlign practices use natural body positions and eliminate the linear right-angled poses that seem to define yoga and many styles of fitness and training. The straight-leg and heel-pressing, right-angled position shown in **Fig. 1.3B** has permeated fitness training and culture for far too long. YogAlign seeks to open a discussion with each individual about how they are using their body and why. It is not about taking orders or instruction from others, but more about developing discernment, awareness, and education about the innate design of your body/mind. YogAlign is a self-healing system that is questioning orthodoxy, making anatomical sense, and empowering the practitioner in the way that traditional yoga classes empower the instructor.

Natural Alignment for Life

I've had literally hundreds of people come into my studio seeking to re-establish the natural curve of their lower back and sacrum. Many have sacral injuries caused by overstretched ligaments from endless hours of chair-sitting and/or from practicing unnatural exercises in yoga or stretching classes. The sacrum is a shock absorber and has a natural tilt in it that protects the hips and knees from compression forces when we walk or sit. Tucking it under or stretching the ligaments that keep it stable lead to long term pain and joint destabilization.

With the increase of yoga injuries, many teachers are coming to understand that forward bends are dangerous if you have disc injury. Yet many will still say it is safe for the non-injured to practice these bends, as long as they hinge from the hips, stretch from the hamstrings, and pull in the lower belly muscles to keep the lower back safe. When the lower belly is pulled in, what happens? The action of drawing the navel towards the spine shortens your front body, compresses the front of your discs

Three Simple Tests Determine Whether a Pose Serves the Human Design:

1. *It should allow the spine to maintain its natural curves.*

2. *It should not restrict the ability to do deep, full, rib-cage breathing.*

3. *It should have a real-life correlation to functional movement positions.*

YogAlign *encourages proper body alignment, builds strength, and increases mobility.*

YogAlign *can add longevity to your life by providing a template for the body to follow, allowing it to be functional and highly mobile well into old age.*

YogAlign *emphasizes maintaining natural body position and the natural curves of the spine, and only utilizes positions that mimic functional movement.*

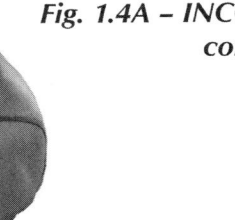

Fig. 1.4A – INCORRECT: Forward Bend with compressed spine.

Fig 1.4B – CORRECT: Forward Bend with decompressed and aligned spine.

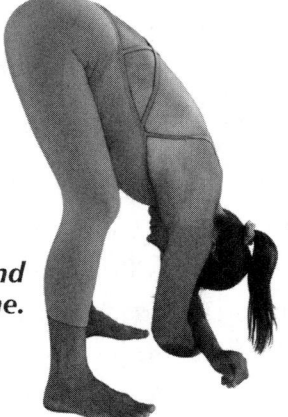

in the lower back and puts excess strain on the sacrum, leading to more pain and discomfort. Pain is the body saying "I don't move this way." The pose in **Fig. 1.4A** is quite likely one of the reasons that sacrum injury and destabilization is the one of the most common of all yoga injuries.

In YogAlign we believe in honoring the way each body is uniquely coded, and don't impose ideals like keeping a "straight" spine when clearly our spine functions as it was designed—with curves necessary for shock absorption. In YogAlign, students learn anatomy from a holistic perspective—that all parts affect the whole—in order to protect the structure of their bodies.

GETTING THAT "KID BODY" BACK

Getting your kid body back with YogAlign begins with learning to do deep, functional inner core breathing. Maintaining natural spine alignment is the key to breathing from the inner core, where one can access all of the respiratory muscles. Engaging the psoas/diaphragm connection frees the spine when breathing, creating more of the kid body feeling. YogAlign also encourages using daily self-massage to bring blood flow to our tissues, and sensory awareness to our nervous system. We "re-code" the movement centers of the brain for better postural patterns, training our muscles to carry less tension, and freeing the fascia web to support a better posture from the inside out.

We will explore all of the techniques and concepts discussed in this chapter more in-depth throughout the rest of this book. By the end you will see that YogAlign is easy, fun, simple, and fascinating. More importantly, when you begin to feel its effects through your practice, you'll see that it just makes sense.

—

YogAlignMent Principle #1

To cultivate the art of self love,
practice *ahimsa*, or non-violence, in
all yoga poses or positions.

—

YogAlignMent Principle #2

Pay attention to how your body
feels, and remember that all poses
should feel steady and comfortable.

CHAPTER 2: FREE YOUR FASCIA

YogAlign focuses on attaining good posture, not performing poses.

> **"**The muscle–bone concept presented in standard anatomical description gives a purely mechanical model of movement. It separates movement into discrete functions, failing to give a picture of the seamless integration seen in a living body. When one part moves, the body as a whole responds. Functionally, the only tissue that can mediate such responsiveness is the connective tissue.**"**

Feitis and Schultz, *The Endless Web*

Simple, fundamental movements shape our body on a daily basis. Fascia is the underlying determinant of the quality of our movement—and therefore our lives. Rather than being made up of separate parts, the human body is a continuum where all parts affect the whole. Any movement that we make reverberates throughout our entire body.

Your Posture Is Determined by Your Fascia Lines

Fascia is the stretchy web of connective tissue that permeates all of your muscles and organs, and lines every cell, providing an internal support system for your structure. Making up 20 percent of the weight of your body, fascia resembles the cellulose substance found inside citrus fruits. Think about the shape of a grapefruit and how, when you peel away the skin, you will see that the circular shape of the fruit remains intact, retained by the white cellulose matrix that holds the fruit together like a wrapper. If you pull apart the sections, you will see more of the white cellulose material separating the juice of the grapefruit into distinct sections spiraling from the center. If you continue to look at each smaller and smaller part, you will see that there are tiny little juice buds that are encased in a wrapper of finer cellulose. If you then looked with a microscope, you would see the cells that make up the grapefruit also have a membrane that makes up the wall of every cell. All of the juice in the fruit is contained by the cellulose structure, and creates all of the distinct sections.

The outer myofascia of the human body is like the white cellulose of the grapefruit, which continues to hold the shape of the grapefruit even after it has been peeled. Fascia in the human body is made of elastin and collagen protein strands. Our fascia runs in long lines from head to toe, and also in bands that encircle the body, mitigating movement and supporting our entire structure. These lines form a stretchy net surrounding the entire body, and if our skin were to be peeled away, our shape would be held in place by this web of connective tissue. Fascia holds up the skeletal structure, attaching it to our muscles and organs, and attaching those muscles and organs to each other. As such an integral part of our bodies, it's no wonder that the balance of tension in the fascial structure defines our movement, our posture, and even our moods.

Similar to the tent image in Chapter 1, our fascia is organized in directional lines of pull that can also be compared to the rigging on a sailboat, with our spine as the mast. The myofascial lines are the stays and the rigging that hold the mast in position. If the mast is out of alignment, or the rigging is pulled too tightly on one side and too slack on the other, the boat is off-center. There will be no fluidity when the boat is moving and you will be unable to sail until the rigging is properly adjusted. Like the boat, in order to find balance and become graceful in our movement, we must balance our fascia lines.

Fascia is everywhere, and like the white marbling you can see in a cut of tenderloin steak, these tissue lines permeate the muscles. The strands of fascia running the length of our bodies direct muscles along their pathways, and connect them in distinct lines of movement. Because of this webbed structure, no muscle can contract in isolation; every movement, every contraction, reverberates throughout the entire body beginning with the movements of the diaphragm and its fascial connections to our internal organs at the deep core. Most pain and misalignment problems stem from a lack of integration in our core even when pain appears to be more superficial. Tuning the fascia and balancing the muscles begins by awakening our breathing process, which happens in the center of our body

> **"**Muscle itself is spongy, able to expand and contract and so exerts pressure and friction on its surrounding fascial bed. Muscle tissue is similar in consistency to taffy. Connective tissue gives it shape, direction, and organization, much as the candy wrapper shapes the taffy. Because it is continuous throughout the body, connective tissue generalizes local muscle action. For example, as the biceps move, the whole arm moves, including the shoulder and neck.**"**
>
> Feitis and Schultz, *The Endless Web*

Many people believe that the skeleton is our main support structure, but our bones are more like spacers that are part of the connective tissue or fascia web system. Bones are composed of a highly mineralized substance that makes up the densest part of the connective tissue system. Ligaments are fibrous connective tissues that connect the bones and form joints. Tendons are connective tissues that connect muscles to bones, and are supported by the cartilage that makes up the fascia system. Our brain and spinal cord are also enveloped by connective tissues called meninges, and connective tissue tubing surrounds every nerve and vessel in the body. Connective tissue or fascia even divides the heart into chambers, and the liver into lobes. Fascial tissue is everywhere in our body down to the tiniest cell where the wall or membrane is made up of connective tissue.

FASCIA IS THE ORGAN OF POSTURE

The conventional ideal of body alignment places body masses (head, trunk, etc.) atop one another like a stack of blocks, lining them up so that gravity's axis runs through their centers, relying upon the bony skeleton to sustain their weight. The problem with this traditional model is that a stack of blocks doesn't move. Instead of blocks, the body is more like a spiraling continuum of balanced tensile forces.

> **"**_For a model that is more in accord with the fluid nature of the body, we borrow from the insights of engineering visionary Buckminster Fuller. He is famous for inventing the geodesic dome—the lightest, strongest, and most cost-effective shelter yet devised. Using pliable materials, Fuller used tension rather than compression to sustain his structures. He called his design system tensegrity._
>
> _If we apply Fuller's model to our bodies, we can see that it is the tensional force of our softer tissues that keeps us erect, not the compression strength of our bones. Floating within a sea of fluid tissues, bones are internal spacers for the body rather than beams that resist compression. The length and tension of connective tissue adapts to the changing orientation of the bones and distributes gravitational forces through our bodies as we move._**"**
>
> Bond, _The New Rules of Posture_

THE ENTIRE BODY IS INTERCONNECTED

Ideally, balanced tensile forces in our fascia and musculature structures work together to support our body with movement that is comfortable and efficient. However, by adulthood, dysfunctional alignment and faulty breathing can become ingrained in our neuromuscular patterning, making this ideal hard to realize. When these bad habits are adopted, people work themselves to exhaustion just moving through the day, because it takes double the effort to slouch that it takes to stand and move from the center of their bodies. Culture and lifestyle reinforce these weaknesses, because it has become commonplace to sit and exercise with misaligned, compressed spines.

The body is never static—even when we are sitting—and particularly not when we are slouching. It takes much more effort to have poor posture than good, as poor posture forces muscles to work extra hard at functions for which they are not designed. Unfortunately, very few people have posture that enables them to move their body in balance, with the spinal column supported equally on all sides of the body, and the skull balanced on top of the spinal column. The most common consequence of misalignment is "forward head carriage," in which the skull is held forward of the rest of the body, causing pain and strain in the back, hips, knees and shoulders. When the head is being held correctly, the center of our ear should be aligned with the middle cap of the arm at the shoulder. Common corrections for this misalignment are sucking the belly in and trying to support the head from the upper shoulder, neck, and lower back muscles; or forcefully pulling the shoulders down, straining the neck to support the head. These actions are superficial band-aids, and don't address the underlying problem, which is weak and/or dysfunctional breathing habits.

In YogAlign, we use our muscles and breath consciously and economically, allowing the fascia web to mitigate movement throughout the entire body without strain. Good posture is effortless, arising from deepening of the breathing process, the balance of tensile forces, and relaxation in the nervous system.

FREE YOUR FASCIA

Massage brings blood flow and sensory awareness, and establishes a relaxation pattern in the nervous system. Massage and Rolfing by a skilled practitioner is very helpful for changing the structure of the outer myofascia that can be palpated from the outside of the body. Rolfing was invented by Ida Rolf, and is now a popular form of body work involving strong manipulation of the body's soft tissue to realign and balance the body's myofascial structure. However effective, bodywork alone is not enough to change structure at the nervous system level. It must be combined with breathing and movement re-patterning exercises that affect the deeper layers of the body. Breathing movements facilitate fascial re-organization at the inner surface of our ribcage and the lining of our pelvic floor and diaphragm; areas that are not palpable by human hands. YogAlign uses the inner movements of deep breathing to bring blood flow

MORE FASCINATING FASCIAL FACTS FOR THE ANATOMICALLY CURIOUS

The Fascia Trains Theory has been developed by Rolfer and somatic educator, Thomas Myers. Myers is the author of *Anatomy Trains* and a set of supporting videos, and has also penned over 60 articles for trade magazines and journals on anatomy, soft tissue manipulation, and the social scourge of somatic alienation and loss of reliance on kinesthetic intelligence.

According to Myers, "The traditional mechanistic view of anatomy, as useful as it has been, has objectified rather than humanized our relationship to our insides. The deeper premise underling the fascial trains anatomy theory is a more thorough and sensitive contact with our 'felt sense'—that is, our kinesthetic, proprioceptive, spatial sense of orientation and movement. The progressive deadening of this 'felt sense' in our children, whether through simple ignorance or by deliberate schooling, lends itself to a collective dissociation, which leads in turn to environmental and social decline."

"We have long been familiar with mental intelligence (IQ) and more recently have recognized emotional intelligence (EQ). Only by re-contacting the full reach and educational potential of our kinesthetic intelligence (KQ) will we have any hope of finding a balanced relationship with the larger systems of the world around us."

Myers, Thomas W., *Anatomy Trains*, 2nd ed. 2009
Edinburgh; New York: Churchill Livingstone Elsevier. www.anatomytrains.com

and fascia-opening where it would be otherwise impossible to palpate or massage our structure. The YogAlign combination of specialized breath work, self-massage, and movement re–education can be very effective. YogAlign reaches every part of the body during each practice with massage, deep core breathing, functional body positions, and kinesthetic awareness exercises.

Ideally, bodywork needs to be combined with a permanent change in movement patterning so that we can develop efficient, balanced fascia tensional integrity, or "tensegrity." This work happens in YogAlign by using breathing and re-patterning of posture. An actual "re-wiring" of movement is essential, or the fascia will return to its original state. This is why often people receive deep bodywork resulting in immediate good posture and relief from pain, yet within a few months their body returns to its previous habituated dysfunction. There must be a change in the neuromuscular codes that direct our movements, or fascia thickening and poor posture patterns will return.

The case of the most common type of poor posture — slouching, or a shortening of the front body — shows the head pulled forward, the shoulders rounded, and the lower back flat with no natural curve. While the front body slouches, the back body is strained and sore in response to the over-contraction of the front. The tightness in the front leads to a thickening, or an overgrowth, of fascia concentrating in the upper back, especially between the shoulder blades. The fascia system lays down more tissue in the back in order to stabilize the shortening of the front body. This thickening is the body's response to habituated muscle patterns that ingrain positions like sitting posture, even if those positions are not ideal. If a person becomes habitually stooped in posture, the thickened fascia will eventually slow the metabolic rate of the back muscles and lead to chronic pain and stiffening. By correcting alignment patterns that cause excessive muscle effort, excess fascia will actually dissolve from the inside out, similar to the way scar tissue dissolves away from an injured area.

Combining core breathing and natural spine alignment body positions, we acquire a powerful tool that balances our fascia web and postural patterning from the inside out. In this way, the practice of YogAlign enables us to move and breathe freely and effortlessly in all of our activities.

Your Brain Makes Maps of Your Body

Visualizing allows us to sense more of our body. What we can sense, we can change. Having an image in your mind of how the myofascial lines run through your body helps you to sense them and then consciously change what has become unconscious. The anatomical drawings of muscle connections and fascia trains in this book will help you visualize the optimal balance that we seek. Once you have this visual map, you can begin to practice body and sensory awareness from an inner perspective that allows you to truly feel the body. You will actually *sense* the fascia and the muscle pathways as you move and practice functional breathing.

Note: The YogAlign Postures Chart begins on page 341 and provides an easy reference to each pose and the Methods directions.

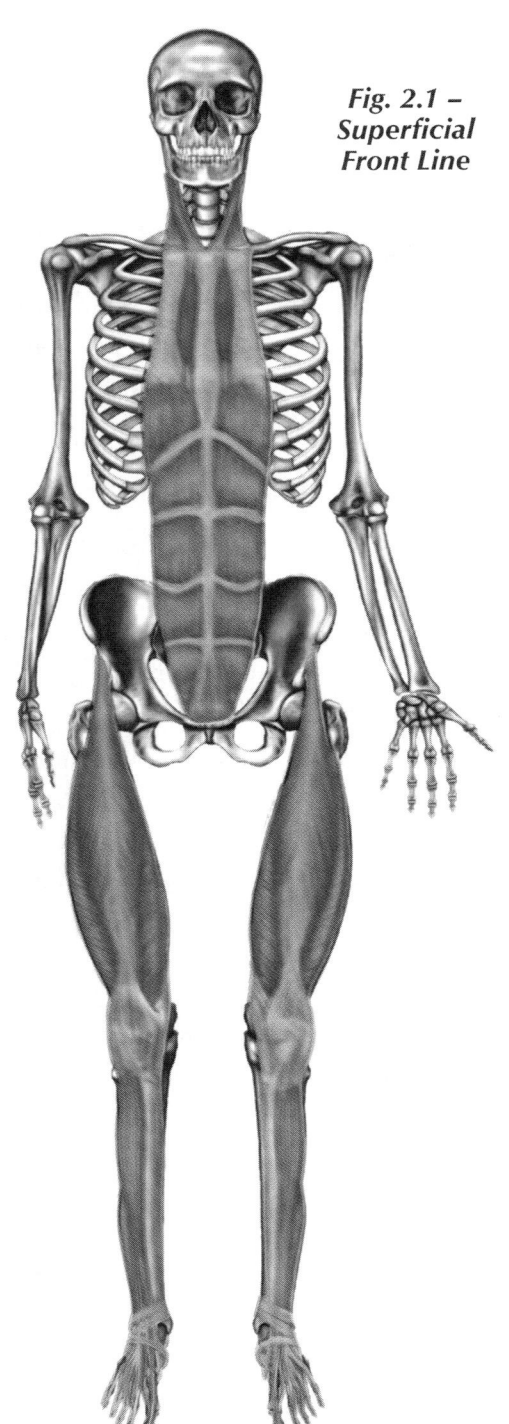

Fig. 2.1 –
Superficial
Front Line

Redrawn from *Anatomy Trains*
by Thomas Myers

SUPERFICIAL FRONT LINE

The superficial front line of fascia is close to the surface of the body and is easily massaged or palpated via the superficial muscle structure (**Fig. 2.1**). The line of fascia connects the top of the toes to the mastoid process of the skull. Exercises that over-emphasize the tightening of the six-pack muscles reinforce muscle patterning that pulls the ribs down towards the pubic bones, shortening and tightening the entire front from head to toes. This shortening effect compresses the hips, knees and spine, while also causing a restriction of the rib cage's breathing movements.

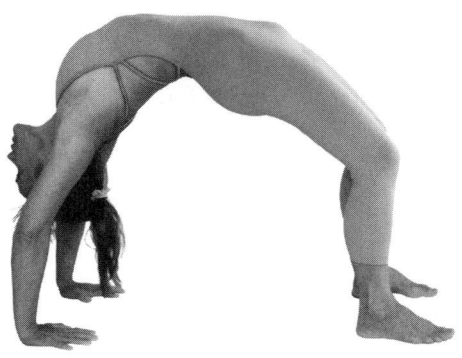

Stretching the superficial front line.

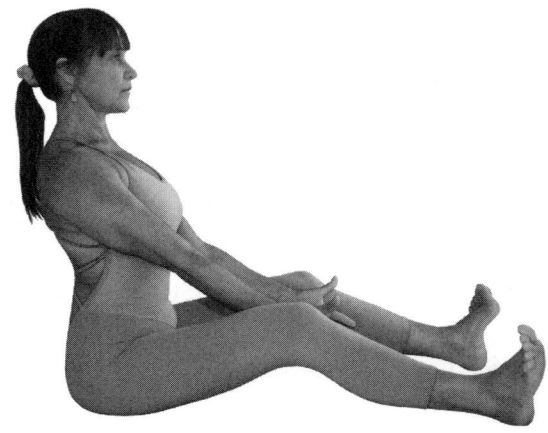

Contracting the core muscles of the body, including the muscles along the superficial front line.

SUPERFICIAL BACK LINE

This line of fascia extends all the way from the top of the eye sockets to the underside of the feet. This line goes over the top of the skull, along the back of the neck, and down the back, connecting along the sacrum, and lower leg to the underside of the foot (**Fig. 2.2**). In many people, the muscles and fascia along the back line are in a chronic state of over-stretched tension. Chronic back and hamstring pain is the result of the muscles of the superficial back line locked out long in tension forces drafted to balance the weakness or tightness of the core and front body.

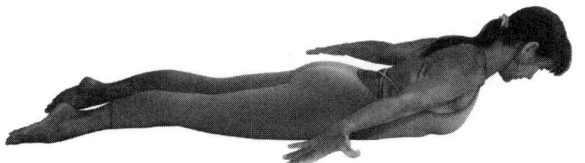

Contracting the back line.

Sitting in chairs and slouching with bad posture creates the structural imbalances that lead to the inevitable sore back and neck. The relief of lower back pain and tight hamstrings is not found in doing exercises that shorten the abdominals and compress the spine in the process of stretching the tension out of the back body. Instead, the source of the pain is located and relief is found using YogAlign's deep functional breathing process, which brings power to the deep core and equilibrium to the disparity between the tight and/or weak front, and a back or side body locked out in tension.

Stretching the back line.

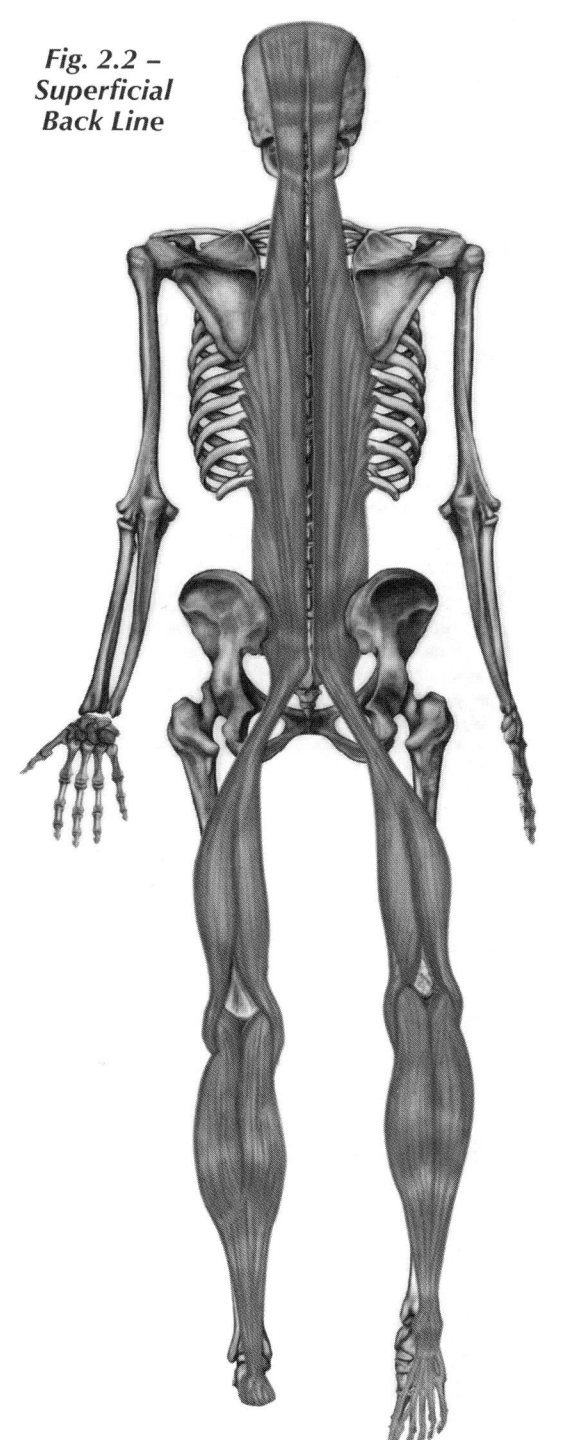

Fig. 2.2 –
Superficial
Back Line

Redrawn from *Anatomy Trains*
by Thomas Myers

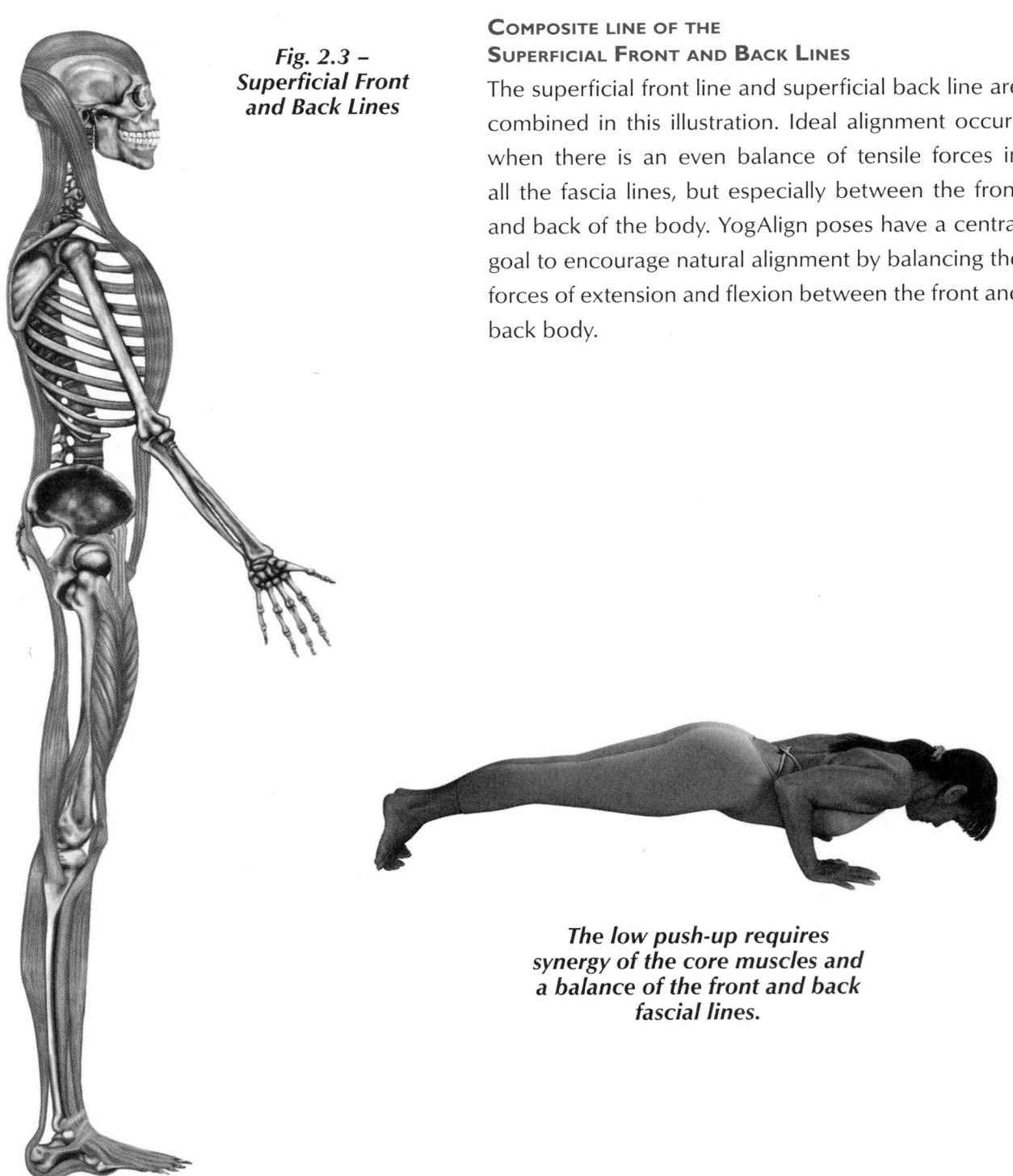

COMPOSITE LINE OF THE SUPERFICIAL FRONT AND BACK LINES

The superficial front line and superficial back line are combined in this illustration. Ideal alignment occurs when there is an even balance of tensile forces in all the fascia lines, but especially between the front and back of the body. YogAlign poses have a central goal to encourage natural alignment by balancing the forces of extension and flexion between the front and back body.

*Fig. 2.3 –
Superficial Front
and Back Lines*

*The low push-up requires
synergy of the core muscles and
a balance of the front and back
fascial lines.*

Redrawn from *Anatomy Trains*
by Thomas Myers

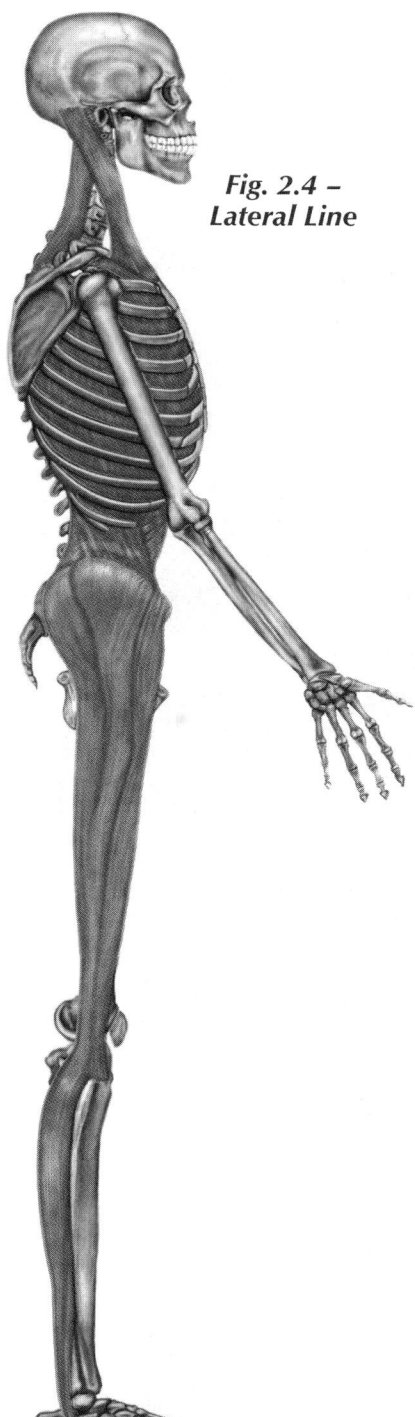

Fig. 2.4 –
Lateral Line

Redrawn from *Anatomy Trains*
by Thomas Myers

LATERAL LINE

In **Fig. 2.4**, notice how the fascia pathways of the lateral line crisscross several times helping to stabilize the body in all sideways and lateral movements. The lateral line runs from the strap muscles of the neck to the intercostals between the ribs, to the large gluteus muscles and lateral stabilizers of the leg and foot. Poor breathing habits that initiate breath from the neck or upper shoulders can cause fascial thickening that can sabotage movement and fluidity in the muscles and fascia of the entire lateral line, from the skull to the foot.

Fig. 2.4B

Stretching the lateral line.

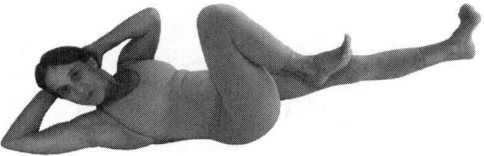

Contracting the lateral line.

EXPERIENTIAL EXERCISE #3

The Lateral Line

Stand holding one of your wrists or elbow area as shown in **Fig. 2.4B**. Leaning to the side slightly, create an action of trying to stand upright without actually doing it. Keep your arm pulling back towards your trunk while spreading the fingers of your extended arm. Keep your knees slightly soft to avoid hyper-extending the back of your knee while keeping your ribs over your pelvis. Press into your feet and take a deep breath through your mouth as though sipping on a straw. Notice the feeling of energy through the entire lateral side of your body from the fingertips to your foot. After doing this for a few seconds, bring your arms down to your sides and then lift both arms together experiencing the difference in length between the two sides of your body.

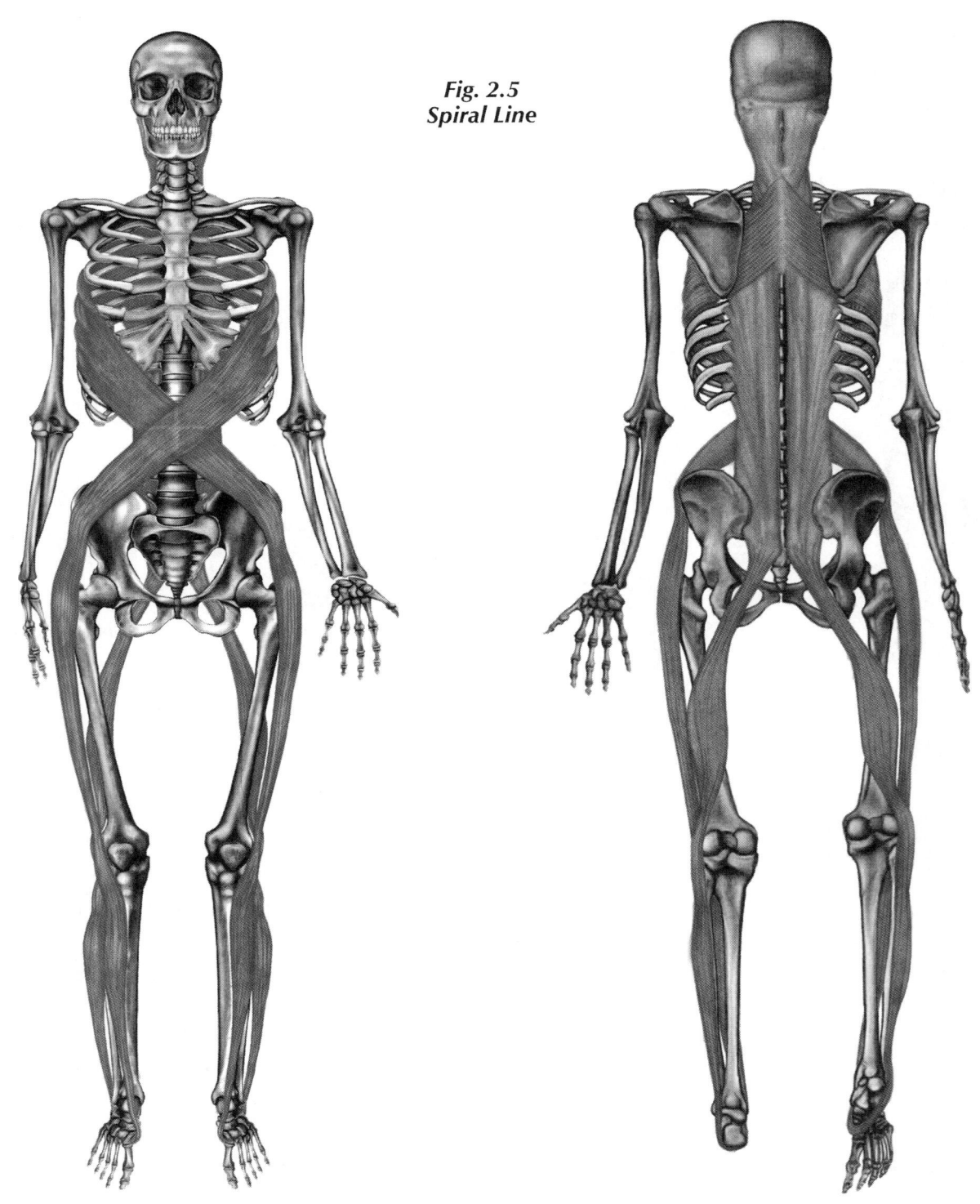

Fig. 2.5
Spiral Line

Redrawn from *Anatomy Trains* by Thomas Myers

SPIRAL LINE

This line helps to create and mediate rotations in the body (**Fig. 2.5**). The spiral line begins in the occiput region (base) of the skull and travels under the shoulder blade around to the lateral abdominals in the front body, where it crosses back to the hip area. Traveling down to the outer knee, it then stirrups under the foot, and intersects up the leg in the back body to join the superficial back line. A balanced spiral line will ease twisting and remove tension in the muscles of the hip, neck, and scapula. Imbalances in the spiral line often cause pain in the top of the upper shoulder which then radiates under the shoulder blade and down around the front of the body and back to the hip, causing knee misalignment and foot pain. Tight neck muscles can become prisoners of their fascial envelopes. Any tension that forms along a fascia line can tug on distant connections of the web, and affect posture all over the body.

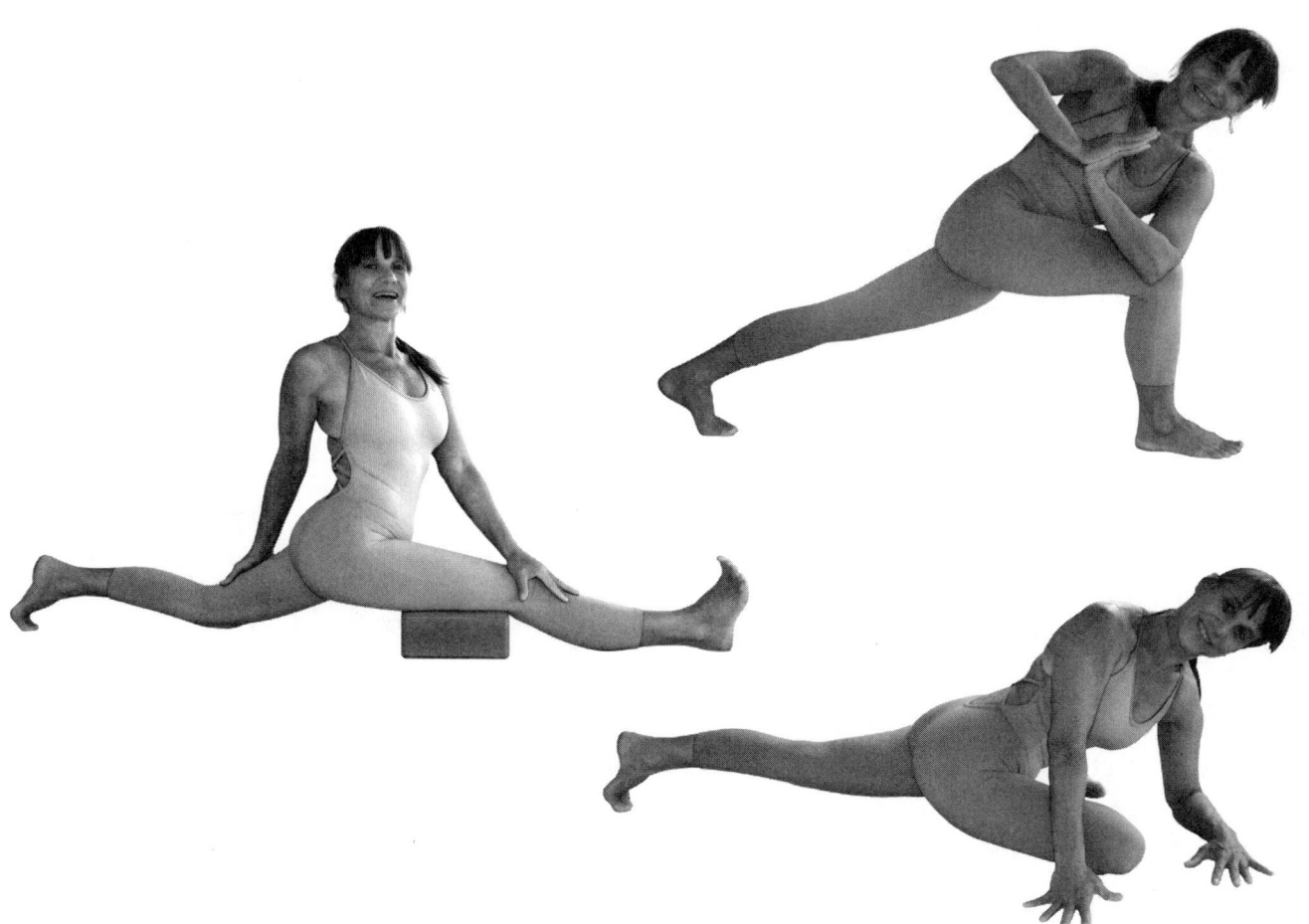

Twists and rotation poses engage the spiral line of fascia.

Fig. 2.6 — Arm Lines

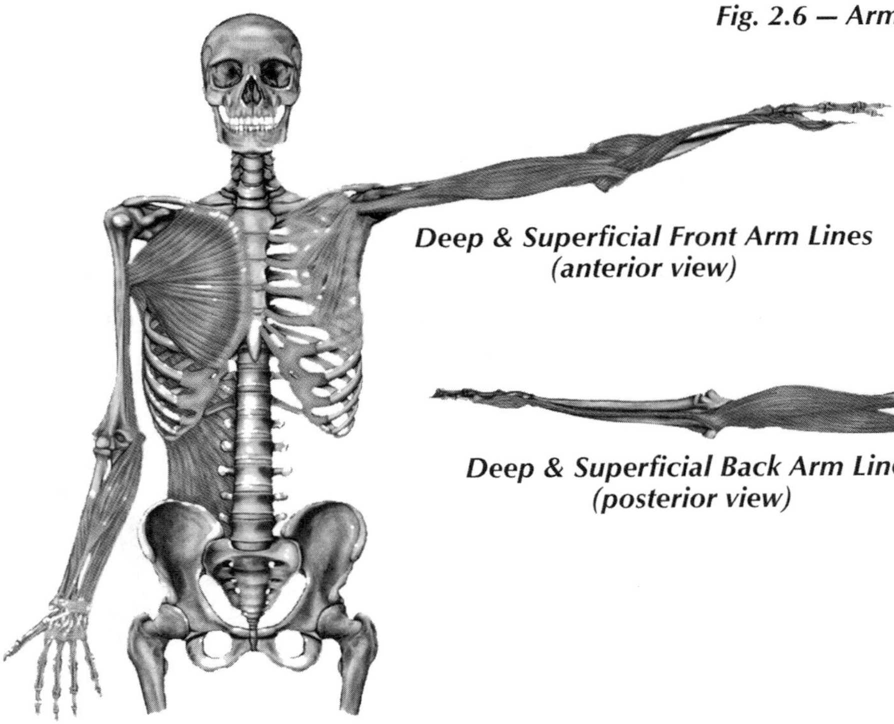

Deep & Superficial Front Arm Lines
(anterior view)

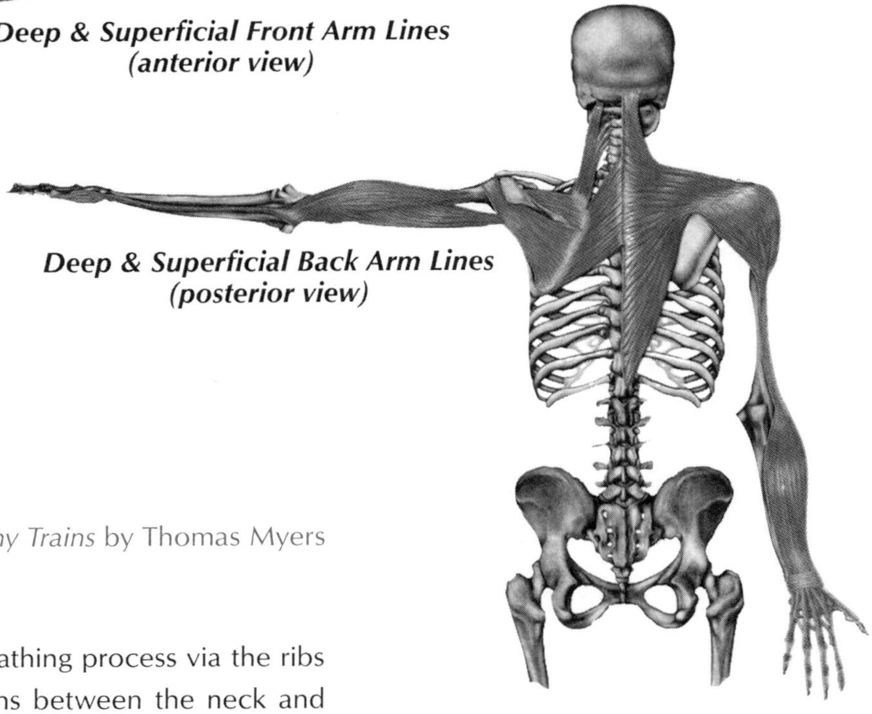

Deep & Superficial Back Arm Lines
(posterior view)

Redrawn from *Anatomy Trains* by Thomas Myers

ARM LINES

The arm lines connect to the breathing process via the ribs **(Fig. 2.6)**. Notice the connections between the neck and the arms in the back, and between the arms and the chest in the front. Thumb movement is connected to the front of the shoulder and the pinkie finger is connected to the lateral border of the scapula. The arm lines are seamlessly connected to the rest of the fascia lines, and any movement of the arm affects the body as a whole. Learning to engage arm line connections from the deep core helps to stabilize joint function, and prevent injuries in the extremities. Many people are disconnected from the ability to sense and move from the deep roots of the arms that extend from the back, hip, spine, diaphragm and chest muscles. YogAlign techniques balance the actions in the front and back arm lines, reestablishing movement patterns that arise from the center of your body.

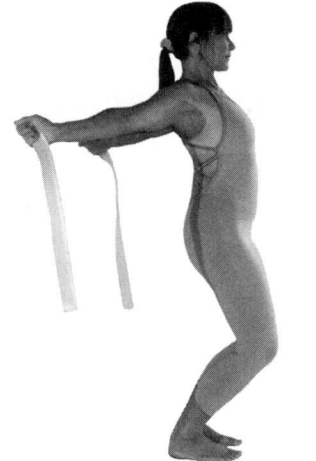

Circumduction of the shoulder joint involves contraction and stretching of the arm lines.

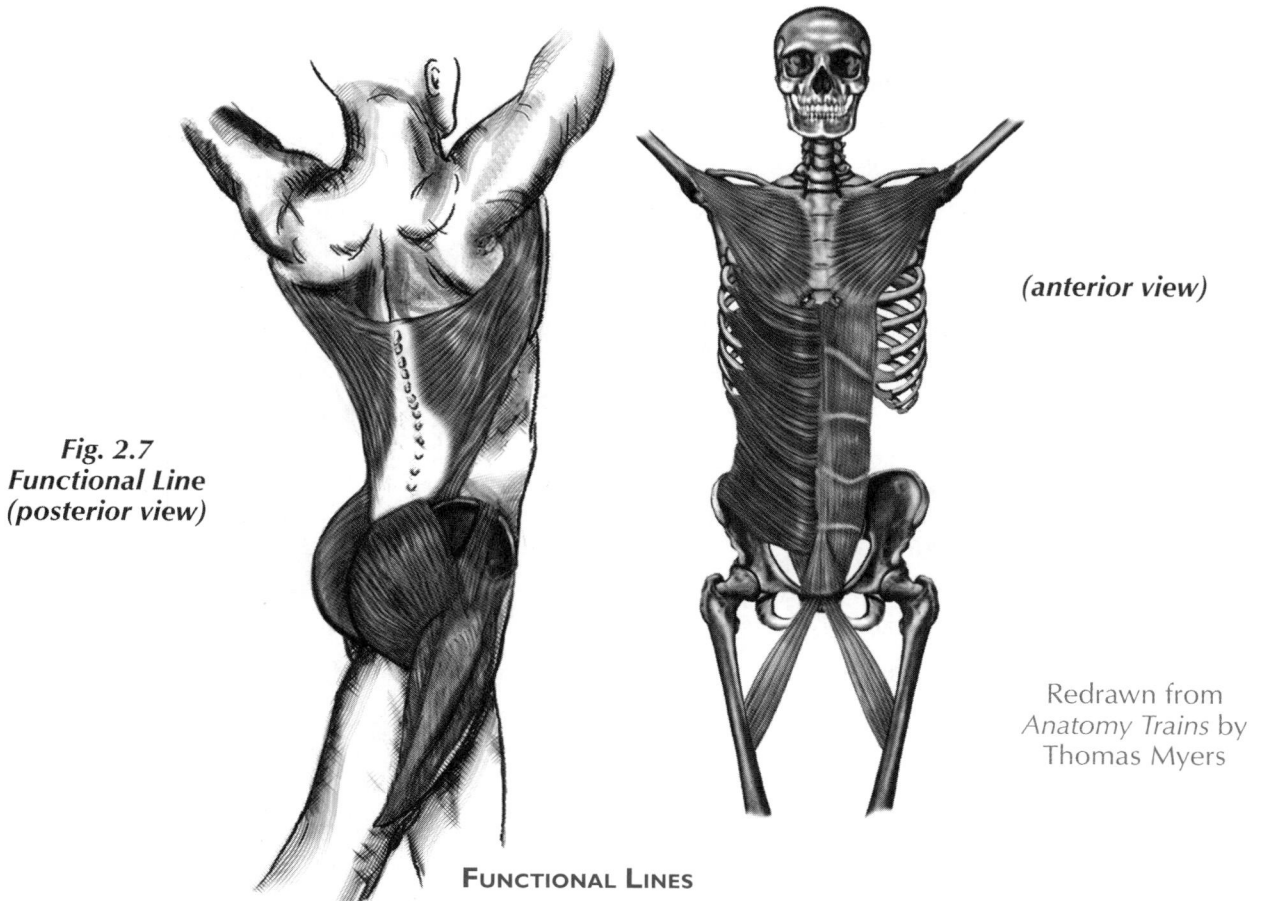

Fig. 2.7
Functional Line
(posterior view)

(anterior view)

Redrawn from
Anatomy Trains by
Thomas Myers

FUNCTIONAL LINES

These lines include the buttock muscles, inner thigh, outer core, chest and lats or latissimus dorsi muscles (**Fig. 2.7**). The functional lines of fascia connect the arm lines to the surface of the trunk and to the front and back of the legs. They help to link the arms to each other through the front and back of the body, and to opposite sides of the buttocks. These lines do not come into play in normal sitting or standing movements, but are activated in sports activities where they assist in—and counterbalance—deep movements supported by the inner core, such as hitting a tennis ball. Since many people do not breathe or move from the center of their body, they do not have a well-defined, functional fascia connection, resulting in shallow breathing and poor movement skills. In YogAlign we focus on activating and engaging the muscles along the functional line even in our regular daily movements.

The "Twisted Tree" pose engages the players of the functional line.

Deep Core Line

Notice how this deep core line runs from the side of the skull through the deep neck and continues all the way through the inner visceral body to the soles of the feet **(Fig. 2.8)**. This is the line most closely associated with the actions of the breathing apparatus and the "core of the core" muscle group: the psoas.

> **❝**The fascia of your diaphragm and lungs is connected with fascial sheets that lie along the inside surface of your spine and descend through your pelvis and groin. The fascia in turn is continuous with tracks that run down your inner legs to your feet. When, during inhalation, the descent of your diaphragm pulls down on the fascia around your lungs, it sends bio-electric signals all the way to your ankles.**❞**
>
> Bond, *The New Rules of Posture*

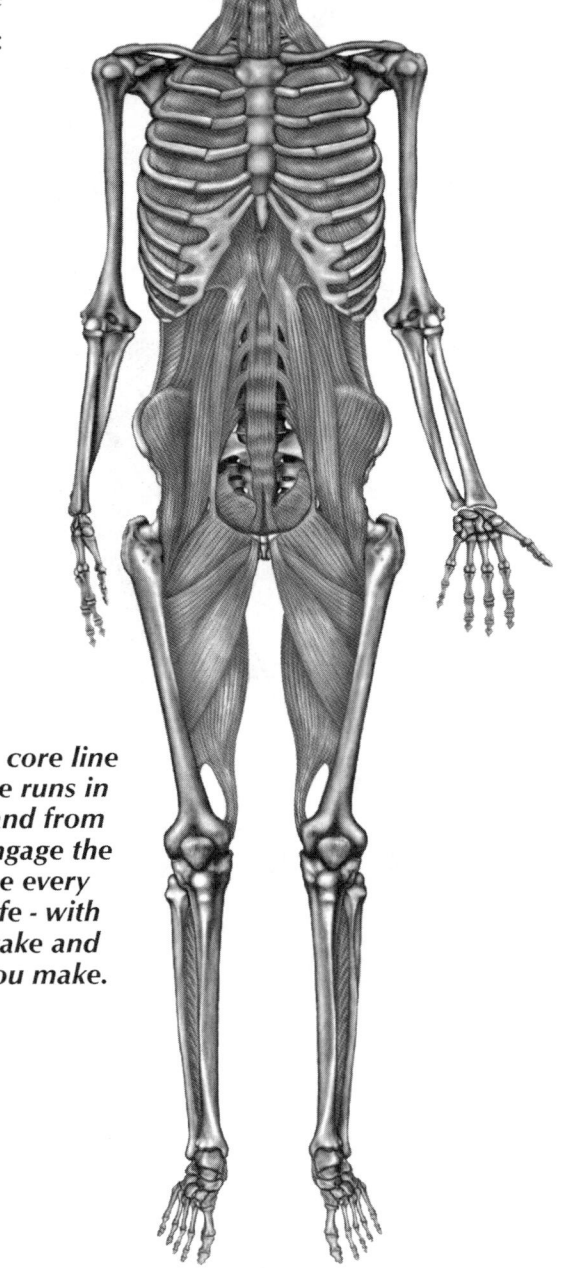

Fig. 2.8 — The deep core line of connective tissue runs in one continuous band from head to toe. You engage the actions of this line every moment of your life - with every breath you take and every movement you make.

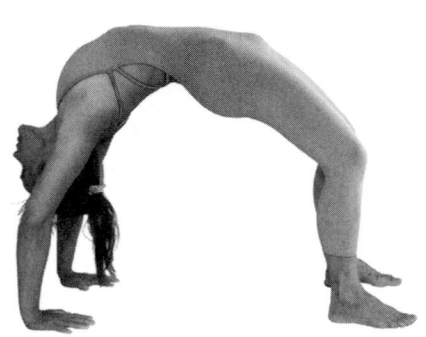

"The Wheel" pose stretches and opens the deep core line.

Redrawn from *Anatomy Trains* by Thomas Myers

In an aligned body, the forces of the deep front line support core-centered movement and natural alignment of the curves of the spine.

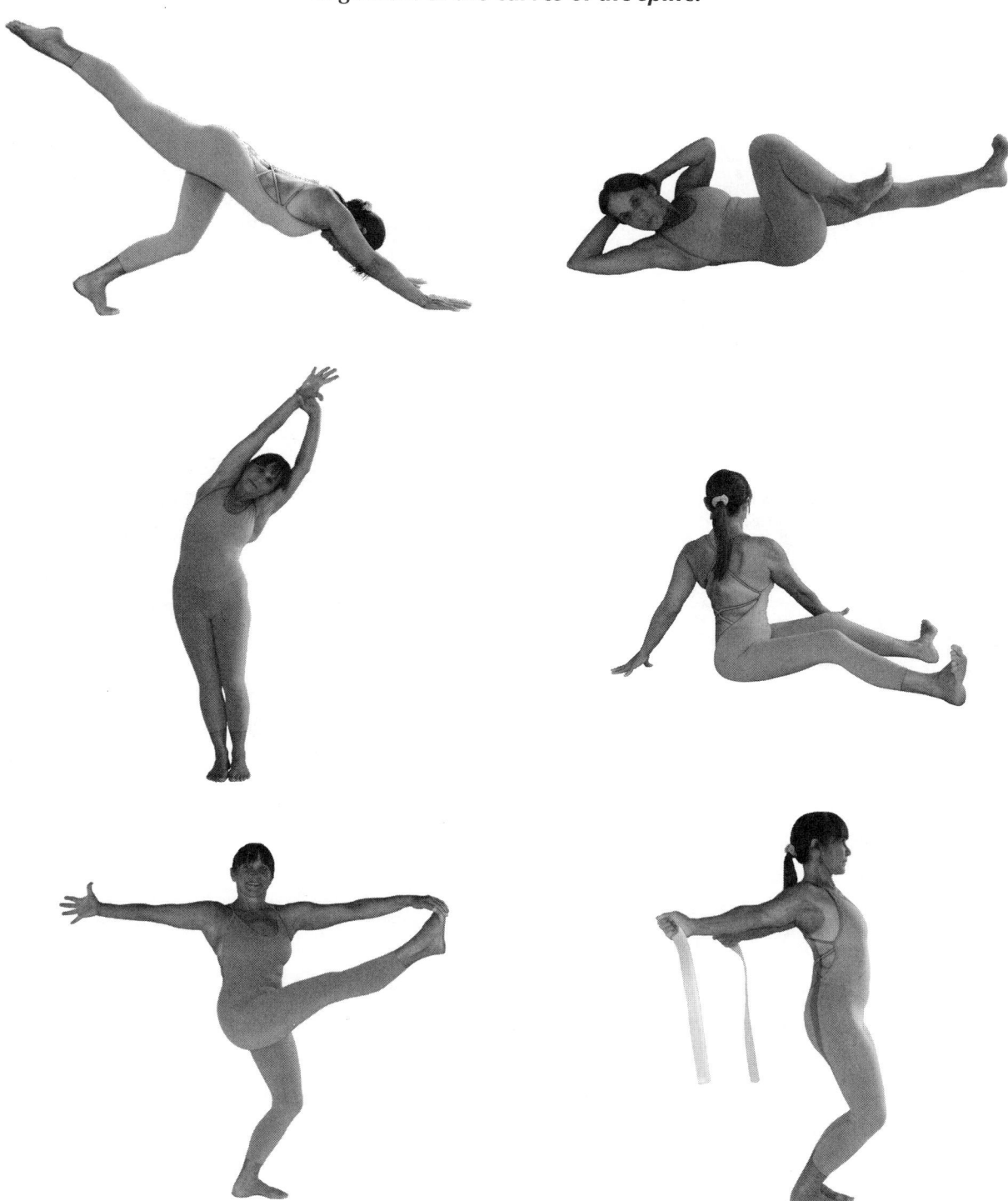

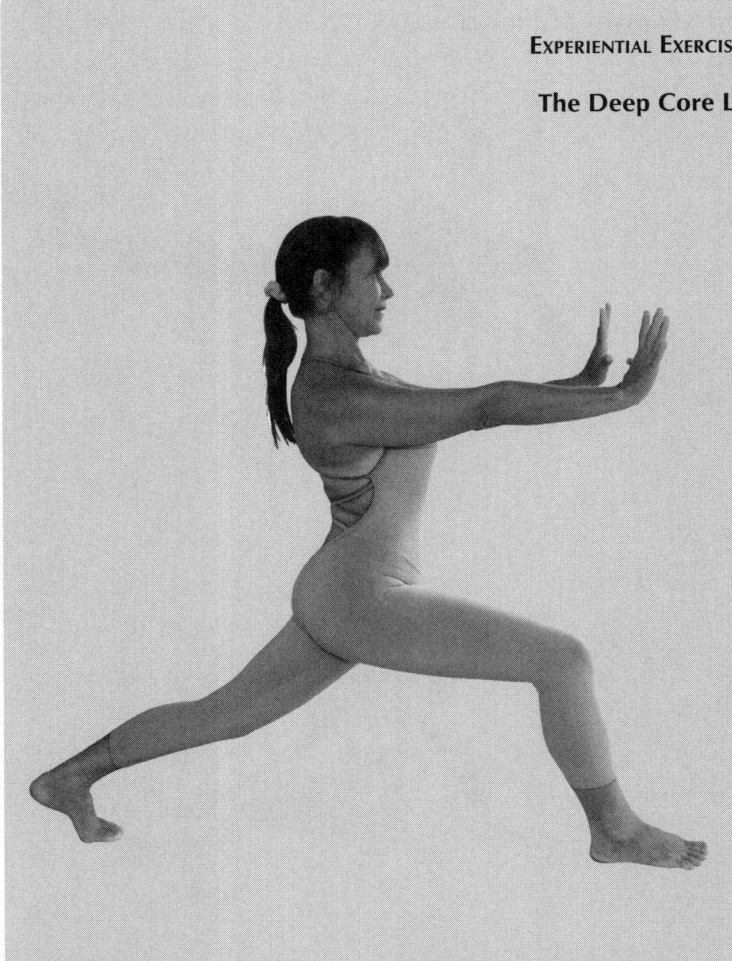

EXPERIENTIAL EXERCISE #4

The Deep Core Line

Stand in a lunge as shown here in the picture. With your shoulders level, place your hands out in front of you as though you are pushing a wall. Stay on the ball of your back foot with your hips squared up as shown in the picture. Keep your back knee slightly bent and your front knee over your ankle. Your front shin should be at a right angle to the floor. Pull the tips of your shoulder blades down and breathe in like you are sipping on a straw. This small hole in your mouth creates resistance—like weight training for breathing muscles. The sucking inbreath creates an elongated strengthening of the trunk, or waist.

Notice how the movement of the breathing process seems to pull a string that goes down through the groin and inside of your back leg. Some people even feel the pull of the fascial line going all the way to the foot. Make sure that your spine has its natural curves and that you are not flattening your lower back by tucking under your "tail."

FASCIA IS SHAPED BY OUR MOVEMENT AND OUR BREATHING HABITS

When we engage a muscle, an electrical charge signals the body to lay down more fascia along the lines of pull, in support of that movement. We need these fascia lines to organize and direct our body. However, if we continually put the body in unnatural positions, muscles begin to contract excessively and send out strong signals, causing us to develop fascial lines that hold us in these tense and rigid positions. When there is a shortness in our front body from sitting and employing weak breathing habits, our back muscles and fascia become strained and thick. Over the years, the muscles will become hard and ropey, and there will be excess fascial development reinforcing bad postural habits. This is how people wind up stiff and bent over with conditions like the dowager's hump so commonly seen in older people.

Fascia overgrowth is simply the fascia doing what it is designed to do, which is to support the structure in our habituated positions and movements. Freeing the fascia to be functional and balancing the tensile lines is the key to changing our inner and outer shape. When we get rid of habituated muscle tension, fascia can be directed to dissolve to a more fluid state from the inside out. On the other hand, unnatural movement and extended sitting or uncomfortable exercise positions can lead to the over-development and thickening of the fascia lines, and the patterning of poor movement and externalized breathing.

How we breathe is the most basic of our movements, so breath patterning is a huge determinant of posture and fascial health. Postural patterns are the forces that shape the ongoing development of our individual fascia. Improper alignment of our body hardens the fascia and we lose fluid, lubricated support in our movements and structure.

> **"**_Our bodies, then, contain a three-dimensional web of fascia with pockets and tubes for our various organs and muscle and microscopic compartments for every cell. Connective tissues are everywhere. In fact they make up about 20 percent of the body's weight. Anatomists have determined that were they to remove all other tissues from a body—liver, lung, brain, muscle, blood, fat, nerve, etc.—they would be left with a recognizable human form made of connective tissue._**"**
>
> Myers, _Anatomy Trains_

YogAlign poses are defined by the active and conscious release of habituated muscle tension. This engagement leads to balanced fascia lines that develop from the inside out, creating fluid lines of dynamic tension in the fascia web. All movements in YogAlign are focused on freeing our fascia and supporting healthy connective tissue all over the body. Excess muscle effort, such as poor posture, encourages detrimental overgrowth of fascia. If you keep the spine in natural alignment, neuromuscular action will support that alignment, and fascia will organize supportively. Our fascia patterning directs our every movement, therefore freeing the fascia is the key to being pain-free and aligned.

YogAlignMent Principle #3
Balanced connective tissue keeps you supported and
suspended in a web, allowing kid-like flexibility.

YogAlignMent Principle #4
Practice poses that emphasize equalized fascial tension
throughout the entirety of the body.

CHAPTER 3:
THE ANATOMICAL ROAD MAP OF YOUR CORE

*The psoas is
the core of your core.*

❝*When we speak of the body, we can't ignore the fact that we consist of bones, joints, muscles, organs, nerves, vessels, energy flows and much more. These elements are integrated into a functioning, ingenious whole and are subject to certain rules. If we don't know these rules, or ignore them, problems will occur sooner or later.*❞

Franklin, *Pelvic Power*

WHERE AND WHAT ARE YOUR PSOAS?

Many of us know more about the hard drives in our computers than we know about our own human anatomy and function. Yet the human body is more fascinating and more complex than any computer.

Do you know where your psoas muscles are? "No" is the usual answer.

The psoas muscles are one of the wonders of our anatomical structure, yet few of us have any idea of where they are and how they function. Often overlooked, misunderstood, ignored, and deactivated, the psoas muscles are located posterior to (behind) layers of abdominal muscles, and anterior to (in front of) the back muscles. As such, they lie at the very core of the human body **(Fig. 3.1)**. As the deepest of core muscles, the psoas connect the spine, diaphragm, and pelvis to the legs. They originate at the lower spine, attaching to all five vertebrae and discs in the lumbar spine, up to T-12 (the lowest vertebrae of the thoracic spine). Acting like two guy-wires, these deep groin muscles connect our upper body to our lower body, running from the spine to their connections at the inside of the upper leg bone.

The psoas muscles cannot be seen or felt directly, so most people have no idea that they exist, and therefore lack the bodily awareness necessary to sense the muscles' actions. The renowned body worker, Ida Rolf, believed and taught that the psoas muscles are *the* most important muscle group in the human body. The psoas are "the core of your core," and learning to engage, activate, lengthen, and relax this muscle group is key to living pain-free and from the "core."

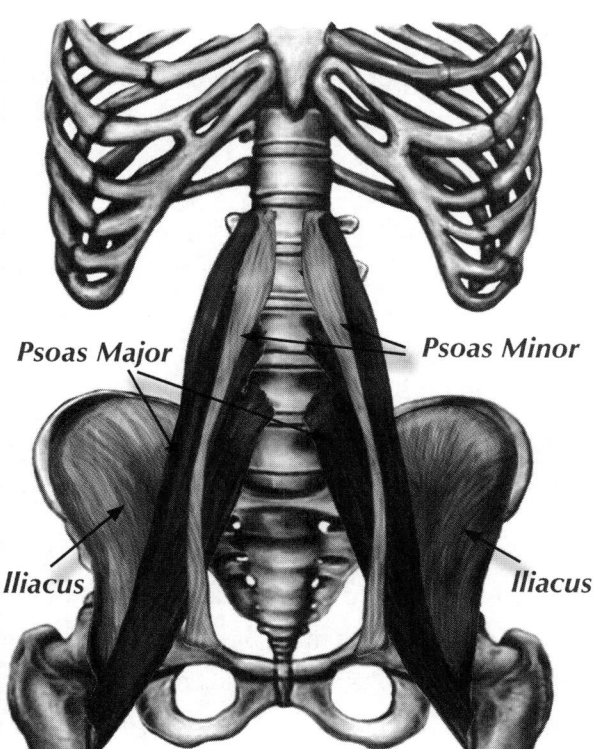

Psoas Major *Psoas Minor*

Iliacus *Iliacus*

Fig 3.1 – The psoas muscle group

Psoas Activation: Waking up the Core of Your Core

The psoas are the "jack of-all-trades" muscles, playing many roles in body movement and core stabilization. They are a hip flexor, act as a guy-wire, and function as a pelvic stabilizer. They initiate forward movement of the legs, assist in downward movement of the diaphragm for inhalation, stabilize the spinal curves, support abdominal organ structure, and even connect our body to our emotions. The psoas also work as an antagonist to the six-pack, balancing the lower back and the hip rotators.

The psoas are actually three different muscles that are known collectively as the *iliopsoas group*. The *iliacus* lines the inner part of the hip, and joins the *psoas major* at the pelvic brim in front of the hip socket, at a connection called the conjoint tendon. From that point, the fibers of the iliacus and psoas major converge and insert at the upper inner-leg bone. The intricate segments of the psoas which insert on the lumbar spine—all the way to the lowest thoracic vertebrae—are called *fascicles*. These fascicles connect to the transverse (lateral) and spinous (posterior) processes of the lumbar vertebrae and discs.

The psoas major and the iliacus flex the trunk towards the thigh, and tilt the pelvis forward, or anteriorly. The psoas major is shown in deepest red and the iliacus in the medium shade of red in **Fig. 3.1**. The third part of the group (shown in the lightest color of red) is the *psoas minor*, which is a muscle/tendon considered absent in 60 percent of the population, although this fact is subject to speculation by some anatomy teachers. It can be surmised that the psoas minor may be a ligamentous structure in all people, but only be developed with an actual muscle body in 40 percent of the population. The psoas minor tilts the pelvis posteriorly, and acts as an antagonist to the actions of the psoas major and iliacus, which tilt the pelvis anteriorly.

If constricted and weak, the psoas can not only cause back and hip pain, but also engage the fight–or–flight nervous system, causing feelings of anxiety. When we sit for hours in a chair or car, the back of the chair holds up our spine, causing the core spinal muscles and psoas to weaken and shorten. This sabotages optimal spinal alignment and breathing, and affects nerve and organ function. The psoas muscles also have a crucial role in the positioning of the lumbar, or lower back, curve of the spine, and are a major determinant of the tilt and position of the pelvis. As the only muscles that connect to the discs in the lumbar area of the spine, they are a major factor in the modern epidemic of lower back pain and sciatica.

You cannot feel comfortable in your body and have ease of movement if you don't have a functional psoas group, yet the way most of us slouch in our chairs can actually override the natural functions of the psoas muscles. The psoas will function as a spine stabilizer if we use them, but most of us sit poorly in our chairs, letting the back of the chair support us rather than engaging the psoas in one of its most important functions. Since we sit so much and don't use the psoas for support, they become weak and tight and remain contracted even when we stand up. A tightened psoas group exerts a lot of force on discs, compressing nerve signals along the anterior spine. To relieve back pain it is essential to create a program for restoring good function and awareness of the psoas group, in harmony with other muscles of the pelvis, lower back and abdomen. Functional movement, yoga poses, and sitting in chairs all need to be done with psoas awareness. When we are functional in our posture, our psoas and its related fascial structures are healthy and our movement is fluid and efficient. The key to reorganizing the fascia lines of the body to support natural alignment is activating the psoas/diaphragm connection. By using the movements of inhalation at the moment when the psoas contracts, one can create synergy and stabilization of the core among the abdominals, psoas, pelvic, floor, and back muscles.

> ❝*The psoas group and the core lower back muscles—the quadratus lumborum, or QL—connect to the diaphragm and spine providing the deepest core support of the body. Though the QL is palpated from the back, it is considered the deepest muscle of the abdomen.*❞

> Biel, *Trail Guide to the Body*

THE REAL CAUSE OF BACK PAIN

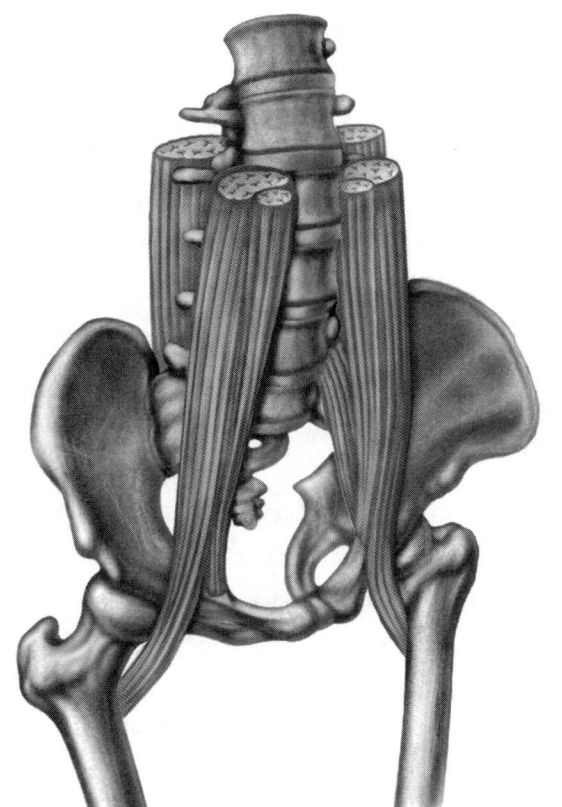

Fig. 3.2 – The QL and the psoas

While the Quadratus Lumborum, or QL, originates on the posterior hip crest and inserts at lumbar vertebrae—as well as the posterior of the bottom rib—it is indeed significantly related to core abdominal and back support. Often called the hip hiker, the QL assists in extension of the spinal column as well as lateral flexion, or the ability to lift or hike the hip towards the ribs.

Figure 3.2 shows how the psoas and QL function together to provide balance between the front and back of the lumbar spine. The psoas run along the front of the pelvis connecting to the inside top of the femur or leg bone at the lesser trochanter. The QL originates at the iliac crest of our hip bone (the posterior or back-top of the pelvic bone) and insert on the transverse processes of the first through the fourth lumbar vertebrae to our last rib (**Fig. 3.3**). The psoas and QL muscles also connect to the diaphragm, assisting in the breathing process, in addition to girding core body support.

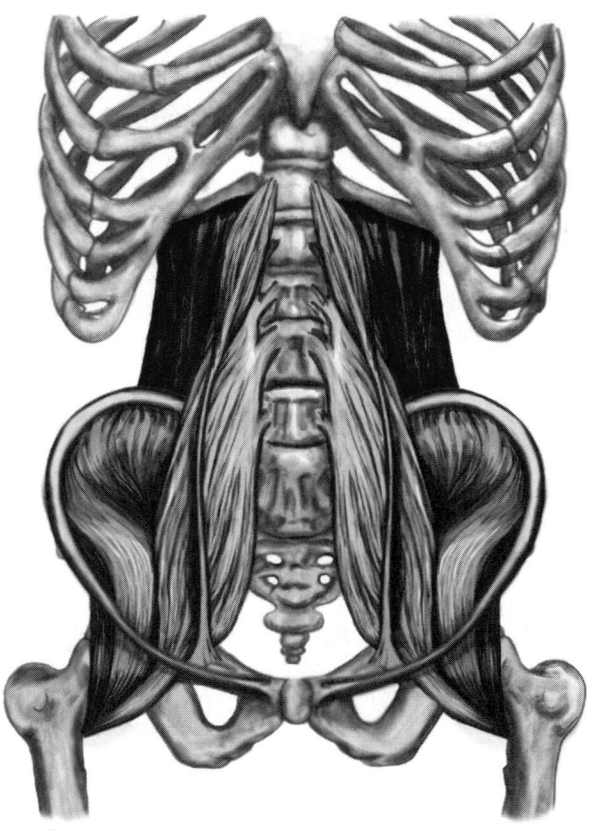

Fig. 3.3 – The quadratus lumborum is the deepest of the abdominal muscles.

When balanced, these two muscles work in synergy, creating core support of our spine and internal organs that develops from the inside out. Exercises that emphasize strengthening core structural support by bringing the breast bone towards the pubic bone over-ride the spine-stabilizing functions of the psoas and the QL. When exercise consists of movements that tighten and shorten the area of our waist, the spine extending functions of the psoas and QL are overridden. In the quest to make the abs tight, the spine and the internal infrastructure are compressed, and become strong yet shortened. The QL and the *erector spinae* (or back extensors) become strained and locked out in chronic tension by the shortening of the abdominals in the front body. Training the muscles of the belly to become tight and short inhibits the movements of breathing, overall body movement, and even emotions — creating a tense muscular lockdown running from head to toe.

In this situation, the lower back muscles can feel like tight cables, with tension extending to the neck and shoulder area via fascia lines and postural patterning. People in this situation are imprisoned in an exhausting downward spiral of tension, misalignment, and pain that can adversely affect the entire body inside and out.

Many people become trapped in this muscular vice grip by the popular idea that tightening the stomach muscles will fix a sore and tightened back. When psoas and hip imbalances start to result in lower back pain, there is a common belief that the remedy is to strengthen the ab muscles to support the back. People head for the gym, and practice those famous abdominal crunches, or other similar fitness exercises, all of which focus on keeping the navel pulled *in*. During these exercises, people with weak and/or tight psoas and diaphragm muscles compensate by using the neck, shoulders, upper back, and tightened belly to support their posture and breathing functions. These tightened, pull-your-navel-towards-your-spine exercises create holding patterns that override optimal alignment and breathing, and frequently exacerbate back pain in the process.

THE CENTER OF "FIGHT OR FLIGHT"

The psoas group is sometimes referred to as the "fight-or-flight" muscles. When we feel fear or stress, these deep muscles respond instinctively by tightening and drawing the limbs and organs together, creating a shield for our internal organs. The psoas muscles, along with the diaphragm, attach to the lumbar spine in the area of the body's center known as the *solar plexus.*

The solar plexus is also called "the second brain", or abdominal brain, because it is here that we store our gut feelings and intuition. There is a powerful relationship between the psoas, diaphragm, organs, and nerve ganglia that originate in this body center. Breathing, all core and lower body movement, and the activation of our gut feelings are all centered in this solar plexus area.

When we are constantly bombarded with stress, the psoas may stay unconsciously and chronically semi-contracted, exerting force on our spine, even pulling up on the lower leg attachments, causing a condition known as "short leg syndrome." Very few people have one leg bone shorter than another, however, a tightness in the psoas on one side can pull up on the leg bone at the psoas attachment site, causing an unevenness in the leg length. A shortened and weak psoas, combined with tight back muscles, can also either overarch or flatten the lumbar or lower back spinal curve, depending upon the angle of the pelvis. This altered spinal curve can disrupt the proper alignment of the hips, causing the pelvis to tilt too far forward or too far back. Down the road this disruption of the pelvic angle can, and frequently does, lead to disc malfunctions and chronic back pain. Scoliosis sometimes develops when one side of the psoas muscle is stronger, weaker, or more contracted than the other. Sport activities like golf and tennis, with strong engagement on one side of the trunk, can imbalance the psoas group, and misalignment in the hips can migrate pain and compression all over the body. Feet, knees, the lower back, and even the neck and shoulders are all affected by hip displacement, which has its root in psoas imbalance. Intelligently activating your psoas can synergize movement from your core, aligning your spine, and relaxing your mind.

PSOAS IMBALANCE AFFECTS THE ENTIRE BODY

If one is balanced, the body will function without pain. When the psoas is either weak or contracted, moving, breathing, feeling, and good spine alignment are all compromised. An imbalance of the psoas muscles can cause pain and misalignment over the entire body, affecting not only movement but emotional patterning as well. The traditional method of training our abdomen and trunk muscles to primarily cause flexion rather than extension of our spinal column is anatomically questionable, as it can create this undesired imbalance.

The psoas, the QL and the other muscles of our trunk can instead be trained in synergy to extend the spinal column, which is the most beneficial application of our trunk muscles. Keeping tight abs restricts movement all over our body, particularly breathing, which is our deepest movement. Short, tight trunk muscles restrict diaphragm movement and the vitally important psoas stabilizing functions. YogAlign techniques enable practitioners to consciously develop the connection between the psoas and the diaphragm, where the fundamental movement of our legs begins.

In **Fig. 3.4**, you can see how the psoas and the QL connect to the structure of the diaphragm, as well as how all of our major wiring and tubes connect through the diaphragm. Some of the structural tubing that passes through the diaphragm includes the Vena cava foramen, esophageal hiatus, abdominal aorta, spinal column, the psoas muscles, and the quadratus lumborum. **(Fig 3.4)** as seen from beneath the rib cage, looking up towards the head, the spine is at the bottom center, with the psoas major attaching on either side, and the QL

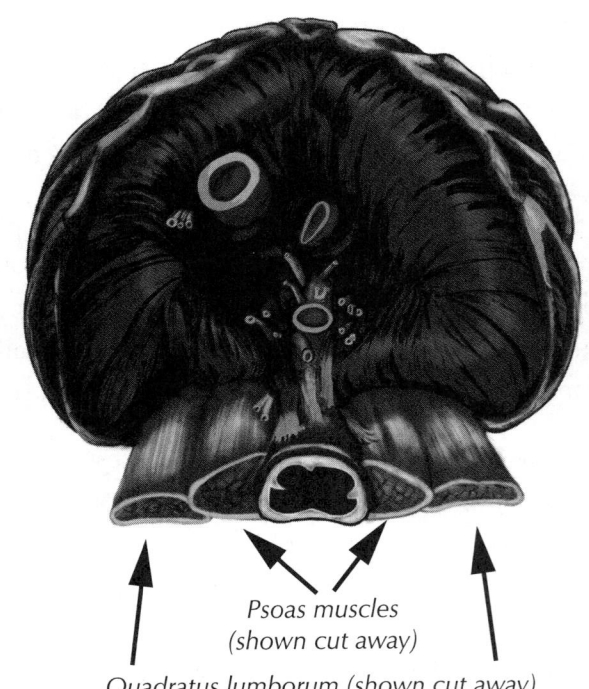

*Psoas muscles
(shown cut away)*

Quadratus lumborum (shown cut away)

Fig. 3.4.

flanking the psoas on each side of the spine. The psoas and the QL provide support on either side of the lower spine and contribute to the movement of the diaphragm when functionally activated together as synergists. The psoas is the connector muscle from the diaphragm to the legs. Using inhalation while contracting the psoas as a hip flexor will bring tone and length to the muscle.

We really can "breathe into our legs" using this diaphragm-to-psoas-to-femur connection. One of the most fundamental exercises in YogAlign is shown in **Fig. 3.5**, the "Core Connector." This exercise uses the breath to bring stabilization to your core, and strength and flexibility to your psoas, extending all the way down into your foot. The unique inhalation process used in the "Core Connector" strengthens and lengthens the psoas at the same time. One begins to feel how the movements of the legs originate at the diaphragm level which leads to core-centered movement abilities.

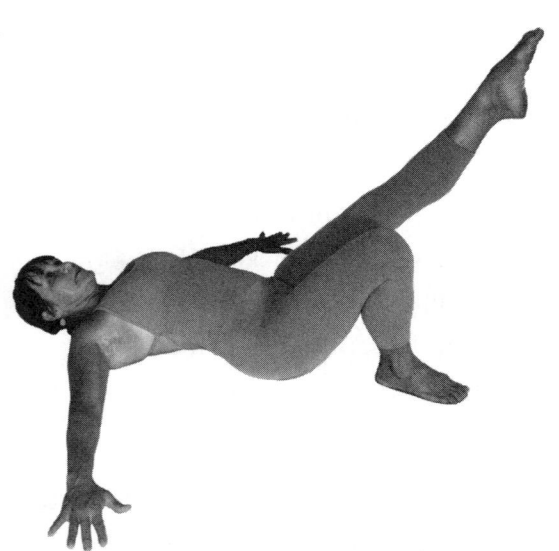

Fig. 3.5 – Core Connector

A chronically tight, weak, or shortened psoas can also lead to upper body destabilization, pulling the head and shoulders forward. In this condition, secondary breathing muscles (the neck and shoulders) become primary breathing muscles, inhibiting proper breathing. When one begins to breathe from the upper body, the shoulders become lifted and the neck is over-tensed. People with a weak or tight psoas group may also overuse the muscles in the neck and upper back to keep the weight of their head from jutting forward. Along the spine, back muscles can become chronically locked in a tight and long position that reduces the length and extension of the front while exerting unnatural force on spinal discs and nerves. This tightness also signals the fascia to thicken, leading to rigid posture patterns.

Remember These Important Points about the Psoas:

- **The psoas muscles are "the core of your core," connecting your upper body to your lower body and your inner body to your outer body.** Your psoas muscles emerge from the connective tissue of your diaphragm, acting like roots that connect your spine to your legs. They stabilize the actions in your spine, help you to breathe, and initiate forward leg movement. Without your psoas muscles, you would be unable to take even one step forward.

- **The psoas muscles support your internal organs and affect the position of the pelvis.** Tension in the psoas can invoke a fear-reflex that can keep you in a continual state of low-level anxiety. Learning to relax the psoas is the key to finding freedom in your spine, peace in your mind, and ease in the breathing process.

- **Effective muscle patterning involves initiating movement from the psoas muscles.** When you activate the psoas functionally, your body responds quickly and easily, and you will have a vital, pain-free, and flexible body.

- **Attempting to strengthen your core without functional knowledge of your psoas muscles can cause more pain and misalignment in your body.** Understanding and activating the psoas muscles is the key to effectively using the core of your body.

- **Chair-sitting weakens and shortens the psoas muscles.** Because the back of the chair becomes a substitute for the spine stabilizing work of the psoas and extension actions of the deep intrinsic postural muscles along our spine, these muscle groups can become weak and problematic through lack of proper functioning.

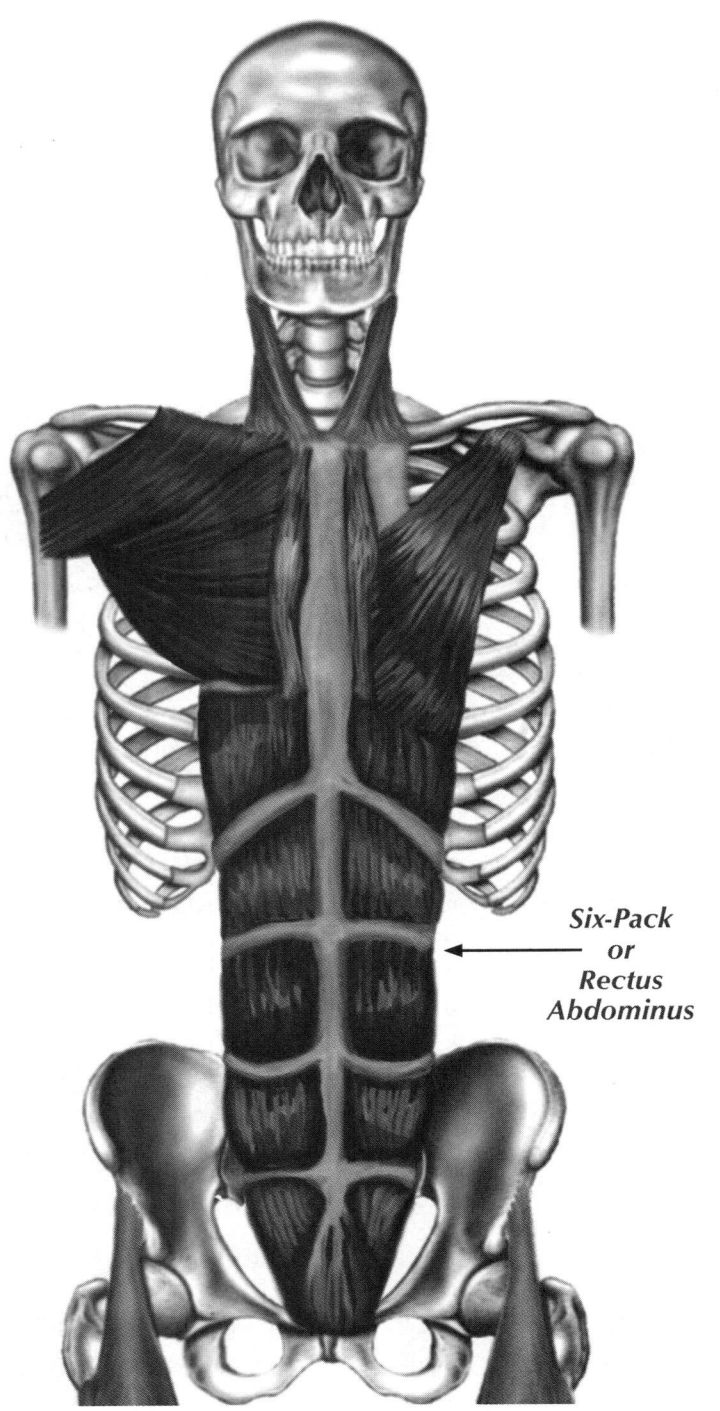

Six-Pack
or
Rectus
Abdominus

Fig. 3.6 – The "six-pack" (rectus abdominus) connects from the lower rib cage and breastbone to the pubic bone.

YOUR "SIX-PACK" MUSCLES

The *rectus abdominus* muscle is the poster child in our culture for core strength and sex appeal. Connecting from the ribs and breast bone all the way down to the pubic bone, this "six-pack" muscle is worshiped as the icon of fitness in our modern culture. In reality, this muscle should be toned, but not tight, and this gold standard of sexiness may actually be detrimental.

The rectus abdominus connects through the fascia lines from the *pectoral* (chest) muscles, shown here in **Fig. 3.6**, and out to the arms. A strong but shortened six-pack can pull the arm forward and result in shoulder and rotator cuff injuries. No muscle, not even the six-pack, acts in isolation. When you think of the rectus abdominus, remember the fascia and how it controls muscle engagement in lines of pull that extend all over the body. The fascia of your belly connects into your ribs and out into your arms, literally causing a forward pull on arm movement if the abdominals are chronically engaged to be tight and hard. Via the superficial front line of fascia, the outer belly is actually connected to the jaw behind the ear, to the arms, and to the top of the feet (**Fig. 3.7**), making tightness in this area something that can affect the entire body.

You might have glamorous six-pack

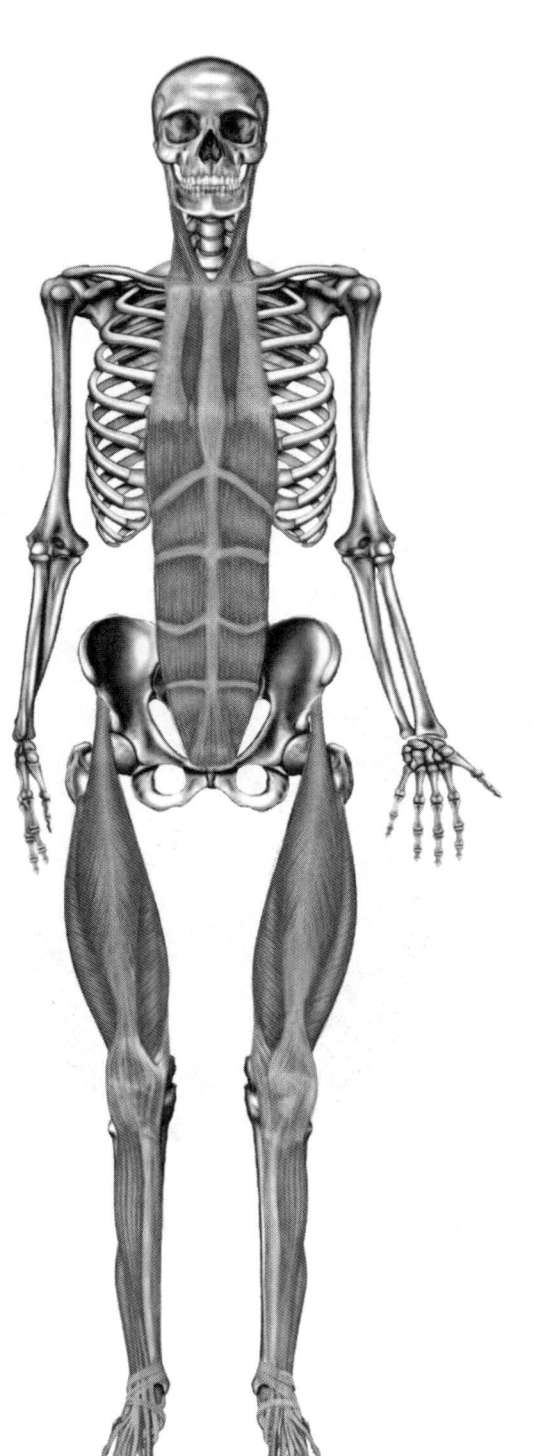

Fig. 3.7 – The superficial front line

abs, but in actuality they may be working against you. The tight belly can lock down the movement of your ribs, and constrict the movements of your diaphragm, while overriding the functions of your psoas. Tight abs and a weak and/or tight psoas group can contribute to compressed spinal curves that negatively affect organ and nerve function, and even cause back pain. When the belly is wired to be tight in a way that keeps the navel chronically pulled towards the spine, lines of tension radiate throughout the entire body, sabotaging ease and mobility. Over-tightening of the six-pack area simultaneously creates contraction in the pelvic floor. A tight pelvic floor locks up movement all over the body from the hips to the head and down to the feet. Too much tension or tightness in the muscles of the pelvic floor can cause back and foot pain, as well as tightness in the hip flexors. These restrictions then travel down or up muscle/fascia pathways, exerting a fascial pull on inner thigh, which can then imbalance the hinging actions of the knee, potentially causing pain or serious injuries.

The body is a continuum and we are connected in a fascia web — no muscle engages by itself in isolation. Muscles are all part of a "gang," contracting in groups that are directed by lines of pull in the fascial structures. Our entire body is connected seamlessly and held in balanced tension through the fascia web.

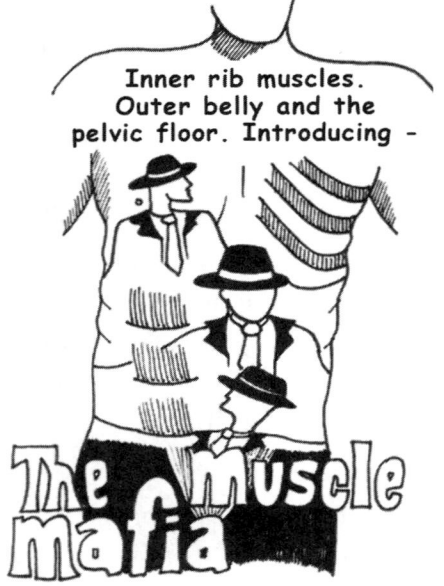

When we pull in our belly, we affect our body from the jaw to the pelvic floor and beyond. It's like a "muscle mafia," where the boys know what is happening all over the neighborhood, keeping tabs on one another, and even stabbing each other in the back.

There are more players in the abdomen beyond the six-pack muscle. An important stabilizer of the spine and one of the deepest core muscles is the *transverse abdominus*, or TA, (**Fig. 3.8**). It is the muscle that narrows the waist and provides horizontal support for abdominal organs. The fibers in this muscle run horizontally between the ribs and the hips. The TA is primarily involved with exhalation, abdominal compression and lumbar stabilization. A toned TA provides a muscular ring of support for the lumbar spine and protects internal organs. Further described in Chapter 4, YogAlign's specialized breathing exercises engage the TA, abdominals, and intercostals (rib muscles) in stabilization, concentric, and eccentric muscle actions. An emphasis on keeping extension in the body while contracting the abs encodes the core area to elongate and stabilize the spine as its primary muscular action.

Figure 3.9 shows the *external* and *internal*

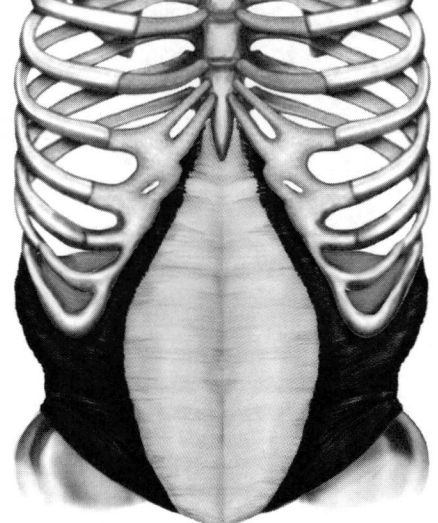

Fig. 3.8 – Transverse Abdominus

obliques, which lie between the six–pack and TA. The *external obliques* flex the spine laterally and rotate it, as well as assist the *external intercostal muscles* of the ribs in the inhalation process. The internal obliques have similar actions of rotating and flexion of the spine, but assist in the exhalation process. The internal oblique muscle fibers run in the same direction as the *internal intercostal muscles* of the ribs, and extend their actions of exhalation. YogAlign teaches unique variations of abdominal exercises that tone and lengthen the intercostals, and

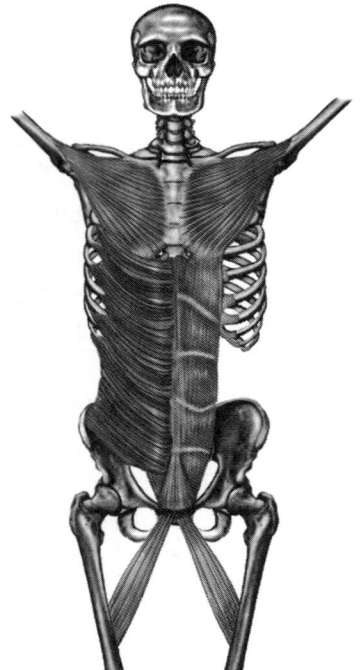

Fig. 3.9 – The external and internal obliques are shown here on the left side of the trunk.

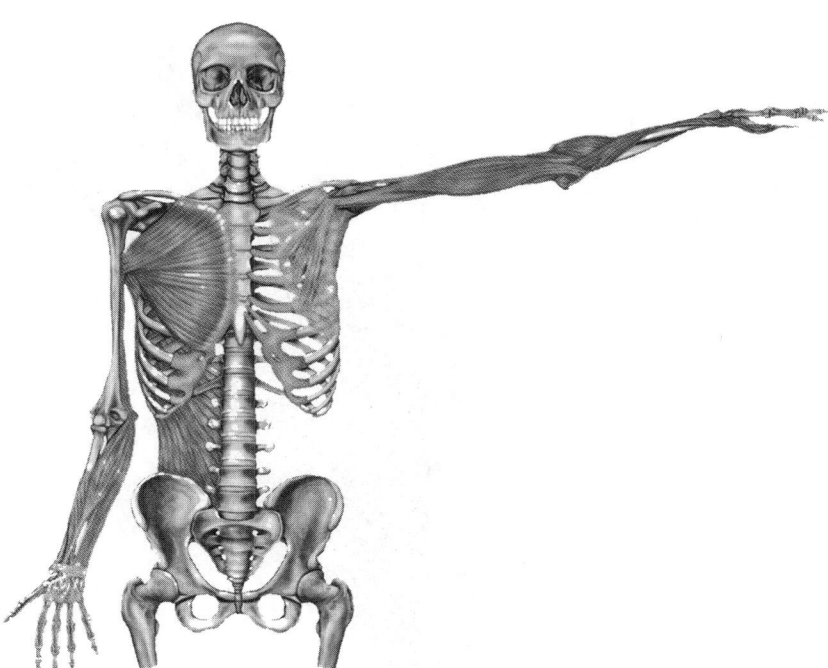

Fig. 3.10A – Fascia Arm Lines (Front)

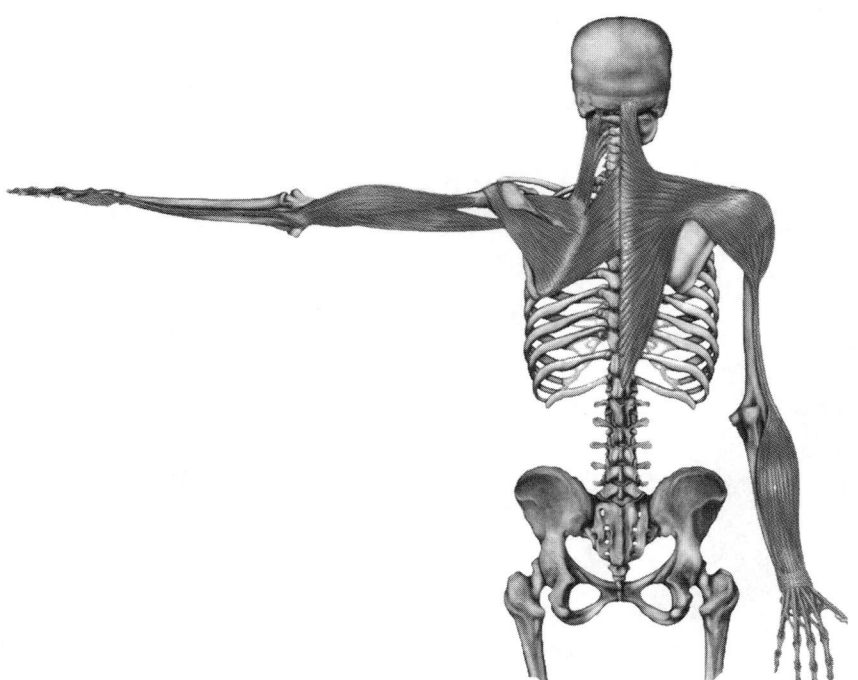

Fig. 3.10B – Fascia Arm Lines (Back)

the internal and external oblique muscles, freeing movement of the rib cage and stabilizing the spinal column.

ARMS, SHOULDERS, CHEST AND BACK

If you were asked to name where the muscles of your arm originate, you might point to the cap of your shoulder. In truth, your arm is attached to the center of your body, with movements connected to the breast bone, belly, hip, sacrum, spine, and back ribs.

Figure 3.10A shows how the arm originates at the pectoralis connection to the rib cage in the front of the body. The thumb area has fascial pulleys that connect the movement of the arm back to the front of the shoulder and the middle fingers to the cap of the shoulder, while the foundation of movement for the little finger connects to the back body at the lateral border of the scapula. The arm is directly connected from hand to hip and spine, and from spine and hip to the feet, via the fascia and muscle pathways.

Lats (**Fig. 3.11**) are an important foundation for arm movement, and they help in deep breathing and lateral rotation.

Figure 3.12 demonstrates engaging the lat muscles the YogAlign way. Notice that the natural curves of the spine are visible, and there is no compression or pull on the sacrum. Here you can practice opening the front body at the same time that you stretch open the side, and strengthen the extensor muscles along the back line of fascia. Deep breathing in YogAlign positions creates a strong inner stretch, and develops elasticity in the inner lines of fascia that cannot be massaged or palpated from the outside of the body.

In the front of your body, the biceps brachii and pectoral muscles connect the movement of your arm to your sternum and breathing process, then extend into lines that connect to the abdomen. The arm muscles are connected to the core via fascia lines that run down the center of the body (**see Figs. 3.10A & 3.10B**). Your arm spirals

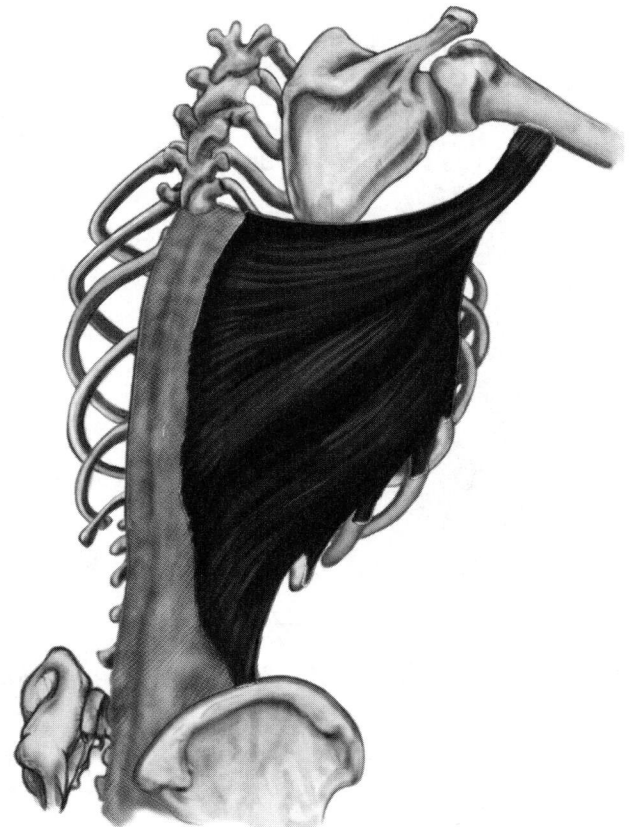

Fig. 3.11 – The Latissimus Dorsi muscles, or "lats."

out from the center of your body, and good support begins with strengthening and toning from your navel to your fingertips. The large pectoralis major is another culturally glamorous muscle often referred to simply as "the pecs." A connection with the functional line of fascia here integrates cross lateral movements, which are common in sports, connecting pectoral contraction to the opposite leg.

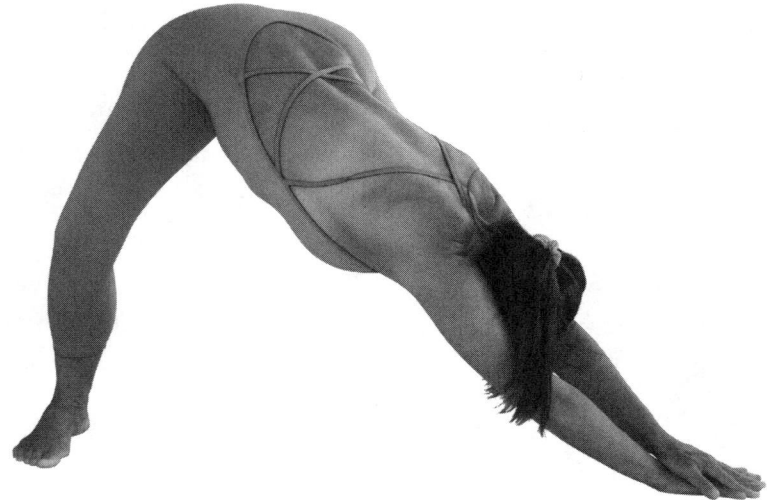

Fig. 3.12 – Lattissimus dorsi strengthening: Surfer Stretch.

The *pectoralis minor* (**Fig. 3.13**) lies below the glamorous pectoralis major muscle. This "little muscle that could" is actually a major player in the position of the scapula, or shoulder blade. The pectoralis minor attaches to a small, bony, finger-like projection called the *coracoid process* which is part of the scapula in the back. The coracoid sticks out under the collar bone in front, almost to the start of the shoulder. It serves

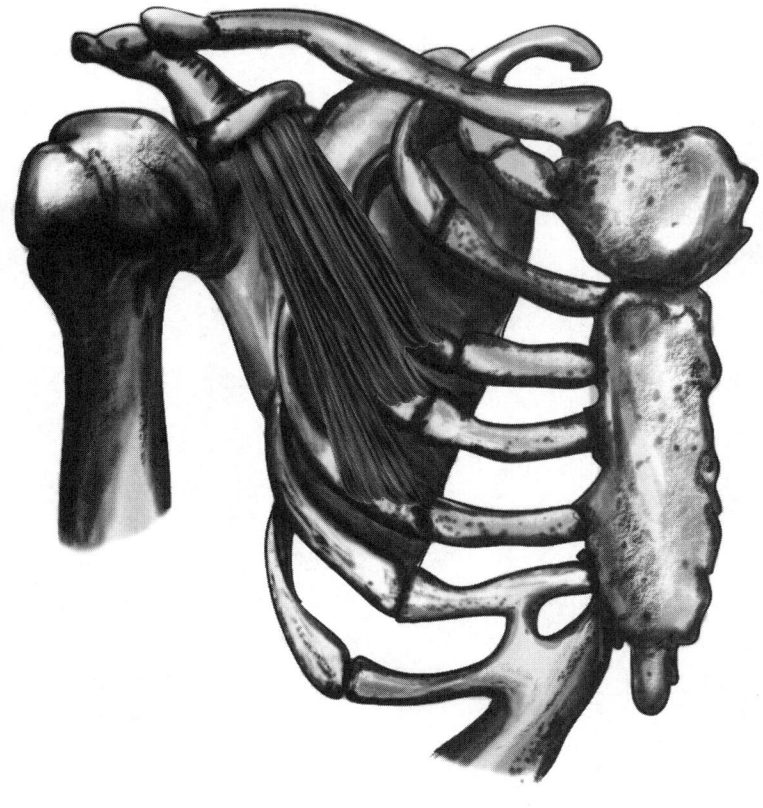

Fig. 3.13 – Anterior (front) view of the body: the pectoralis minor muscle attaches to the coracoid process and ribs.

as an attachment site for the bicep brachii arm muscles (**Fig. 3.14**), the smaller *coracobrachialis*, and the pectoralis minor muscle. A primary nerve bundle called the *brachial plexus* lies under the area where these muscles attach to the coracoid process. Many injuries in this area occur when there is tightness or a lack of tone in the pec minor and upper costal rib cage muscles. Practicing deep breathing with full upper rib expansion is very beneficial to posture and arm function, and creates space in the chest and shoulder joint providing support for the nerve pathways to the arm.

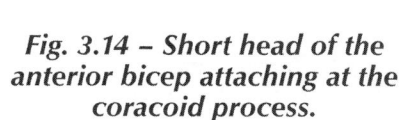

Fig. 3.14 – Short head of the anterior bicep attaching at the coracoid process.

EXPERIENTIAL EXERCISE #5

Find Your Coracoid Process

Here is a self-massage technique to help you find and massage the muscle and tendon attachments at your coracoid process.

Using your right fingers, massage the left side of your collar bones from the center of the body, out towards the shoulder.

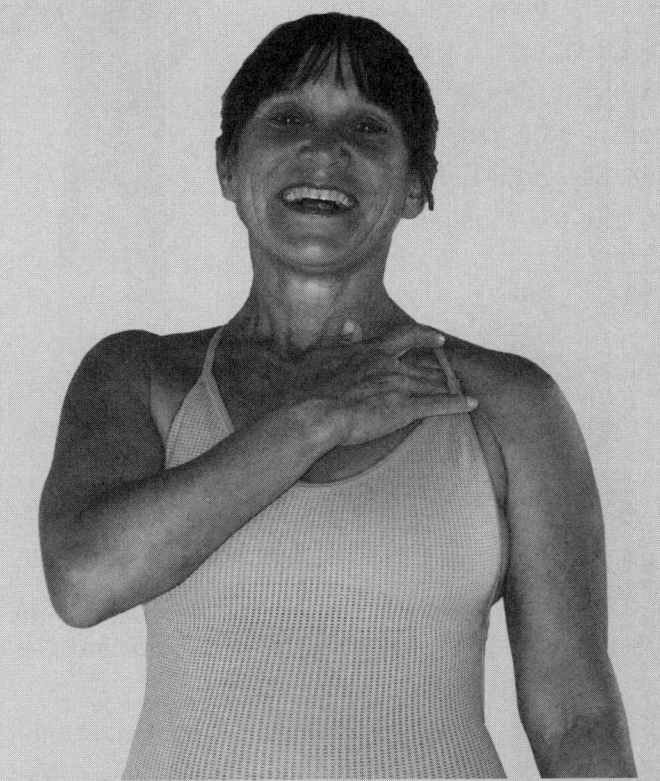

Massage along the top and bottom of the collar bone, simultaneously moving towards your shoulder on the left side of your body. Underneath the collar bone at the end towards the left shoulder, you should feel the coracoid process sticking out like a little knob. These can be deep in some and hard to palpate, and quite close to the surface in others. For many they will quite possibly feel sore. Spend a minute or so massaging this area, working deeply and firmly.

Massage the left upper rib-cage muscles and the intercostal muscles between these upper ribs. Massage the deltoid, or cap of the shoulder, as well, and then roll the left shoulder up and back a few times. While standing, allow your arms to hang by your sides. Notice if the left arm feels differently than the right arm feels.

Now massage your right chest, arm, and shoulder in the same way as you did your left.

After massaging both sides, stand with your feet hip-distance apart, keeping your knees soft. Notice how your shoulders and chest feel. You may feel a huge lift from your top ribs—as though you are suspended from above—as your shoulder blades float down the back, releasing your neck muscles from unnecessary tension.

Figure 3.15 shows how the scapula is a floating bone held in place by a complex roundhouse of intersecting muscles, and fascia with competing vectors of tension and pull. It has only one bone-to-bone ligament connection, at the *acromion process*, located at the end of the collar bone. The shoulder is a delicate non-weight bearing joint with a huge range of motion. The position of the shoulder blade is a huge determinant in the health of the shoulder joint and the posture of the upper body. The scapula is intricately involved with the breathing process, because it is connected to the spine and the ribs via muscles involved in breathing and spinal stabilization. When postural patterns include an elevated scapula held up by excess muscle tension in the neck and upper shoulders, the breathing process

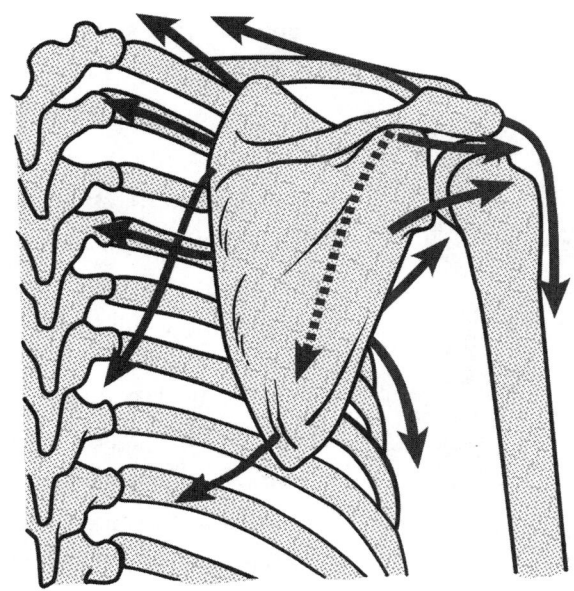

Fig 3.15 – An optimal balance of the muscular actions affecting the scapula stabilizes the shoulder joint and reduces chronic pain and injury.

is constricted, and the shoulder joint is rolled forward in a risky, non-functional position. When both scapula are stable and balanced, the rib cage is expansive and breathing is deep, which frees movement in the shoulders, neck, and arms.

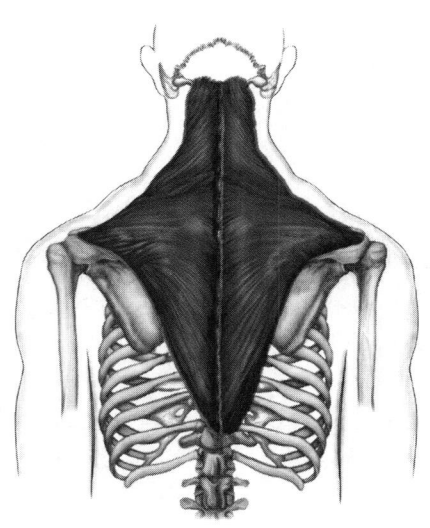

Fig. 3.16 – The trapezius muscles

Stabilizing the scapula involves activation of the rhomboids, serratus anterior, and lower trapezius muscles attached to the shoulder blades in the mid-back. Stabilizing the scapula involves activation of the rhomboids, serratus anterior, and lower trapezius muscles **(Fig. 3.16)** attached to the shoulder blades in the mid-back. Drawing the scapula downwards helps open the chest, allowing the engagement of the pec minor **(Fig. 3.13)**, located in the front upper rib cage, as a breathing muscle that elevates the ribs. (These actions can be viewed in the accompanying YogAlign DVD during the Breathing Segment.) Learning to engage these essential breathing muscles improves posture, releases neck pain, and functionalizes shoulder alignment. Keeping the scapula grounded in a functional position while focusing on breathing techniques is one of the essentials of natural alignment in YogAlign practice.

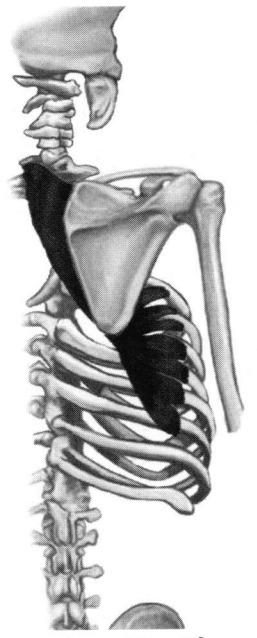

Fig 3.17 – The rhomboids and the serratus anterior (or the "banana bunch" muscle) are major players in stabilizing the scapula.

The rhomboids and the serratus anterior—or superhero muscles (**Fig. 3.17**) — work together as important players in the positioning of the scapula and the movements of breathing. The serratus anterior wraps around the body from the back to the front, attaching to the surfaces of the upper eight or nine ribs as well as to the anterior medial border of the scapula. Most of it is concealed (except a portion beneath the armpit); some of it *can* be seen on the front of the lower ribs in a lean muscular body. Viewed from the side, it looks like a small bunch of bananas.

The rhomboids adduct, or draw in, the scapula, and the serratus abducts, or pulls away, the scapula from the midline of the body. When balanced in their actions by working as synergists, the rhomboids and the serratus anterior provide a structural sling support for the scapula. When the scapula is engaged downward by actions of the rhomboids and lower trapezius, the serratus anterior becomes an accessory muscle of inspiration (or breathing muscle), providing more power and support to the entire trunk area. The serratus anterior also provides a strong, mobile base of support for positioning the scapula optimally, generating maximum efficiency in actions such as raising the arms overhead.

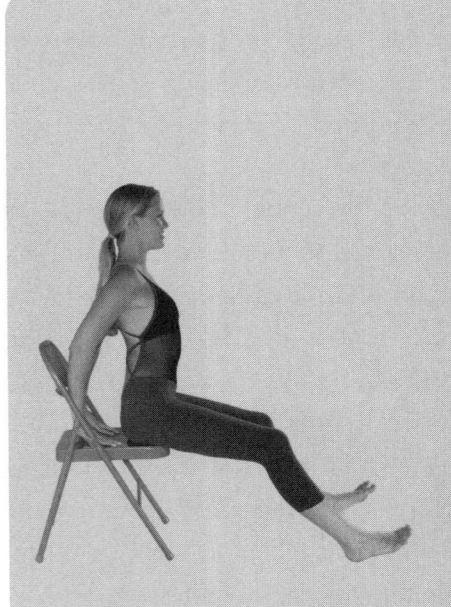

EXPERIENTIAL EXERCISE #6

Breathing Awareness

Sit in the position shown at left. Make sure that your fingertips are pointing in towards your hips, and keep the shoulder blades drawn down along the backside of the body. Inhale slowly and feel how the muscles that connect to the coracoid process in the front of the body are activated from the inside out. Inhale with a small mouth opening, as though you are sipping through a straw, and notice how your arm lines seem to stretch open. Continue to keep your shoulder blades pulled down in the back. As the arm lines open, the neck will relax so your head can simply sit on top of your spine with no effort. Practice turning your head from side to side, using a mirror to make sure that your head is perfectly balanced in the center of your shoulders.

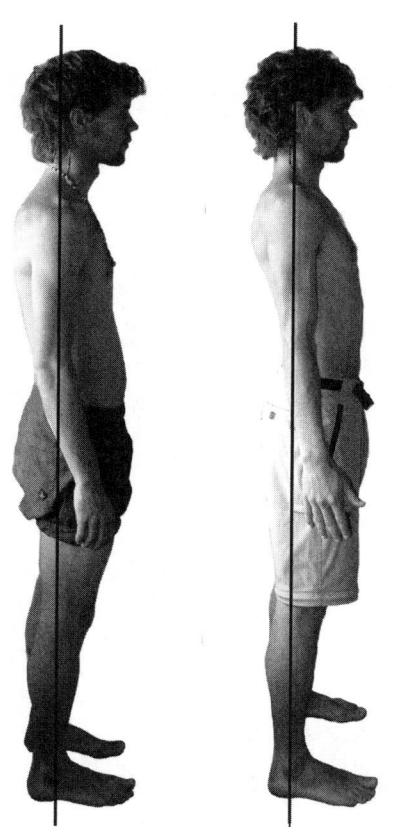

Fig. 3.18 – A rock climber who was "pulled forward" changed his posture after only four days of YogAlign.

The deep front arm line connects from the coracoid process of the scapula, to the pectoralis minor, out to the biceps and into the thumb. Keeping the shoulder blade stable is an essential part of toning the fascial pathways in the arms. The YogAlign process of bringing natural alignment to the neck and shoulder girdle reduces forward head carriage and pain in the neck and back, as well other postural problems such as kyphosis. Kyphosis is excessive rounding in the upper back and is very common in the elderly, office workers, cyclists, students, and rock climbers.

Shoulder blades that are chronically lifted push the head forward, and alignment crumples like a house of cards, with one muscle causing another to engage in a dysfunctional way, all the way down the line. When the shoulder blade is elevated, we have no foundational strength in our arm movements, and muscles in the neck and arms begin to perform functions they were not designed for. These imbalances create tension all over the head, neck, jaw, back, and shoulder region. Standing or sitting in a naturally aligned position while breathing deeply from our core enlists muscles in the area of the rib cage that foster good posture patterning.

The importance of releasing the over-contraction of the muscles and fascia of the front body and strengthening the muscles of inhalation and spinal extension cannot be overemphasized. Self-massaging the upper rib/collar bone area, including muscles that attach to the coracoid process, helps activate the breathing muscles in the upper chest. These muscles provide support to the skull by keeping the upper rib cage in a functionally aligned position. To correct a frozen, tense shoulder blade positioning that strains the neck muscles and pulls the head forward, we must learn to breathe from the source: the psoas/diaphragm connection, in combination with expansive fluid movements of the entire rib cage. Practicing core breathing in chest-opening positions will help balance fascia lines from the upper ribs and arms to the pelvic floor. Focusing on the muscles used for deep breathing while stabilizing the scapula can balance the arm lines as well as other fascial lines, freeing chronic tension patterns all over the body.

❝*At almost no other place in the body than in the first rib is there such a concentration of meridians, blood vessels, nerves and muscles. The neck muscles alone consist of seven layers, which go over the first rib at the back. The windpipe, the gullet, the carotid artery, and the thyroid gland, which controls the cell metabolism and the carotid body gland (the organ that measures oxygen concentration in the blood) are neighbors of the first rib. If one becomes aware of the lively energy and the substance transfer around the neck and the first rib, it is almost impossible to have bad posture. However, if the posture is slouched, sunken or depressed, this area is tense and our awareness is turned off. The pelvic floor (in turn) reacts with blockage; the pressure from above is more than it can take.*❞

Franklin, *Pelvic Power*

EXPERIENTIAL EXERCISE #7

Body Awareness

From a standing position, imagine that your trapezius is like the lead apron your dentist requires you to wear before taking an x-ray. The lower part of the trapezius extends the flow of the muscle downwards and helps to stabilize the shoulder blade in the back body. Feel its denseness and heaviness. Now imagine that the center line of your trapezius is like a water fountain shooting up from the bottom where they meet in a V. The fountain of water is supporting your head allowing your neck muscles to relax. Your head bobs in the fountain with no effort from your neck or shoulder muscles. Imagine the trapezius at the shoulder blades is like a muddy wetland. With ease, feel your collar bones sinking down into the mud now that you don't need to tense your neck muscles in order to hold them up. The lower part of the trapezius now pulls in at the outside of the V shape, like two lines tethering a boat to a buoy.

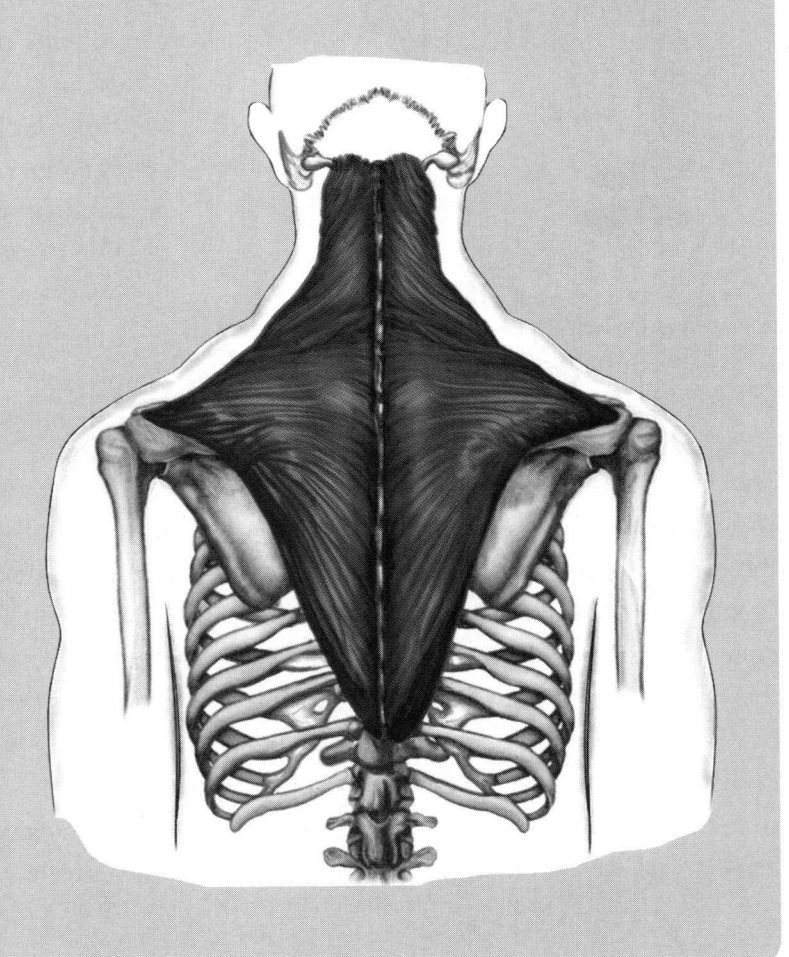

When we sense our body, it is helpful to visualize our muscles flowing in rivers instead of seeing them as dense, separated parts. Many adults have imageries or internalized statements that do not assist their innate functioning. Statements like "I am old," and "I am stiff," or even seemingly innocuous assertions like "My knee is bad," obstruct more beneficial positive imagery. Some of the words used to describe conditions can actually make people internalize imagery that slows down the healing process. For instance, when someone is told they have a frozen shoulder, they may hold the arm and shoulder region rigid, ingraining the feeling and visualization of "being frozen." By using metaphors that assist function, we can encode our thought patterning with positive visuals, and language that supports our healing from the inside out.

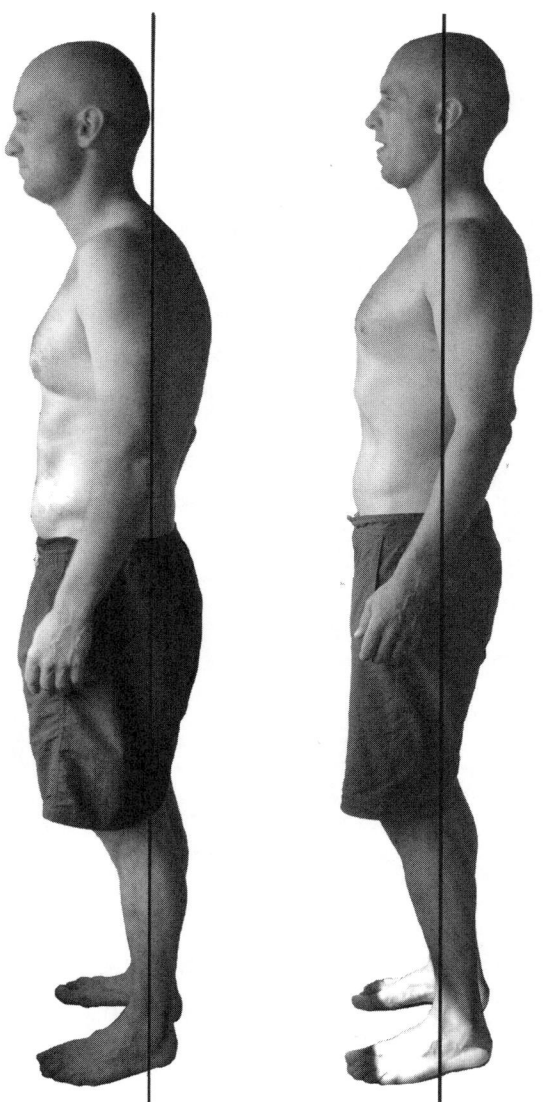

Fig. 3.19 – An organic farmer and skiing guide released the muscle tension in his front line and activated the deep core line after only four sessions of YogAlign.

YogAlignMent Principle #5
Know your anatomy and practice
self–massage and deep breathing every day.

CHAPTER 4: BREATHE FROM YOUR CORE

🕉 *Why Do Deep Core Breathing?*

🕉 *To Live Means to Breathe*

🕉 *Poor Breathing Ages Us*

🕉 *Anatomy of Breathing Muscles: Diaphragm and Intercostals*

🕉 *Put It All Together*

🕉 *Keep the Gift of the Lift: Inhalation Creates Extension, Exhalation Creates Flexion*

🕉 *Inhalation Gives You the Gift of the Lift*

🕉 *Secondary or "Fight or Flight" Breathing Muscles*

🕉 *Core Connections of Breathing*

🕉 *Going to the "Motherboard" with Conscious Breathing*

🕉 *Poor Breathing Can Affect Your Body and Your Mood*

🕉 *Your Breath Gives You Life and Longevity*

Breath is your life.
If breath is inhibited, so is
your life.

"Yoga is as much a practice involving the breath as it is involving the body."

T.K.V. Desikachar

"On one hand, breathing is mostly unconscious and automatic. It influences our actions and our emotions and at the same time is influenced by them. On the other hand, it is an action that one can influence in a conscious, voluntary manner, by changing it in various ways, with consequences on many different levels."

Calais–Germain, *Anatomy of Breathing*

WHY DO DEEP CORE BREATHING?

A consistent practice of deep breathing can balance, align, elongate, and tone your body. Deep breathing can correct poor posture, align the spine—our body's shock-absorbing mechanism—and eliminate pain and muscle tension. Deep breathing can jump-start our metabolism, massage our organs, help us develop endurance, and even make us better at lovemaking. Learning to breathe from our inner core can help us live our life in the present, while freeing our mind from negative patterns of fear, anxiety, and depression. Deep breathing can help us experience true vitality, and feel the power of the life force that keeps every cell of our body functioning.

Breathing is an exercise that is at the center of all actions in which we engage. It is the most fundamental of our movements, bringing in oxygen and removing wastes from our body. How we do it affects every system and every part of our entire being. Since most of our breathing occurs unconsciously, we often take it for granted, despite the fact that as human beings we breathe approximately 15,000 to 20,000 times each day. It is the most frequent movement that we make, and it determines our structural alignment, directs our nervous system responses, and defines our emotional wellbeing. Whether we are consciously directing breath into our body or not, breathing is happening at every moment in our lives. In YogAlign, learning to breathe from our core—using our primary breathing muscles, and balancing the muscles of respiration to free the rib cage—is the most important skill we can learn.

For optimal health and fitness, we can learn to breathe effortlessly with depth, power, and fluidity. Weakened and constricted breathing muscles prevent us from being able to function in a relaxed, efficient manner, affecting the entire body from the inside out. Many aches and pains, and even some serious chronic conditions, arise from weakness and misalignments developed from poor breathing habits. It is not just those who are out of shape who can have problems breathing; some people who are very strong and tight may have dysfunctional breathing habits as well.

Strong athletic people often have overengaged abdominal muscles, which can inhibit functioning of the muscles of inspiration, including the intercostal muscles between the ribs and the diaphragm. Since the arms connect to the abdominal region, tight sexy abs can even restrict shoulder mobility. Chronic tension in the belly also compresses the internal organs, affecting digestion, elimination, and our ability to breathe, laugh and feel relaxed.

Both abdominal tightness and core weakness can adversely affect postural patterning. Have you ever noticed how people with a strong and tight six-pack muscle often have head and shoulder alignment that is pulled forward? Weakness in the abdominal muscles can cause a pot belly from a weak or short

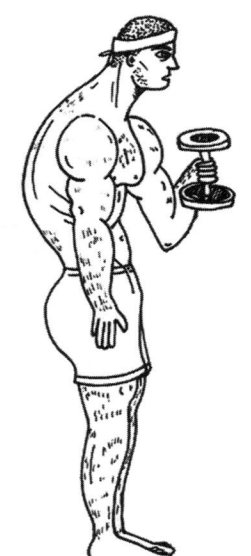

waist line that causes internal organs to protrude. Both tight and weak abdominal muscles can reduce the length of the trunk, leaving little space for our internal organs, while at the same time creating a fascial pull that draws the head and neck forward of the spine.

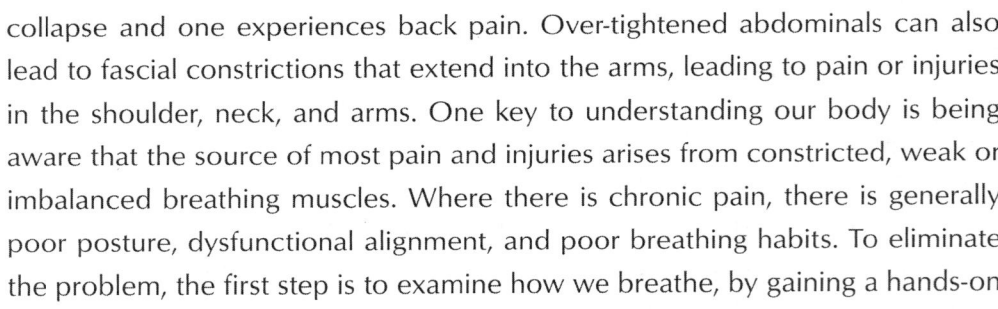

When the front body is weak or tight and pulled forward, fascia forces call on the back to support the collapse and one experiences back pain. Over-tightened abdominals can also lead to fascial constrictions that extend into the arms, leading to pain or injuries in the shoulder, neck, and arms. One key to understanding our body is being aware that the source of most pain and injuries arises from constricted, weak or imbalanced breathing muscles. Where there is chronic pain, there is generally poor posture, dysfunctional alignment, and poor breathing habits. To eliminate the problem, the first step is to examine how we breathe, by gaining a hands-on experiential and mental understanding of the anatomy of our breathing apparatus. Awakening the power of breathing can connect the emotional body to the physical body, and create an open and joyous ability to feel and move deeply, without restriction.

To Live Means to Breathe

The movement of our breath and the beating of our heart combine to form the rhythmic core of our lives. There is no moment in life when we are not involved in the breathing process. Whether asleep or awake, we breathe, like every other creature and organism on the planet. Breathing is one of the most subtle, yet important, bodily processes. It provides the fuel and foundation for living. Even the process of breathing itself massages the heart and our internal organs. How we breathe from moment to moment defines our fascial balance, which ultimately defines our movements, our structure, and the quality of our life in general.

We don't have to tell our body when or how to breathe. The body instinctively keeps the breath going without any conscious prompting at all. From the time we are born and start voluntary movement, our neuromuscular system begins programming our own unique codes, which become our habituated way of moving. Breathing is one of the most basic movements of the body, and as such is generally unconscious and directed by the autonomic nervous system. However, our postural patterning and our sitting/ movement habits greatly affect how well our innate system of breathing can perform its job. Small babies and children breathe and move freely, yet few adults in the modern world have breathing and movement codes that are fluid and efficient.

Since breathing can be a conscious movement as well as an unconscious one, we can use conscious breathing as a powerful tool to create a new way of being. The primary focus of YogAlign is to use conscious breathing to "breathe your way" into natural, neutral alignment. By practicing conscious breathing in combination with movements and yoga positions that are designed to support optimal body alignment, we can learn to re-establish positive patterns and habits that will support our body's natural design. As posture improves, so will unconscious, effortless, and optimized breathing.

Look at the people around you, and you will see many examples of shallow breathing, poor posture, and weak spines. Poor posture has, unfortunately, become the norm in the Western world. Even dysfunctional posture and movement patterns—along with persistent aches and pains—can begin to feel familiar and normal after a while. You may feel yourself trapped in a painful, contracted body with limited abilities to move fluidly or breathe deeply. Poor posture is part of a domino effect in which dysfunctional breathing habits create poor posture, which in turn further inhibits breathing. It's as though your own body patterns are working against you.

When you observe stiff, elderly people, you are seeing the effects of poor breathing habits that have, over a lifetime, created a brittle and contracted rib cage area. In old age, fascial patterning restricts the simplest movements of the arm, or the ability to open the mouth wide enough to take a bite from an apple. The path to a pain-free life and aging with vitality is learning how to efficiently exercise the breathing muscles, keeping you supple and joyful. The good news is that you *can* change your breathing habits for the better by paying attention to how you breathe, consciously redirecting your breath until effective breathing occurs automatically. In this chapter and later on in Part 2, you will find simple and concise techniques that can help you profoundly and quickly change your breathing habits.

Remember: Breath is life, and freeing your breathing process will free your life.

Poor Breathing Habits Accelerate Aging

It has become commonplace for most people to get shorter as they age, and our culture has begun to accept that aging inevitably means shrinking. In this case, the abnormal has become the norm. This appearance of shrinking often occurs because people have stopped strong movements of inhalation which can increase the forces of extension in the body. When the breathing muscles are not engaged deeply, the physical result will be an overall reduction in pulmonary elasticity of the lung tissue and severe shortening in the muscles and fascia in the superficial front and deep tissues of the body. Gravity, poor breathing habits, and chronic belly and neck tension pull the whole body forward, making one "shorter." The fascial lines contract and thicken, leading to poor posture, stiff movement, chronic pain, and joint and organ dysfunction. Perhaps it is not aging itself creating these afflictions, as much as poor breathing patterns that contribute to everything from a slouching posture, to bad knees, to the need for hip replacements.

YogAlign clients have been able to reverse these ailments without pills, pain or surgeries by learning to practice breathing with their inner core muscles and allowing their body to do the rest. No matter what age you are, YogAlign poses support optimal posture lines that assist in fluid breathing. These poses eventually re-pattern the body/mind system into balanced and supportive alignment, mitigating the effects of a lifetime of poor breathing and posture.

ANATOMY OF BREATHING MUSCLES: DIAPHRAGM AND INTERCOSTALS

The lungs are the organ of respiration, and the main place where our blood absorbs fresh oxygen from the incoming air. The right side of the heart pumps venous blood full of carbon dioxide into the lungs. Here, the blood is enriched with oxygen, and this fresh arterial blood flows back into the heart where it gets distributed throughout the entire body.

During inhalation, the various breathing muscles and connective tissue forces (discussed in the previous chapters) pull open the lung tissue, changing the pressure in the thorax which causes air to fill the empty space in the lungs. The tissue of the lungs has specialized fibers that, during exhalation, retract back to their pre–inhalation shape using what is called "pulmonary elasticity." Our primitive brain is wired to keep the diaphragm expanding and contracting 24/7, without our conscious involvement. With conscious attention, however, breathing can become a strong exercise in and of itself, and exhalation can be done with conscious force of focus, in addition to the basic pulmonary elasticity. Conscious deep breathing affects the entire body, bringing it into a state of maximized oxygenation, spine extension, and fascial opening.

Normally, the breathing process happens unconsciously through the autonomic nervous system. But by using conscious breathing techniques with focused inhalation and exhalation, we can develop stronger and more powerful muscles that supercharge the expansion of the lungs, and the intake of oxygen into our cellular structures, toning the abdomen through the movements of exhalation. In order to achieve these powerful breathing movements, we have to effectively engage the diaphragm muscle at the center of our body by using real-life body positions that allow it to function without restriction.

The Diaphragm

The diaphragm (**Fig. 4.1**) is a large but thin muscle, with a fibrous wall that connects to the ribs and the lower spine, creating a transverse shelf between the thorax and the abdomen. The diaphragm has a fibrous center which is called the central tendon, around which muscular fibers are arranged in a sunbeam-like fashion. Because the fascial web connects the diaphragm to the heart, lungs, and even the throat, there is really no separation of the thorax and the abdomen. Looking like a parachute (or a jellyfish), the outer fibers of the diaphragm attach to the entire inner circumference of the bottom of the rib cage. The diaphragm attaches in the front at the sternum level, and extends down nearly to the waist in the back, inserting into the third lumbar (L-3) vertebrae. The diaphragm acts like a pump or piston at the base of the lungs, and is integral to the power and

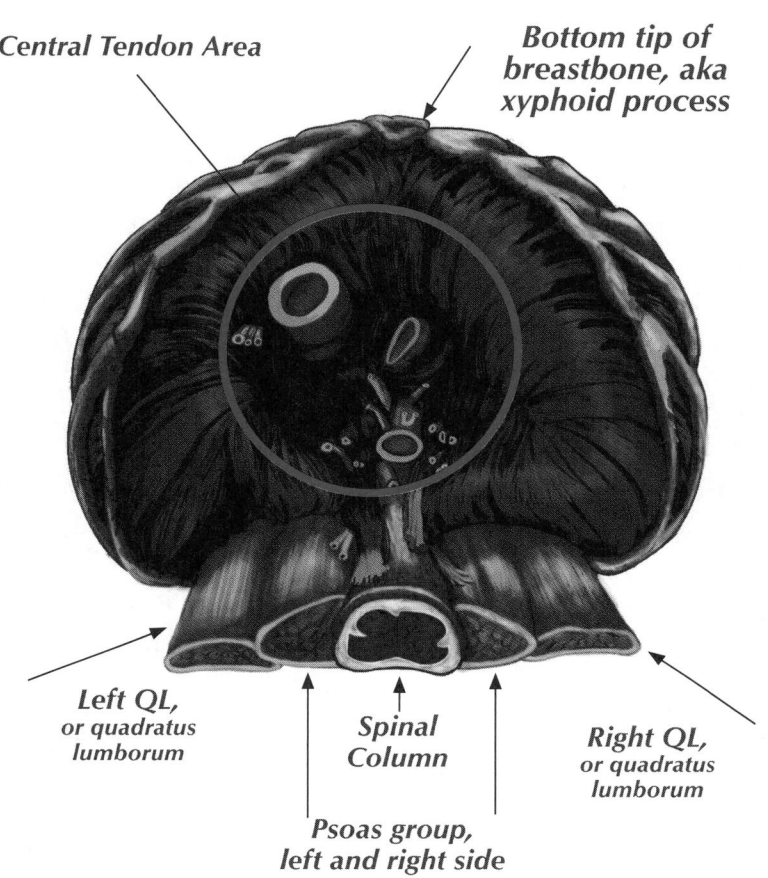

Central Tendon Area

Bottom tip of breastbone, aka xyphoid process

Left QL, or quadratus lumborum

Spinal Column

Right QL, or quadratus lumborum

Psoas group, left and right side

Fig. 4.1 – Shown above in the central tendon area of the diaphragm is the vena cava foramen, esophageal hiatus, and the abdominal aorta.

longevity of our structure, since breathing is the most essential movement of our being. Movement of the diaphragm creates a massaging action, toning the heart, the intestines and other inner organs. Our spine, esophagus, and main arteries all pass through and are connected to the diaphragm. This inter-connected nature of the diaphragm shows that it is an essential muscle, which we too often taken for granted.

Notice how the diaphragm connects to the inner surface of the rib cage in **Fig. 4.1**. By increasing the expansion capabilities of the rib cage, we are stretching the diaphragm muscle during inhalation. A conscious engagement of the intercostal muscles during inhalation creates a strong outward expansion of the rib cage, causing the diaphragm to lengthen as it contracts downwards into the abdominal cavity. This downward contraction can be assisted to be stretched open at the same time it contracts downward by the psoas muscles. The two psoas muscles function like the roots of the diaphragm, inter-connecting the movements of breathing from the solar plexus area through the spine, and down to the legs and feet. Through the practice of the Core SIP breath (see Experiential Exercise #9), one begins to feel experientially how core breathing can create length from the crown of the head to the arches in the feet. It is this crucial connection from the diaphragm to the legs via the psoas that is *most* important in re-establishing core-centered fluid movement and longevity-boosting extension in the spine.

Every breath you take causes a massaging action that shapes and moves the internal organs. The stomach, liver, kidneys, spleen, pancreas, abdominal aorta, tongue, and the large intestine are all connected to the diaphragm, and are therefore affected by the breathing process. The spine, along with all its essential tubes and wiring—for blood flow, nerve pathways, and intake of nutrients—passes through, and is fascially woven into, the fabric of the diaphragm. The diaphragm is at the center of activity for life itself.

During inhalation, the QL contracts and helps to extend the vertebral column, creating more space and length in the waist. In YogAlign, there is a focus on keeping the extension in the spine even when exhaling which normally causes the spine to shorten in length. Muscles considered to have primary actions as abdominal compressors can, during exhalation, be enlisted to paradoxically lengthen as they contract, providing stability, tone, and extension to the spine, while supporting posture and breathing. Our trunk muscles serve us optimally when their primary action is to stabilize the spine and provide a toned length to our waist area. When exercises or ingrained habits emphasize keeping the belly tightly pulled in, the chronic tension actually weakens the belly as well as brings the breastbone towards the pubic bone. Inside the body, the delicate balance between the psoas and QL is overridden, along with optimal functioning of the diaphragm, stomach, intestines and pelvic floor. Contrary to popularized belief systems, the tighter we make our "belly", the more restriction we create in feeling, breathing, and movement. Because of our fascial pulley design system, the tighter we make our front, the more the back muscles in the superficial back line are enlisted to work. The result of all of this unnecessary tension is back and hamstring muscles that feel chronically tight and sore in response to the shortness in the front body.

Rib Cage Muscles

There are many muscles that connect to the rib cage and assist in breathing and movement of the trunk, but the rib cage muscles *themselves* primarily control the expansion and contraction of the ribs. These muscles, called the *intercostals* (the "spare rib meat"), lie between our ribs. There are *external intercostal* muscles that act on inhalation, and *internal intercostal* muscles that act on exhalation. If one set is weak or contracted, it affects the performance of the other. During inhalation, the external, or outer, intercostals contract and pull the ribs apart, creating more space for the lungs to expand. Conversely, when we exhale, the internal intercostals contract and pull the ribs together, decreasing space in the thoracic cavity, and creating the exhalation. When we exhale, there is a flexion, or shortening, created in the spine that pulls us forward unless there is a conscious connection to staying upright. Keeping extension in our spine and aligned posture no matter what our breathing process is doing is one of the main focal points in YogAlign.

If one were to open up the body, one would see the rib cage muscles connected through a seamless fascia line to the core trunk muscles and to the entire inner structure of the trunk area. The external obliques have the same muscle fabric direction as the external intercostals and act as synergists, assisting the movement of inhalation in the rib area. In the movements of exhalation, internal oblique muscles assist the internal intercostal muscles, pulling the ribs together to decrease the space in the thoracic cavity. Every muscle that attaches to the rib cage is enlisted in the breathing process, and they are all connected to fascial lines that extend all the way out to our fingers and toes, making breathing a movement that reverberates throughout our entire structure. In YogAlign we practice keeping the spine extended, even when exhaling, in order to enlist as stabilizers muscles normally considered as abdominal compressors. These stabilization forces keep the torso long and the spine extended, preserving vitality in our structure.

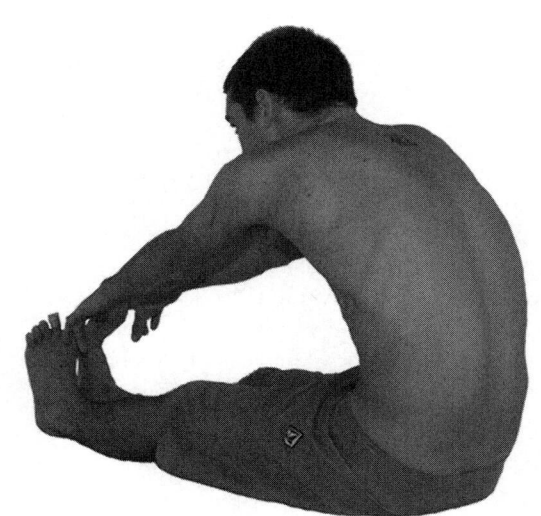

Fig. 4.2

Our goal with YogAlign is to balance and awaken the breathing muscles, teaching them to work in synergy so that they can tone, align, and strengthen the core without inhibiting movement. To do this, we must learn to let go of the idea that we can strengthen parts of our body in separate sections. The body is a seamless continuum, and all parts affect the whole. For instance, even a seemingly remote action like engaging our toes to pull towards our shins causes contraction to occur in our abdomen and rib cage area, and can ultimately restrict the movements of breathing. Leaning forward to stretch out the back (**Fig. 4.2**) compresses the spine and engages the abs to flex the spine which weakens the forces of inhalation and extension. While the knowledge of how to use breathing to change structure and assist function is invaluable, more scientific research needs to be conducted in order to fully understand the breathing process, and how it can be helped or hindered by certain exercises.

Before engaging the body deeply, YogAlign emphasizes using self-massage to awaken the senses and increase blood/oxygen flow in the tissues. Releasing tension from the muscles between the ribs is essential to achieving a full, deep breath and to gaining sensory awareness of our muscles. Self-massage of the upper rib cage and the neck area around the collarbones can eliminate chronic tension that may inhibit the movements of breath. Tension in the neck can *seriously* inhibit the movement of the upper rib cage when we inhale, so it is essential to have the neck muscles relaxed. Ideally, all of the ribs should be able to move freely when breathing.

Put It All Together

The muscles between the ribs have an exquisite natural design and function. Did you know that your rib cage muscles (*intercostals*) are designed to move your ribs simultaneously in three different directions?

EXPERIENTIAL EXERCISE #8

Intercostal Exploration

Stand comfortably with your feet hip-distance apart and avoid locking out the backs of your knees. Practice breathing in slowly and deeply, as though you are sipping on a straw trying to fill your trunk with air, similar to the way a ball inflates from a compressor. Focus on moving your ribs first and then feel how your breathing happens. To help you determine your individual breathing patterning, sense the feeling of breathing and notice where the movement of inhalation stops. Do you feel your belly protruding underneath your breastbone when you try to take a deep breath? Do you feel tension in the tops of your shoulders? Or is there a feeling of overall fullness or expansion? The latter movement is the ideal programming for breathing.

Focus on using a sipping breath (or you can actually sip through a straw) to learn to engage the movement of your ribs first when inhaling. This movement is very different than trying to push out with your belly to bring in air. Ideally, when you inhale, your ribs and belly should expand evenly with an overall feeling of inflation, much like the way a round balloon expands when filling with air. If you experience your breath getting stuck or sense that your rib cage is not expanding at the sides of your body, spend some time examining your breathing process in order to determine how you are actually using your breathing muscles. The beginning movement of your breath creates the quality of your breath, so make sure that you are not first sticking your belly out when you breathe or the breath movement will become stuck under your sternum. In many cases the instruction to "breathe with the belly" actually tightens muscles that restrict the rib cage from moving. Ribs that cannot rotate and move freely inhibit diaphragm expansion and movements all over the body. Sense your entire body as you perform breathing exercises and become aware of the inner sensations created by the movements of breathing.

On the inhalation, feel the contractions of the outer rib cage muscles (external intercostals) and lateral trunk muscles engaging to open the ribs and diaphragm out to the sides.

To explore this dynamic more deeply, stand with your feet hip distance apart and with your index fingers pushing into your intercostal muscles between two ribs in the front of the body under the breast area. Take in a deep breath and hold it. Notice how you can feel the contraction of your external intercostal muscles with your ribs expanded.

Keep pushing the muscles inwards with your fingers and exhale strongly, noticing how the external rib muscles seem to disappear as your ribs now close together. Can you now feel the internal intercostal muscles pulling the ribs together from the inside when you exhale?

Hold these exhaling muscles tight for a moment, feeling how these inner rib cage muscles work with the outer belly muscles to squeeze the air out. Now release the exhalation muscles and begin to inhale noticing again the actions of the external intercostals. The inner and outer rib cage muscles lie right next to each other and are designed to move the ribs in many different directions. In this exercise, we are trying to feel the difference between their two actions.

When you are exhaling, feel your outer abdominals and inner rib cage muscles draw in towards your spine. Stay long in your torso when you exhale keeping the natural curve in your lumbar spine. Do **not** allow your spine to flatten or compress. You must also keep the muscles in your mid-back contracted to keep the bottom tips of your scapula, or shoulder blades, pulled down. This will allow the ribs in your upper chest area to open and lift keeping expansion in your front body. Your intercostal muscles need to be balanced in their relationship to each other in order to have efficient breathing.

These movements include expanding the ribs up and out diagonally, sideways horizontally, and diagonally down and out to the sides. This expansive opening of the ribs, and downward contraction of the diaphragm, makes more space in the chest cavity. This creates a change in air pressure, causing more air to rush in, filling the lung cavity. The Esperiential Exercise #8 will help you experience how the intercostal rib cage muscles do their most important job: expansion in all directions, allowing the lungs to inflate and bringing oxygen into your body.

KEEP THE GIFT OF THE LIFT:
INHALATION CREATES EXTENSION, EXHALATION CREATES FLEXION

Because the contraction forces of the exhaling muscles tend to shorten the body, we must be consciously aware of lengthening at the waist, even while we exhale. By engaging your exhaling muscles to lengthen as they contract, you acquire an inner ring that supports your organs and stabilizes your spine. Your trunk muscles become primarily engaged as spine stabilizers, instead of as spine flexors that pull you forward, enabling your structure to be properly aligned with less effort.

The spinal/trunk extension created when you inhale is what YogAlign practitioners refer to as "the gift of the lift." The Core SIP Breath (SIP stands for "Structurally Informed Posture") informs your body of how to be in good posture by aligning you from the inside out. When you focus your awareness on keeping your structure lifted and extended when you exhale, your body begins to create a new software for your posture, and soon automatically engages the muscular actions of extension that "keep the gift of the lift." By consciously focusing on keeping your trunk elongated, your brain will gradually direct—via the nervous system—the muscle fibers of your core towards stabilization rather than flexion and shortening, making this stabilization automatic. Breathing with the Core SIP inhalation method brings tone, suppleness and strength to your diaphragm as well as to the other muscles of respiration. This creates an ideal support system, radiating out from the very center of your body. No matter what pose you are in or how you are moving your body, practice keeping the elongation that comes from the inhalation process rather than letting the movements of exhalation shorten your torso and neck.

"*Abdominal breathing is often depicted as a pattern in which the abdomen protrudes in front with each inhale. Many disciplines teach a type of abdominal breathing that is anatomically questionable. For the abdomen to protrude in this way, it must shorten when inhaling. This is a learned pattern, one that is mentally controlled. Movements that are mentally controlled lack adaptive flexibility. The tendency is to over-focus on what has been learned. In this case, the abdomen is moved in preference to the ribs.*"

Feitis and Schultz, *The Endless Web*

EXPERIENTIAL EXERCISE #9

The Core SIP Breath

Now that you have awakened the actions of your rib cage muscles, the Core SIP Breath will put it all together and tune up your entire being. Stand with your feet hip-distance apart, knees slightly softened. Let your arms hang by your sides. Gently press into the floor with your feet and notice how your spine responds by elongating. Focus on keeping that lift. Pucker your lips as you would if you were going to whistle and slowly breathe in through your mouth as if you are sipping through a straw. This is called the Core SIP Breath, or simply the SIP Breath; SIP stands for "Structurally Informed Posture."

This inhalation creates an extension in the body, and an engagement of your waist muscles deep in your core. Keep sipping in as you breathe, while you consciously focus on the lengthening of your body that occurs each time you inhale.

When you exhale, practice keeping this length in your spine and waist rather than letting the contraction movements of exhalation shorten your waist or pull your sternum, or breastbone, down.

Use your mid-back muscles to draw the tips of your scapulas down in your back. This action allows your upper chest to expand, creating natural alignment and support in your head, neck, and shoulder region.

Continue with the Core SIP Breath on the inhale, keeping your waist area long and lifted as you as you exhale through your nose or your mouth. As you inhale and your spine and trunk lengthens, you may feel a stretch all the way down into both sides of your groin, engaging a muscle/fascial connection from your diaphragm and psoas all the way through your legs and into the arches of your feet.

Feel what the deep core SIP Breath brings to you while you focus on the internal, front, and back areas of the body. When you sip the breath in, notice that the windpipe feels like a cool tube with air passing through it. Your breathing tubes are not only a passageway for air; they are also a muscular ring that provides support to your spine. As you breathe in, notice how this muscular air tube strengthens, elongates and supports the front of your spinal column. Breathe slowly and sense your breath's inner dynamics. It is important to maintain the elongation that comes from inhalation all the way through the exhalation process. Engaging this core diaphragm breathing creates powerful, fluid posture and movement dynamics that work from the inside out.

With consciousness intention, each in and out breath can be used to traction, align, and strengthen your spine and the muscles that act upon it. Using this breathing process can help you achieve natural alignment that will free your neck and shoulder muscles from the constant strain and overuse that occurs when breathing and posture are less than ideal. Always bring awareness and focus onto how your entire body feels when you breathe.

INHALATION GIVES YOU THE GIFT OF THE LIFT

When doing these breathing exercises, you may have noticed that your breathing muscles tend to automatically engage, and may be difficult to control. YogAlign gives people the tools to reprogram unconscious breathing habits that contribute to pain and misalignment all over the body.

Although it takes focus and concentration, it will not hurt and by doing the YogAlign breathing exercises, you will be able to acquire functional breathing habits that foster a pain-free dynamic structure.

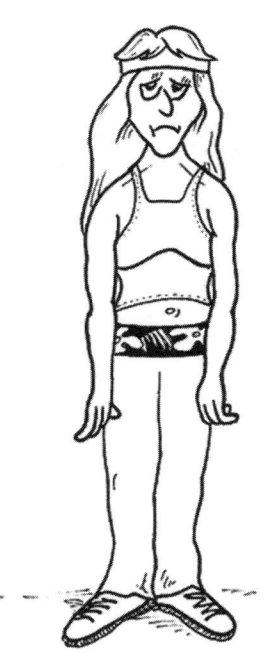

Establishing functional breathing habits will free up your body from performing unnecessary tasks. Breathing can be exhausting work if performed by the secondary breathing muscles in the upper back, neck, and shoulders. If you have ingrained breathing "dysfunction," such as leading with the upper shoulders on inhalation, you are wasting precious energy while working overtime with every breath.

Many people habitually breathe with the secondary muscles of the upper neck and shoulders as shown in **Fig. 4.3.** instead of with the diaphragm and rib cage which are the primary breathing muscles. Forward head carriage and rounded shoulders often result from the inordinate amount of time we have spent sitting in chairs with poor alignment, compressing the spine while inhibiting the vital movements of the diaphragm. Because of poor alignment, the body begins to rely on a secondary breathing system that is ineffective and lacking in fluidity and ease. Perpetuating the problem, when you are not breathing well, your spine collapses along with your diaphragm and you begin to unconsciously engage your upper neck and back muscles for postural support and breathing mechanics.

The upper neck and shoulder muscles are meant to help in the breathing process, but should not be used to initiate breath. When we initiate our breathing process from the secondary muscles, the shoulders round and pull the head forward creating bad posture. These muscles are not primary breathing muscles and should not be asked to hold the weight of our head past neutral, nor should they be initiating the movement of breathing. When posture is not optimal, we can't properly initiate breathing from our center, which further exacerbates poor posture, setting up a cycle of bodily stress and misuse.

Notice the number of people around you who have forward head carriage and rounded shoulders. Because we breathe 15,000 to 20,000 times a day, a pattern of using the upper shoulders with poor posture patterning can easily become habitually ingrained. Continual shallow breathing using secondary muscles creates fight-or-flight responses in the nervous system causing higher blood pressure, muscle tension, and a faster heart rate. Poor alignment holds these secondary breathing muscles in contraction, as in the case with forward head carriage, and can enlist a semi-permanent fight-or-flight response. When neck and shoulder muscles are chronically engaged in dysfunctional positions, serious pain and injuries can and will result. Drafted into action by excess muscle tension, fascial lines will thicken and become rigid, restricting movement, nerve pathways, and blood flow around the joints. The body hardens into a bad posture position, glued in place by thickened fascia in the associated neck and shoulder lines and controlled by software that supports the poor habits.

The overuse of these secondary muscles not only wastes energy but causes pain, stress, bone spurs, arthritis, and wear and tear on your joints. Neck and jaw muscles habitually over-enlisted as breathing muscles become tight, and greatly restrict the movement of the shoulders, resulting in chronic tension and pain in the upper body. (See illustrated example of the muscle players in **Fig. 4.3)**. Fascia lines then spread the tension to other distant parts of the body, which then become players in the folly as well. Tense upper-shoulder breathing ultimately leads to premature aging of the body, chronic pain, and injuries. Over-engaging your upper breathing muscles throws

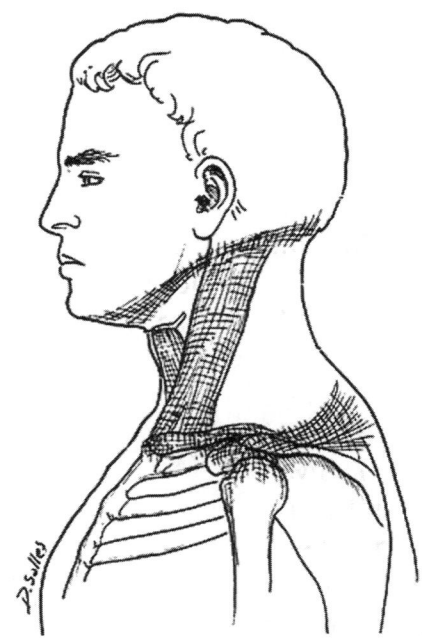

Fig. 4.3 – Fascia that permeates the throat's strap muscles can get thick and glued, creating an inhibition of upper body movements.

off alignment, which inhibits the breathing process. After awhile, it is the old chicken-and-egg routine: Is your posture poor because of the way you breathe? Or does your poor posture create weak breathing? The answer, we find, is both.

So how *does* one change poor posture or poor breathing habits?

Many people would start by taking a pain pill or calling a massage therapist or chiropractor, to get

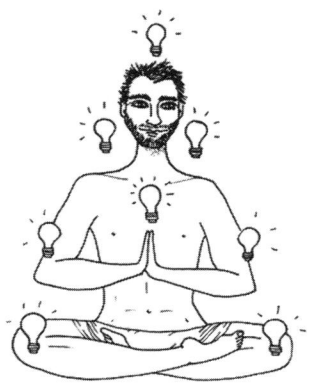

someone else to "fix" the problem. Such treatments may be very helpful in the moment. However, if poor posture and pain is chronic, the symptoms will simply return. Instead of relying on temporary relief, a self-care healing system can give you the tools to be your *own* healer. Like turning off the extra lights in your home, and burning only the lights you need, you can become breath and movement efficient, and conserve energy in your own body by turning off muscle patterning you don't need. With the breathing, movement, and alignment skills you acquire when practicing YogAlign, you gain valuable self-reliance, allowing you to heal and align yourself, and become sustainable within your own body.

Many daily movements—like chair sitting, and even yoga poses and fitness exercises—can set up a pattern of poor postural programming that actually reinforces tension and misalignment patterns we may already have. Why engage the body into spine-compressive positions that go against our natural design? If you feel uncomfortable in your body doing yoga (or anything else), try to take a deep breath. If you feel restricted when you breathe, the body needs to be moved to a more naturally-aligned and functional position, in order to maintain healthy physiology. This next exercise demonstrates how even the smallest movement in the far periphery of the body reverberates throughout the entire body, either assisting or inhibiting our breathing and functionality.

EXPERIENTIAL EXERCISE #10

Breathing Awareness and Body Position

Stand with your feet hip-distance apart, feet pressed into the floor, with your knees slightly bent. Take a deep breath using the Core SIP breathing technique. Draw the bottom tips of your shoulder blades down and maintain this stabilization both on the inhale and the exhale. Notice how long you are able to carry your inhale, and pay attention to how well your ribs expand and contract.

Now stand with your feet together and practice the SIP breathing technique. It can be shocking to discover how keeping your feet together can affect muscles in your core, causing restriction in your breathing capacity. Keeping the feet together engages muscles along the superficial front line of fascia that runs from the top of the feet up through the upper thighs and belly, all the way to the skull area behind the ear. When standing with the feet together, the abs and thighs contract, and this contraction reverberates along the fascial lines, tightening muscles up to the belly/rib cage area, preventing the ribs from expanding and the diaphragm from moving down in the abdomen. Exercises that direct you to keep your feet together will not assist you to breathe well or be well, but will instead train your core muscles to restrict the movements of breathing.

Variation 1: With your feet back in a natural hip-width stance, and the knees slightly bent, lift your arms straight out to the side at shoulder height, palms facing down with your fingers stretched wide open. Draw the bottom tips of your shoulder blades down while keeping your palms stretched and your fingers opened wide. Exhale strongly and then inhale again using the Core SIP Breath technique. Notice the expansive feeling of your rib cage, and the duration and quality of your inhalation process.

Variation 2: This time do not change your foot position but simply tighten and close your fingers together with palms down — a typical maneuver many are trained to do in yoga. Exhale and then slowly begin to inhale using the Core SIP Breath. You may notice how much shorter your inhalation time is. Simply closing the fingers compresses the rib cage, causing a line of pull through your arm lines to your chest, which restricts and shortens the breathing process. This is because the fascia lines in the arms extend from the tips of your fingers all the way to the ribs and diaphragm in the front body.

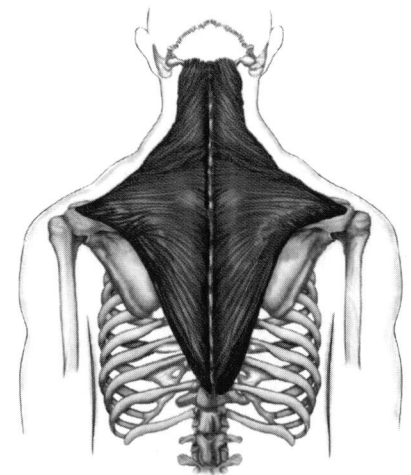

Fig. 4.4 – The Trapezius muscle, like a river, has many currents or directions of movement.

SECONDARY OR "FIGHT OR FLIGHT" BREATHING MUSCLES

It can be rather unsettling to realize that many common moves in yoga and fitness classes are actually creating breathing and alignment dysfunctions, both in the moment and down the line.

For example, one of the most common "rote" yoga moves is hands together above the head in prayer position, with fingers pressed tightly together and often with the head looking up towards the ceiling. This pose is a beginner's pose, not considered to be dangerous or risky, and yet we have found in our work with posture and yoga that these small movements are what ultimately define the big movements. In other words, even a simple movement like putting your palms together overhead may use muscles like the upper part of the trapezius (**Fig. 4.4**) in ways that contribute to an overall dysfunctional postural alignment. When engaged dysfunctionally, the trapezius can become top heavy, forcing the head forward and restricting movement in the neck area.

Touching your hands and fingertips together overhead while looking up is one of those moves that "rob Peter to pay Paul" (**Fig. 4.5**). Touching the hands together in this position improperly engages upper shoulder muscles, and compresses the neck of the spine. This movement is essentially a type of shrugging, yet it is routinely practiced in most yoga classes. The breathing process in this position is compromised, and the head is thrust forward as the upper shoulder muscles tighten. To do the pose requires moving the arms away from the neck and shoulder region,

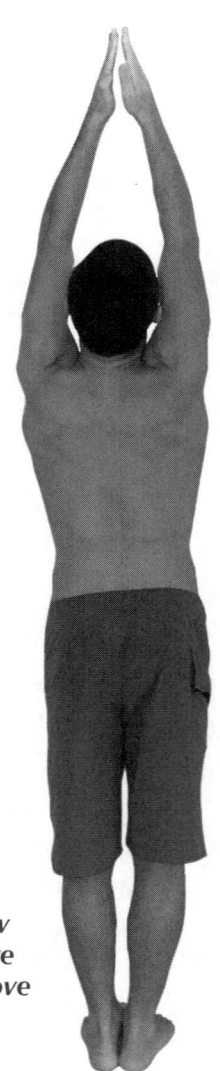

Fig. 4.5 – Zack shows how touching your palms above your head forces you to move from your extremities.

stretching shoulder stabilizing ligaments and creating movement actions that over engage the upper trapezius muscles. In many cases the head moves further out of balance, and the upper shoulders become chronically tight from performing functions they are not designed to do. The tightness in the upper shoulders and neck is interpreted as stress that can trigger the nervous system to activate a low level fight-or-flight response.

All movements in yoga should feel effortless, and promote functional alignment while simulating how the body actually moves in real-life situations. In the end, functional posture is much more important than getting into a "pose." A pose should allow us to be in an ideal postural position, bringing all parts together to form a cohesive whole connected dynamically to our center. All movement should happen expansively from our core, with an equanimity of effort spread evenly throughout our entire body. This fluid movement does not occur by stretching ourselves apart at the seams or by putting our body in spine-compressing, breath-inhibiting positions that have nothing to do with how we actually use our body in our daily life, as shown in **Fig. 4.5**.

Look at the unnatural spine curvature of our model, Zack, as shown in **Fig. 4.6.** Notice the constriction in the abdominal area, and the reversed lumbar (or lower back) curve created when trying to unnaturally

lean over with both legs straight at the same time. When we are moving, it is impossible to go anywhere if one knee does not bend. Straightening both knees and bending over leads to a reversal of natural curve in our lower backs, contracting and shortening of the abdominals, and impeded functional breathing. The diaphragm, which attaches to the lumbar spine, is compressed in this posture. Zack is forced to use the secondary breathing muscles in the upper neck and shoulders in order to breathe while in this pose. Because diaphragm breathing is restricted, this particular pose does nothing to contribute to good posture, or balanced fascia lines. Yet many physical therapists, trainers, yoga, and pilates instructors continue to teach these forward-bend poses with

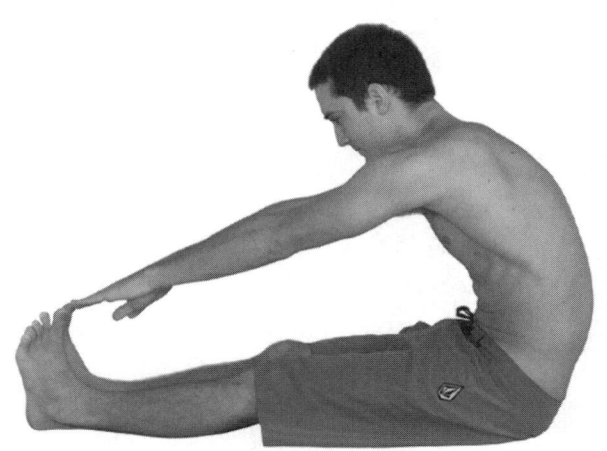

Fig. 4.6 – Leaning forward with your legs straight tightens muscles that shorten the front of the spine, compress the anterior disc area, and inhibit breathing. It is likened to driving with the parking brake on.

straight legs, purportedly to stretch the hamstrings. This is a contradictory effort, creating a contraction of the front body as a means to stretch the back, which has been made sore from excessive shortness and/ or weakness of the core and anterior body.

Not only do such positions cause an inhibition of the breathing process, they can compress spinal discs and overstretch nerves, causing any number of problems. Poses which have little to do with natural movement or balanced fascia lines will actually weaken fitness and function. Poses should balance all fascia lines, imitate good posture and movement, and allow for deep, relaxed breathing. The pose Zack is in feels like trying to "drive with the parking brake on" and is never used in YogAlign. It makes more sense to do poses that keep the body in natural spine alignment, and that assure breathing is effortless and deep. If you cannot take a deep breath, ask yourself, "What is beneficial about this pose and what processes are being ingrained?"

The "Chest Opener" pose (**Fig. 4.7**) is a beneficial breathing pose for Zack, to open his chest and stretch the fascia in the front of his body. This is an excellent pose that will turn on his deep inner core extension and strengthen the back muscles to lengthen as they contract. It affects his entire body all the way from his core center through his arm lines. While opening the front lines of fascia and muscles, breathing into this position will release back tension more effectively than rounding over in a forward bend and attempting to stretch away tightness in the back body. At the same time that Zack is extending his spine with his back muscles, he is opening his chest and arm lines, releasing his neck, and functionally strengthening his core. This expansive breathing position engages his whole body in a balanced dance of flexion and extension.

Promoting conscious awareness of body, mind, and spirit is one of the cornerstone teachings of the ancient art and science of yoga. When you do a yoga pose, ask yourself some important questions and let your structure determine the answer: Are you feeling okay in your body and peaceful in your spirit? Are you present in your mind and senses? Can you feel how you breathe and which muscles and fascia lines engage in the process? Beware of what may seem like an easy or harmless pose. If you cannot take a full, deep, rib-expanding SIP breath, the pose will ultimately bring you more tension and dysfunction by creating ingrained breathing habits that are energy wasters and postural saboteurs.

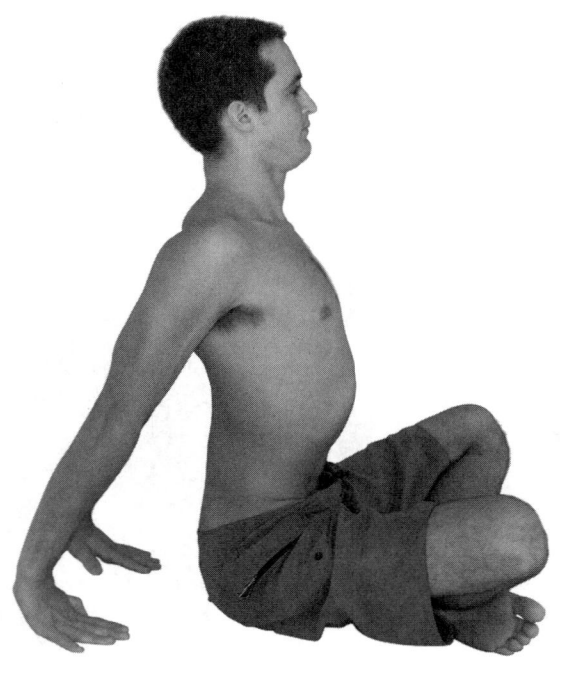

Fig. 4.7 – Chest Opener.
This pose creates length and space in the front body of fascia, while deep breathing enables core-centered strength and stability, revealing the true foundation of the body's structure.

As you will discover when practicing YogAlign, there

is no part of your body that is not involved in the breathing process. Breathing is like a symphony of many musicians, each with an instrument important to the expression of a musical work. To breathe functionally involves the body's inner and outer structure, and affects the health and well-being of the cellular function of the entire body. You can isolate individual muscles in the process, just as you can tune your hearing to the flute or the oboe; but in the end, you must be able to hear all parts of the entire "symphony" at once. Sensing the breathing process as it happens allows us to become deeply attuned to our breathing at the core level, and awakens us to the inner dynamics of our being. This most essential movement of the body can create deep healing experiences in our physical and emotional bodies. By tuning ourselves to our body and its breathing process, we can experience heightened awareness, and enter into the deepest of meditations.

Over the years I have worked with many clients who have healed neck, back, and shoulder pain simply by learning how to breathe from the center of their body, using their primary breathing muscles. Oftentimes it's not just weakness, but chronic tension in the belly and pelvic floor, that leads to constricted breathing patterns. This constriction in turn creates pain that is transferred throughout the body. We have an obsession in our country with making the belly tight and flat, which is seen as an indication of a high level of fitness. In reality, some of the most physically-fit people are not functionally-fit at all, because of patterning that favors tightness in the stomach area and pulls the navel in towards the spine. In the process of tightening the belly, there is a loss of spinal extension and freedom of movement. These people may look and feel good now, but this tightness and the associated inhibited breathing and movement could result in serious consequences over time.

GOING TO THE "MOTHERBOARD" WITH CONSCIOUS BREATHING

So what, exactly, controls the process of how we breathe, when we are not controlling it consciously? Breathing muscles are controlled by programmed codes of movement in our nervous system, which originate in instinctual survival areas in the primitive brain stem. You can create new breathing patterns almost instantly, without painful exercises, by learning to reprogram these neuromuscular codes. After a time, these new codes become innate patterns linked to breathing that happen automatically, and are more physiologically efficient. To make all this happen, you need to learn some techniques that will give you powerful passwords into the "motherboard" of your nervous system. This is the key to re-coding your unique movement patterning. No amount of exercise, yoga poses, massage, or manipulation will change your innate patterning unless you can learn how to utilize conscious breathing and movement at the nervous-system level. In order to become pain-free, we need to re-train our brain by eliminating software patterns that are not beneficial, and instead generate new codes that benefit functionality and the way we move in real life.

Every part of the body's system affects the whole. For example, the autonomic nervous system—which works "automatically'" to keep everything functioning—takes cues from the quality of your breath and the tension in your muscles. Interestingly, the nerves that control the relaxation response innervate the fascia system, allowing us to feel relaxed in our skin. Stress does just the opposite: it affects the body's overall ability to move and breathe with ease because it tightens muscles, raises blood pressure, and even causes the fascia web to contract.

The antithesis of being at ease in the body is the feeling of being "uptight." If we don't have relaxed and open breathing, our nervous system may be triggered into a fight-or-flight stress response. This is especially true for the abdomen, where our core and gut feelings originate, and the reason why stress can lead to

---

CASE HISTORY

A graphic artist and avid gardener booked a YogAlign session with me as a last resort. Having suffered from shoulder pain for years, she had tried massage, physical therapy, chiropractors, and an orthopedic physician, who finally told her that surgery was the only answer. Her shoulder pain was so severe she could not swim, garden or even lift her arms above shoulder level. She was to be married soon, and she and her fiancé planned a honeymoon to Fiji. In our first session, the first thing I noticed was her breathing, which she initiated from her upper shoulders and neck muscles. She was strong and fit but had poor breathing habits, excessively rounded shoulders, and forward head carriage. Through YogAlign she learned to activate her psoas–diaphragm connection and to release her chronically contracted front body and, in particular, her upper shoulders and neck area. Weak rib cage muscles and over-contracted upper shoulder muscles had formed a dysfunctional pattern that gave her arms little support, and kept them rotated forward in the shoulder socket. After a few sessions of YogAlign core breathing and postural rebalancing movements, she was able to alter her dysfunctional breathing habits and muscle patterning. She developed a deeper muscular foundation for her arms which enabled her to move them from the core of her body. She was able to functionally strengthen her rotator cuff muscles and stabilize her shoulder joint. In the process, her fascial arm lines became more fluid and she was able to lift and use her arms without pain. In a very short time, she was able to acquire a pain-free functional life, which included a wonderful honeymoon in Fiji. She told me that no health practitioner had ever watched how she breathed, or drawn any connections between her breathing and her shoulder pain. Using deep core breathing to correct postural misalignment frees up the body, and aligns from the inside out. Muscle tension dissipates, and the fascia corrects itself. The hardened fascia that accompanies this type of habituated muscle tension will simply dissolve from over time if better alignment is maintained.

ulcers. We put our "issues in our tissues." Tension in the mind leads to shallow breathing, which in turn can lead to a sympathetic nervous system chronically dialed in to a fight-or-flight stress response. Be aware that oftentimes the exercises we do to strengthen our core can overengage belly muscles, creating spinal compression, constricting breathing, and igniting the fight-or-flight reflexes.

You are your own teacher when it comes to your breath. Noticing which muscles you use when breathing, and which ones you actually don't need, is an exercise in awareness that will benefit you ten-fold. You can definitely reduce your risk of injury and begin to heal chronic pain by functionally enhancing your breathing muscles. YogAlign has safe and quick ways to healthily re-engage these muscles. By using the exercises described in this chapter, combined with the neuromuscular re-education techniques presented in Chapter 5, you can learn effective ways to add greater functionality to your breathing muscle patterns.

POOR BREATHING CAN AFFECT YOUR BODY AND YOUR MOOD

The tension we feel in our bodies often comes from weak and dysfunctional breath patterning. When our breath is powerful and balanced, it creates a sense of ease throughout our physical and emotional body. When we are not breathing well, our spine is collapsed, and the diaphragm is weakened, so we begin to rely on the neck and back muscles to hold up our structure and help us breathe.

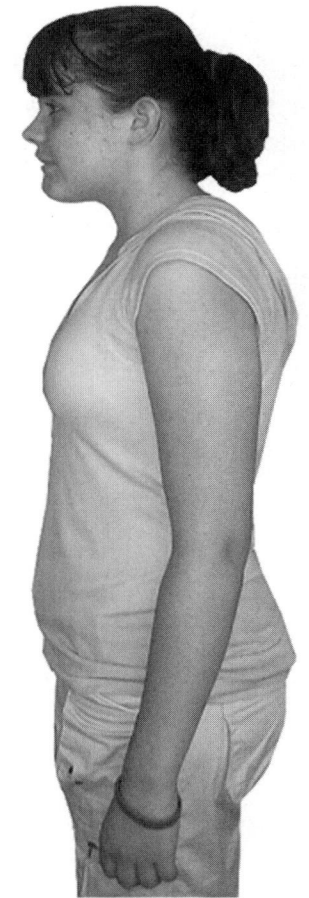

Weak breathing habits lead to poor posture, which cause tightness and tension as muscles assume the burden of functions they are not designed to perform. It is no longer just the elderly who show signs of poor posture, as habitual slouching and poor alignment increasingly affect young people as well.

Observing muscle balance and posture may lead us to conclude that a slouched person might be holding feelings of depression. Are they depressed from slouching? Or are they slouching from depression? If we focus on changing patterns through core breathing, our body will naturally feel light, and our mental energy will be free to express itself. We can become enslaved in a stress cycle simply from poor breathing and the resultant bad posture and negative feelings that this cycle can create. This is an example of carrying "issues in our tissues." When we are aligned and breathing well, it is actually difficult to frown. Conversely, it becomes difficult to smile when one is slouching. Poor breathing leads to poor alignment, which leads to depression, which leads to poor alignment, which leads to poor breathing, and so on. It's easy to become stuck in this stress cycle when our modern lifestyles demand that we spend so many of our waking hours in a chair. Utilizing YogAlign core breathing to align our spine and balance our muscular-fascial web, we can positively impact our reservoir of mental and physical energy and the quality of our thoughts.

Your breath defines your movements, your posture, your mood, and, eventually, determines your life span. Learn to breathe with purpose and passion, in order to re-create who you are.

Your Breath Gives You Life and Longevity

There are some cultures around the world where people stay fully-functional into old age, and movement and posture stays aligned and fluid. Chair-sitting is not part of the daily life of these people; instead, squatting is how these people "sit." In these cultures, people don't need hip and knee replacements, and they are not bound to intense stretching or strengthening programs. When we are aligned in our body, breathing is easy; we don't feel sore and we don't feel tense. There is no force in our movement or strain on joints or bones. When the body is in balance, there is no need to do hours of stretching or intense yoga poses, because we don't feel tight. Having an aligned spine and relaxed open breathing are the keys to health, and they contribute to preserving the integrity of joints and organ function well into old age. YogAlign principles emphasize effortless movement that arises from the center, and requires minimal effort from the extremities. Many people suffer from arthritis in the hips and knees that is caused by chronic compression in the joint areas. Miraculously, extension of the spine and trunk created by the movements of deep breathing can decompress our hip joint and take pressure off of our knees and feet, alleviating the arthritic process. Through practice, you can develop a deep ability to sense your inner body metaphorically as you move. You can envision the breathing muscles assisting the rib cage floating upwards like a helium-filled balloon, effortlessly lifting toward the sky. You can move with your hips swinging free and knees bending without restriction or tension, because they are functionally aligned without compression factors from above.

CASE HISTORY

Gabrielle "Gabby" Reece, is a volleyball professional, model, fitness educator, mother, and wife of extreme waterman, Laird Hamilton. Gabby had a bout of knee pain and swelling that had lasted more than a year and a half. After playing volleyball she would feel stiff, swollen, and sore in her knees. She had to lay off of playing volleyball or working-out for a few days, and she would use ice and rest her knees until the swelling and pain were gone. As soon as she played again, the cycle of pain and swelling would begin again.

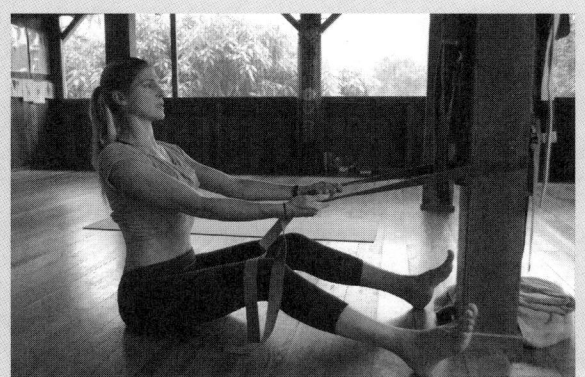

Gabby Reece

Gabby is in phenomenal shape, and yet she expressed that she felt stiff and lacked the ability to comfortably flex or extend her knee. She did not feel flexible nor did she consider herself "good" at stretching. In the first session, she found out that she is extremely flexible when using positions that simulate functional movement. She had strong patterns of tightness in the belly from doing lots of ab work, and these patterns were causing pull in her superficial front fascial line, from her head to her knees.

Using the breathing techniques of YogAlign, she found that the tightened strength of her belly muscles was actually inhibiting her ability to breathe, and therefore move from her center. I taught her how to do exercises with her whole body in alignment, and how to focus on balancing the whole body through the fascia lines, instead of doing compartmentalized exercises that separate the body into parts. She began to gain an understanding of her fascia lines, and was able to eradicate the knee pain and soreness she felt after playing volleyball. She had assumed for years that it was normal to get sore after a hard work-out. She began to use inhalation to create lift and to train her deep-core line of breathing as her power center, so that she was truly moving from her center.

In regards to her experience, Gabrielle had this to say:

"I have done years of exercises that have flexed my body forward. I have suffered greatly for that in my knees. In the first ten days of YogAlign, I benefitted greatly just in relieving pressure off my knee. Inflammation went down and I played volleyball the whole time. It is not like I laid off playing at all. YogAlign gave me a different relationship with my body where I can sense the whole.

I learned there was nothing wrong with my knee as much as my body mechanics and my psoas muscles not working functionally. I used to feel like a heavy mass just clunking around. I have now learned to move around in this lightened floating position when I play volleyball, run or workout. YogAlign just makes sense and it is not intimidating or painful at all."

CASE HISTORY

A young woman in her late-20s booked a YogAlign session with me, complaining of neck pain and low energy. She had been diagnosed with chronic fatigue syndrome and had suffered since her teen years from low energy and depression. She was a singer, and wanted to pursue a career, but found that she lacked the necessary stamina. She felt discouraged about her future. She had taken prescription medicines for her condition but nothing had really helped. When analyzing her posture and breathing, I observed that she had a very weak diaphragm, no curve in her lumbar spine and her head was forward on her spine. Her knees were locked back in hyper-extension and her sacrum and breast bones were collapsed and sagging. She looked unstable and loose in her body, although she said she felt tight. In the first session, she learned to breathe with her diaphragm/psoas connection and did sensory exercises to relax the chronic tension in her back and belly. She learned to support herself from the center of her body using the breathing process and she had more energy immediately. After a couple of sessions, she said the chronic fatigue syndrome symptoms were gone. Her posture was erect, she looked energized and she felt

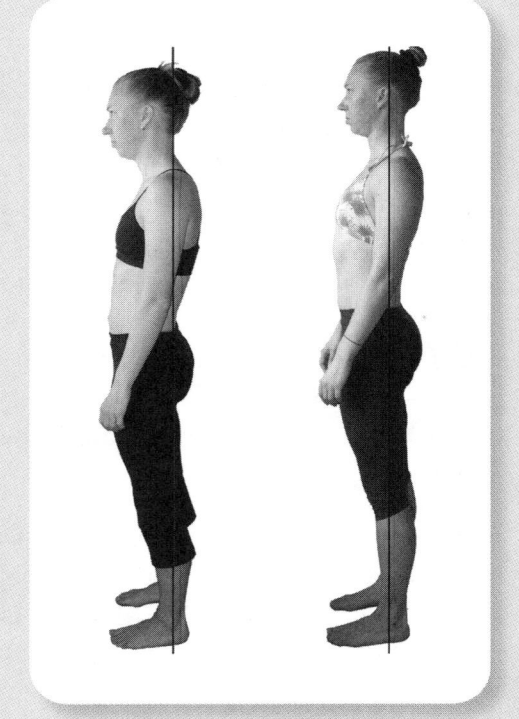

In Fig. 4.8 – After 4 days of YogAlign, this female athlete learned to be aligned with gravity and to use the movements of breathing to support her structure, rather than relying on hyperextension of her knees.

positively about her life and her future. She continued to do the simple posture and breathing tune–ups shown in Part Two of this book, and began to record her songs and compose more music. She told me that no health professional she had seen had ever evaluated or treated her posture and poor breathing habits as the possible cause for the depression and chronic fatigue she had suffered from for most of her adult life.

YogAlignMent Principle #6
Keep the "gift of the lift" by paying attention to the extension created by the inhalation process, and retaining that lift even as you exhale.

YogAlignMent Principle #7
Use the SIP breathing technique to create **Structurally Informed Postural** patterning.

CHAPTER 5: RETRAIN YOUR BRAIN

ॐ *Our Brain Is the Hard Drive for Our Movement and Posture*

ॐ *We Are Not Tight; We Are Tense*

ॐ *We Don't Stretch Because It "Hurts"*

ॐ *Outwit the Stretch Reflex*

ॐ *Train Your Brain with PNF*

ॐ *Natural Alignment and Breathing*

ॐ *Fight-or-Flight Stress Response vs. Relaxation Response*

ॐ *Self-Massage Engages the Relaxation Response*

ॐ *Poor Movement Is More than Muscle Deep*

ॐ *Internal Guided Imagery*

ॐ *YogAlign Neuromuscular Repatterning*

Our bodies are mostly
water and space.
Flexibility happens in the brain.

" *As your muscles gain flexibility you can expect an immediate 15–20 percent increase in strength—without any additional weight training—as well as significant gains in power, speed, and accuracy....You need sufficient strength to contract your muscles maximally when stretching them.* **"**

Cooley, *The Genius of Flexibility*

OUR BRAIN IS THE HARD DRIVE FOR OUR MOVEMENT AND POSTURE

When we get the idea or impulse to move, it's the brain that gives the movement orders to the muscles. The brain is encoded with neuromuscular codes that automatically enable us to perform highly-complex tasks like playing piano while singing, or typing on our keyboards, without thinking about where each individual letter is located. We don't consciously direct every intricate detail of how we move; we are like the drivers of a car in relationship to our body. We can direct the body where we want it to go, just as we direct a car when driving, but we certainly don't make each individual part of the engine perform as we drive.

From the minute details of movement, to the automatic, inner workings of our body that control digestion, elimination or heart rate, our body knows how to move without our conscious involvement. The body does it all on its own, using the nervous system to direct the muscles in complex patterns, with nerve signals firing muscle contractions in fractions of a second. An organ in our brain called the *cerebellum* (Latin for "little brain") is the master calibrator of our posture and is the "director" of our unique movements, posture, and muscle tone. The human brain contains approximately 100 billion neurons, with an estimated 60 to 70 billion located in the cerebellum, making this fist-sized organ nothing less than the hard drive for the whole brain. All data output from different centers of the brain is sent to the cerebellum, including our emotions, memories, attention, and language. The cerebellum fine-tunes our posture, and holds the codes for the individualized ways that we move, think, emote, and breathe. All of our movements originate with signals from the brain that are sent to our muscles, and the muscles then contract according to the codes that have been sent. In order to change our posture, we must rewrite the way these automatic neuromuscular codes direct the complexity of our posture and movement. This is made possible by methods that directly affect our innate patterning on the unconscious level, where our posture "happens" (hopefully in a functional way) without us even thinking about it.

The importance of good posture cannot be overemphasized, and the task at hand is to achieve good posture in a natural, enjoyable way that allows fluid, balanced, and flexible movement from a core-connected infrastructure. Repatterning the nervous system to re-calibrate our posture from the inside out involves addressing how our internal software directs the fundamental basics of our breath and movement. Daily habits are cumulative, and the quality of our movements can increase or decrease the health of our joints, organs, and emotions, as well as almost all other systems of the body. Since the body/mind/spirit connection is a continuum, YogAlign uses several approaches to re-pattern the codes that determine our individual posture and movement; these codes ultimately define the quality of our health and determine our longevity.

What differentiates YogAlign from other practices is its focus on the rewiring of real-life movement patterning, rather than confusing the body with poses that do not necessarily simulate real-life function or movement. As part of the rewiring process, YogAlign concentrates on poses which stimulate the entire body in harmonized natural alignment, and uses powerful techniques that educate our nervous system to retain revised sensory information. YogAlign practitioners are given explicit anatomical road maps, and a consciousness- and sensory-based experience of how the body is interconnected and moves as a whole. For example, sensing the fascia web that connects your arms and legs to your core gives you an experiential map that guides you to move from your center. Your ability to experience, sense, and feel the body as you breathe and move is the moment where impressive changes begin to happen. To be able to "sense the body in its entirety" is a deep meditation that enables you to expand awareness of your inner body, and consciously change movement patterning that has become rote and dysfunctional. Much of our chronic pain comes from a lack of connection to, and awareness of, how the body in its entirety engages in the daily movements of life. Focusing on the whole, and using the body in a continuum shifts old patterning, freeing up your inner "kid body," which is connected, spirited, light, and powerful.

What you can sense, you can change. Proprioception is our sixth sense, and it gives us the ability to sense and feel our structure. It is the acute awareness of the mechanics of how we move. This sensing ability allows us to be physically aware of our body's position in three dimensional space. By developing a more precisely intricate proprioceptive sense we can begin to move with minimal effort, revealing our innate natural alignment patterning. After a period of directed and focused attention, this ability to sense our patterning becomes second-nature, like learning to drive a car. In YogAlign, we program the nervous system to imprint naturally aligned positions—"new code"—to keep us in alignment with only the necessary effort. Any tightness or inflexibility can be alleviated by cultivating whole body awareness while engaging deliberate muscle contractions, by way of proprioceptive neuromuscular facilitation (PNF).

> ❝*Proprioception is the summation of our physical history into the moment of present activity. Every physical act reverberates through the whole body, and this can be consciously felt. Proprioception, then, is sensing the mechanics of movement. When there is a gap in proprioception, there is a habitual inhibition of movement. This is anchored in the flesh by loss of elasticity in the connective tissue and a reduction in its ability to stretch and then return to its original shape. Releasing these contractions in the connective tissues is a matter of physical or mental awareness.*❞

Schultz and Feitis, *The Endless Web*

So, where do these ingrained patterns come from and how exactly can we change them?

Embedded movement patterns are created from the time we are born, and build in complexity as we grow and develop. Coded muscle-lengths and movement patterns, or "muscle memories", enable us to engage in complex, multi-muscle functions such as sports, playing an instrument, or even talking and singing. We develop and encode these muscle patterns in the brain from birth when we begin to move our bodies. Without these encoded patterns, it could take us over ten minutes to direct every single muscle fiber to lift our arms. Muscle memory eliminates the need to tell every single muscle what to do and how to do it, which makes living and moving easy and automatic. From the moment we are born, we develop nerve commands, which become deeply-encoded instructions for complex movement patterning that go far beyond isolated muscle engagement. Individual muscles do not exist in isolation; rather they are grouped in fascial lines that direct our movement and define our posture, gait and even our moods. As we first learn to breathe, walk, and speak on our own, our nervous system is memorizing codes that will become the software for our distinct way of doing things. Have you ever noticed that you can recognize a familiar person by their unique way of walking and moving, even before you're close enough to see their face? This is due to their individual encoded patterning, which makes them move like no-one else. Unfortunately, many of us have movement patterns that are not beneficial, and they have become habituated and innate. We cannot just stop following these patterns, because they have become automatic. We must download new software, and reboot to alter our ingrained codes.

Poor posture is deeply entrenched and physiologically inefficient, and it creates abnormal tension loads throughout the body, which in turn cause joint pain and a lack of core structural integrity. Poor alignment from too much chair-sitting becomes ingrained and begins to feel "normal." Teens with slouched shoulders and adults with abnormal forward head carriage have become a cultural norm. These are poor habits imprinted on the nervous system's control panel of our movements. Many people habitually keep their neck or belly tightened, which hinders their movement and breathing; this hindrance creates poor alignment, which in turn leads to chronic pain and organ dysfunction. Because so much of our movement and posture is unconsciously programmed in our brain, we must use what we can consciously control to establish beneficial neuromuscular patterning. Increasing our proprioceptive sense allows us to access our programming, reboot, and install new movement software in this re-programming process.

The body is like a dense representation of our mental energy, and our movement patterning is therefore affected by our thought, beliefs, and emotions. For those who hold unconscious tightening in the pelvic floor, or in the jaw, or any other place that harbors emotional or trauma issues, poor movement and posture codes are locked up by their emotions and memories. Belief systems, in addition to emotions and memories, can also shape how we move and carry ourselves. How we engage in our body is affected by culturally-ingrained ideals of how we *should* look, feel, and act. For example, many women are inhibited about their breasts, and in the process of trying to hide them, they unknowingly round their shoulders creating poor posture in the process. Many men and women hold the belly in, in order to look more fit, hide feelings, or to appear to be slimmer.

These poor patterns can be recalibrated directly through a focused awareness on the breathing process and how it affects movement. For instance, excess tension in the pelvic floor creates a restriction in our breathing, which inhibits movement in the hips and legs, causing patterning that inhibits movement and joint functions all over the body. It's like a domino effect, with tight pelvic floor muscles affecting the muscles leading down to the feet, resulting in poor knee tracking, resulting in knee pain and injuries. Feelings of inadequacy caused from having weak knees can lead one to round the shoulders, which develops tension in the pelvic floor, further affecting the function of the knees. A cycle of tension, pain, and feelings of depression then becomes chronic and rote. The way to break this cycle is to focus on the movements of breathing and remove the excess tension in the pelvic floor which may be inhibiting breath and movement all over the body. Tension can be eradicated by changing the signals that give rise to it, and by staying in natural, functional alignment positions.

We Are Not Tight; We Are Tense

The resting length of our muscles is what determines our flexibility. Flexibility in the body can be accomplished by training our nervous system to reset the resting length of our muscles. Since tightness or tension of muscles is directed by the brain, it is important to know that our muscles are not actually *tight*, they are *overly tense*. Muscle tissue is about 67 to 72 percent water, making muscles watery in consistency. Because of this consistency, muscles cannot physically *be* tight or dense, they are simply engaged in a state of over-contraction. YogAlign involves mastering the art of easing muscle tenseness via the brain, to create functional flexibility. In this process one begins to feel and *know* the fluidity of the human structure.

Sometimes lifelong patterns of ingrained muscle tension, or repetitive, intense athletics keep muscles contracted and unable to release. Forced exercises like sit-ups are goal-oriented toward creating a hard and tight belly. In many cases, after engaging in such exercises the belly *remains* tight and does not release to a more functional resting length. If muscles don't release to a comfortable resting length, they inhibit opposing muscles from engaging. Many athletes are wired strong but tight, and these belly, back, and leg muscles are encoded to stay over-contracted even when not exercising. Over-contracted muscles lead to joint compression, stiffness, injuries, chronic pain, and an overall waste of energy. Posture is affected, and years down the line arthritis and other chronic health problems can develop.

Developing functional posture happens in the nervous system, and using YogAlign techniques, you can gain the tools to encode new patterns and fix the "vehicle" of your body. Then you will no longer be dependent upon an endless stream of body mechanics, or be spending time and money ingesting pain pills.

WE DON'T STRETCH BECAUSE IT "HURTS"

Fitness magazines inform us that to be healthy and youthful, we must stretch or do yoga. Health practitioners advise engaging in these activities to help a sore back or to calm the nerves. To many people, yoga and/or stretching means one thing: pain. A bad experience, an injury, a position that didn't feel good to the lower back, stiffness the next day—these things might convince us that we are stiff and dense, and perhaps always will be. When the association with yoga and stretching is pain and discomfort, it's easy to procrastinate doing stretching, exercises, or yoga, or avoid doing them altogether. Maybe we persevere, but our body still feels inflexible and we believe that we are "bad" at yoga.

Maybe you don't believe it is possible for you to be flexible—or more flexible—at this time in your life. Flexibility is important for maintaining ease in movement, and is the key to being pain-free and aligned. Yet many people dislike stretching, because it often hurts and brings discomfort. For many of us, the pose shown in **Fig. 5.1** is not "fun" or comfortable, yet we persist in spite of how bad it feels. Notice how compressed Zack's spine is when he tries to keep his legs straight and his heels pressed towards the floor. Look at the rounding in his upper back and how the body is in a poor postural position.

Because many of us define ourselves as "not flexible," we have a belief that getting flexible involves enduring pain while stretching. We welcome this pain as a sign that we are working hard, and that the suffering means we are "getting somewhere." We have been trained to believe "no pain, no gain," and "pain is weakness leaving the body."

YogAlign changes these beliefs, and assures us that there *is* a way to gain flexibility, quickly, with no pain, while increasing strength at the same time. It is exciting to see how YogAlign practice can quickly develop people's flexibility, and change their structural and postural habits. For some, this new way of moving and "being" happens very quickly, even if previous movement patterns are deeply-ingrained from a life's repetition of movements. The resting length of muscles can be re-trained quickly, releasing to a longer length, which maximizes flexibility and initiates the release of old habits of tightness.

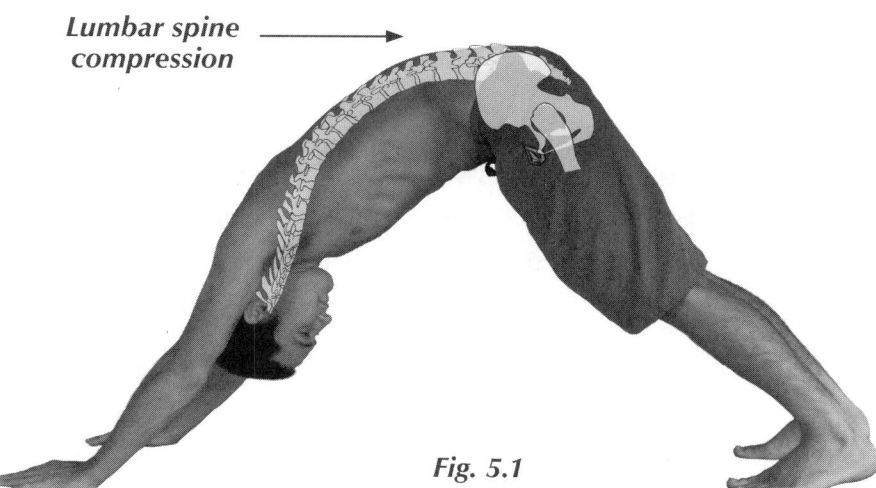

Lumbar spine compression

Fig. 5.1

Let's also look at the concept of stretching to get flexible. The resting length or flexibility of a muscle is hardwired in the nervous system, and the signals to tighten do not actually originate from the muscle itself. We cannot stretch muscle tightness away by force, because it is the nervous system—not the muscle—that is determining the muscle's length. In fact, overstretching can engage something called the "stretch reflex." This reflex is also called the "spinal cord reflex arc," and it keeps muscles and ligaments from tearing and joints from dislocating whenever we move into a position out of our normal range. The pain we feel when doing certain yoga poses is the body's way of telling us that we're pushing the body too far; the muscles we are trying to stretch are regulated at a defined length, and our built-in stretch reflexes won't allow a deeper muscle stretch for our own protection. When you stretch a muscle like your hamstring until it becomes uncomfortable, the brain engages the stretch reflex automatically, tightening the hamstring to protect it from tearing. The muscle is just following orders from the brain. These signals are necessary to protect our joints by stabilizing the muscles around them, literally keeping us from falling apart. To foster flexibility, we need to work *with* these signals, going back to the source (codes in the nervous system) while making sure the body feels safe in the process.

OUTWIT THE STRETCH REFLEX

The good news is that changing the codes in the nervous system is a lot easier and more fun than fighting the body's stretch reflexes. Understanding that our brain controls muscle tension is the first step towards increased flexibility. YogAlign's method of using conscious breathing and self-awareness to train the body, while in naturally-aligned positions, is a safe and quick way to become flexible and strong, with no pain involved. The method's easy and comfortable techniques make your muscular system toned and flexible at the deep, nervous-system level. Yoga and stretching don't have to be painful; you just need to learn to use fundamental body positions that imitate real, functional movements, and learn to re-code flexibility from the brain. You can do this by practicing "tightening what feels tight" with PNF exercises. This conscious tightening of your muscles will help you become both flexible *and* strong simultaneously.

TRAIN YOUR BRAIN WITH PNF

Being flexible is crucial for effective mobility, since tight muscle patterning is often what causes poor alignment and leads to restricted movement, pain, and injuries. The usual suggested remedy for tightness in the muscles is stretching. However, as we have seen, traditional ways of stretching are often counter-productive and even unsafe. YogAlign utilizes proprioceptive neuromuscular facilitation—or PNF—as a powerful, self-guided technique for changing muscle tension in the brain and gaining flexibility.

The PNF technique essentially outwits your habituated stretch reflexes, and resets resting muscle length, which is what determines your level of flexibility. By consciously tightening a muscle past its normal contraction, or "tightening what is already tight", during normal exercises, the nervous system throws a switch that opens us up to more flexibility. PNF allows you to become strong and flexible at the same time, and this occurs quickly, with no pain or strain to muscles or joints. When you add bodily awareness, and conscious, efficient breathing to this tightening, you suddenly have the power to change your movements and posture, essentially creating a new structure or body.

When doing PNF exercises, we engage a muscle in order to stimulate what is called the *golgi tendon organ* or the GTO. The GTO is a sensory receptor located where muscle and tendon join and it detects changes in tension of the area. When tension is greatly increased, the GTO sends a sensory nerve signal to the spinal cord which responds with a motor nerve signal telling the muscle to relax to protect the tendon. An afferent (towards the brain) nerve signal is then sent to the cerebellum from the spinal cord with information about the new resting length of the muscle. The information gets calibrated at that point into your nervous system as the new resting length. So the simplicity of getting flexible happens by tightening muscles while stretching and coding the nervous system to rewire it. Many times when people attempt to stretch without engaging PNF (tightening muscles as you stretch), they wind up just fighting the stretch reflex and never actually rewiring the muscle for a longer resting length or for flexibility.

Consciously contracting muscles during stretching exercises is an example of active muscle engagement, and this active engagement is a key to strength. Active engagement can happen in a variety of ways, including isometrically, concentrically, and eccentrically, with some engagements more beneficial than others.

Muscles are engaged *isometrically* when the body is held in a static position. Isometrics are a type of muscle contraction in which muscles develop contraction or tension without changing length. To better understand this, try this simple exercise: stand in front of a wall, and push your arms out parallel to the floor, using your hands to press against the wall. Notice that although your arm muscles are generating force, and muscles are contracting, there is no change in the length of your arm muscles. Being static, isometric engagement is not as effective as muscle engagement that involves the body in movement, because it doesn't simulate how we move in real life.

Muscles engage *concentrically* when the bones are pulled-in more closely toward the body; these actions typically occur when we lift any sort of weight. Muscles also can be engaged *eccentrically*, in which they paradoxically lengthen as they contract, usually in response to releasing a weight.

Take, for instance, the common exercise known as the bicep curl. The motion of lifting the weight in this exercise causes the muscle fibers in the bicep to shorten and contract, in order to lift the weight and move the bones closer together—this is a concentric action. When the weight is lowered during a bicep curl, the motion becomes an eccentric muscle contraction; as the weight is returned to its down-position in a controlled manner, the bicep muscle fibers remain contracted, but lengthen at the same time.

Most of our daily movements in life contain both eccentric and concentric muscle actions. When walking up a flight of stairs, our thigh muscles engage *concentrically*, and on our descent the thigh muscles engage *eccentrically*. Picking up a child or the laundry is a concentric action (lifting weight), and lowering the child or the basket requires eccentric muscle actions (controlled release). Since concentric and eccentric movements are at the heart of how we move in real life, you can see how isometric contractions would be less effective than the natural combination of concentric and eccentric muscle engagements that we use in YogAlign.

An example of a classic concentric exercise is the abdominal crunch. Most people do these crunches with an exhalation, which causes the spine to compress and the belly area to shorten. In YogAlign, we modify this exercise by engaging the movements of inhaling first, and then contracting our abs to lift the upper body from the floor while in the inhalation process. The internal inhalation process engages the entire core synergistically, creating an eccentric lengthening of the trunk muscles, and internal resistance that strengthens us from the inside out. As the trunk of the body is lowered to the floor, the muscular movements of exhalation protect the spine and lower back from hyperextension. The eccentric engagement caused by inhalation allows the core muscles to lengthen as they contract, which leads to a toned and lean waist; more space for the internal organs; and less pressure on the spinal column and joints. Using concentric to eccentric muscle engagement with focused breathing effects a synergized balance of flexibility and strength and a release of chronic tension and holding patterns.

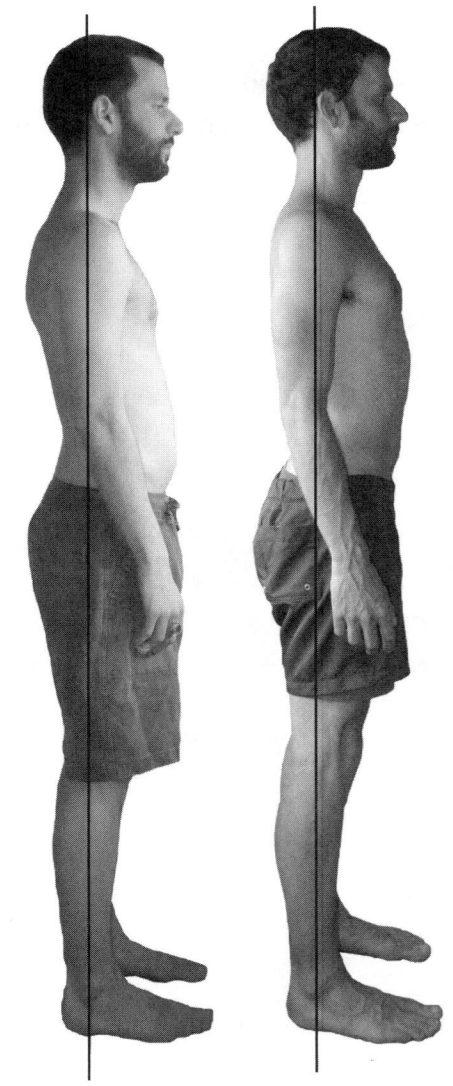

This next simple Experiential Exercise connects breathing to movement, and erases tense and tight neuromuscular patterning all the way back to the brain level. When you do this exercise, you become toned, strong, and flexible all at the same time. Remember: because of fascia connections, every movement you make affects lines of pull that resonate throughout the whole body. Done correctly, the entire superficial back line of fascia, from feet to head, is involved in this exercise — meaning not just the hamstrings but the entire back side of the body is reset in terms of muscle tension.

EXPERIENTIAL EXERCISE #11

PNF Hamstring Lengthener

Lie on your back with your knees bent and your feet hip-distance apart. (If you are now pregnant, you may not want to lie on your back for extended periods of time.) Bring your neck and lower back into a neutral position, with the natural curves intact. Do not press the lower back into the floor. Keep your chin and forehead at the same level. If there is strain to the front of your neck or if your chin is higher than your forehead, use a small pillow to slightly elevate the back of your skull. Lift one of your legs towards the ceiling and with straight arms interlace your fingers behind the back of your leg, either above or below your knee. Press the ball and heel of your foot towards the ceiling with your toes spread wide. **Caution!** If your lower back compresses to the floor, bend your knee until the lower back curve releases from the floor. Keep your arms straight and your shoulders drawn away from your ears, keeping your back and neck in a neutral position.

Retain the natural curves in your neck and lower back. Inhale using the Core SIP breath technique. Hold your breath gently, and consciously increase the contraction in your muscles created by the further extension of your heel and ball of your foot towards the ceiling. At all times, keep your toes open and spread wide. Don't think; just feel what your muscles are doing and accentuate the muscle contractions (tighten what already feels tight). After about 10 or 15 seconds, exhale with your mouth wide open and your tongue extended out. But keep your toes spread and the foot in the same position. Notice how your flexibility has increased without the pain of normal stretching.

After performing the "PNF Hamstring Lengthener" you may feel that your leg and back are now longer and more flexible. This is your experience of engaging the GTO, and its recalibration of your muscle flexibility via your spinal cord and brain.

After completing one of these exercises, look to see if your elbows have started to bend. If so, slide your hands upward towards your foot until your arms are straight and repeat the exercise. Keep your shoulders down and your neck long, but not flattened. This time, point your toes like a ballet dancer, breathe in, increase the contraction of the muscles and then hold the accentuation for 10 to 15 seconds.

Tighten not just your toes and foot, but your whole leg, your belly and whatever other muscle areas are involved. As you exhale with your mouth wide open, extend your tongue and keep your toes pointing. Stretch your entire body and feel the difference between the side you have just exercised, and the side that has not yet been exercised. Then repeat the exercise on the other side. After you finish, take a moment to enjoy the good feelings of energy throughout your whole body.

EXPERIENTIAL EXERCISE #11 (CONT.)

By contracting muscles consciously beyond their normal rate, you are doing a concentric PNF muscle engagement. When you release deeper without the extra contraction but stay in the stretched position, you are going into an eccentric muscle engagement, where, although muscles are contracting, they are lengthening as they do so. Sense your body in its entirety and you will feel how not just your foot and leg but the *entire back side of your body* feels longer, lighter, stronger, and more flexible.

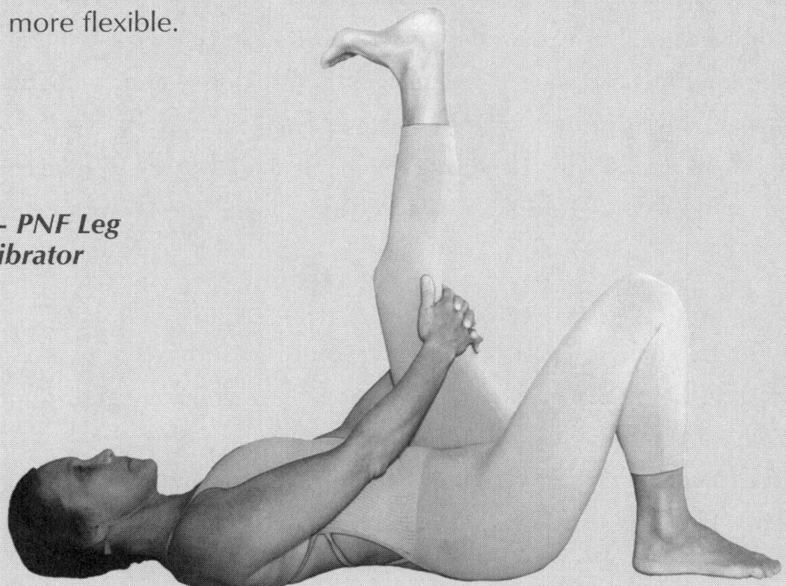

Fig. 5.2 – PNF Leg Recalibrator

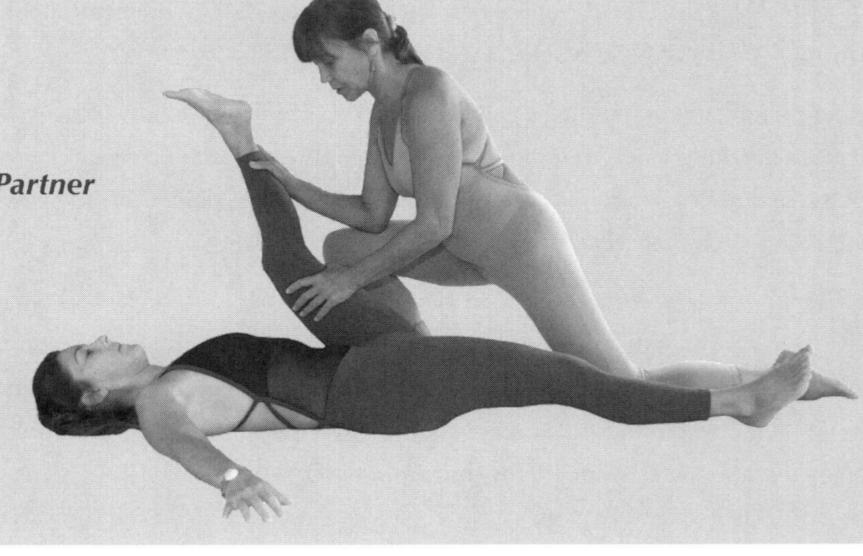

Fig. 5.3 – PNF with a Partner

CASE HISTORY

Sean came to take YogAlign lessons with me to acquire more flexibility as he was very strong but tight. He was motivated to learn PNF YogAlign exercises that he could do on his own. In his mid-30's and very fit, he spent a lot of his time cycling, skiing, running, cross-training, and mountain climbing. Swimming was difficult for him, though, as he felt inflexible and his lack of body fat made him sink like a stone. He had the body of a superhero, but the tension in his muscles was calibrated way too high, and he suffered from frequent shoulder injuries, chronic neck pain, and had several knee surgeries. His upper shoulders were so overbuilt that his head was pushed forward of neutral, causing him to feel constant tension in the muscles of his upper back and neck. His six-pack was impressively tight, and as a result his arms and legs were wired into a forward pulling tension. His magazine cover abdominals were robbing him of precious flexibility and range of motion, putting him at a mechanical disadvantage in his shoulder, knee, and hip joints. I told him to "forget the six-pack and go for the whole keg," meaning that he should focus on exercises that toned and lengthened the muscles that attached and controlled the rib cage area. YogAlign exercises would free the fascia and musculature that was holding his rib cage in a vice-grip, which was adversely affecting his entire body.

He told me how tight he was and how he has "never been flexible." In response, I asked him how his body could be so tight, since he was mostly water and space. He looked puzzled, and I explained to him that his muscles are composed mostly of water, and it is just signals from the brain that have told his muscles to stay contracted when not necessary. It was these brain codes, and not the muscles themselves, that were causing him to feel inflexible. I told him that the methods I would teach him would enable him to go into his brain's computer, and reboot the signals to his muscles, enabling him to feel more flexible that very day. Of course he didn't believe me, but an hour later, sure enough, he was laughing and marveling at his ability to do the splits and other leg stretches he never thought he could do. I showed him how to release the calibration of tension in his pelvic floor and abs, which took pressure off of his knee and shoulders, which had all been sore for months. After our session, Sean was amazed at how different he looked in the mirror, and how much his head alignment had shifted to a more erect graceful position. He thought for sure he would be sore from going so deep in the poses and he was amazed that he felt no soreness or stiffness the next day. He said that YogAlign felt amazing and he felt tuned, toned, relaxed and powerful. He also said that YogAlign was the best workout he had ever experienced. He continues to practice YogAlign today, and has applied alignment and breathing principles to his cycling and climbing. He reported back to me that he now cycles faster and further with no pain and much less effort in his body.

NATURAL ALIGNMENT AND BREATHING

When our breath becomes inhibited, posture and alignment suffer. In turn, poor alignment can inhibit proper nerve-signaling. This is because the nerves that control our autonomic functions lie on the front, or anterior, portion of the spine. Compression of the spine can pinch or compress these nerves, thereby disrupting nerve signaling. Creating space and length through the four natural curves of the spine facilitates uninterrupted and efficient nerve signaling, and elongated and decompressed spinal positions contribute to better brain and spinal core functioning. When your posture improves, your body can then elicit strong nerve signals that improve movement, organ function, and proprioceptive sense.

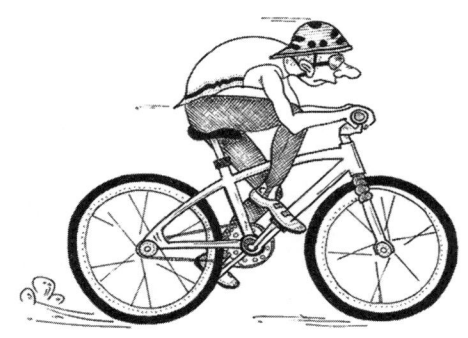

Cycling with poor posture will not make you functionally fit.

When we are standing well, we feel well, and we breathe efficiently and with ease. Our entire being functions better when we are aligned and elongated. Posture and alignment are so intertwined with breathing that it is simply impossible to separate the two. To recode the nervous system we need to breathe well, and optimally align the body to get the nervous system working for us, not against us.

FIGHT-OR-FLIGHT STRESS RESPONSE VS. RELAXATION RESPONSE

Stress can set up a vicious cycle of pain, and engage chronic neuromuscular patterns of poor breathing habits and posture that lead to disease, pain, and depression. This stress cycle can be initiated by depression and negative thinking, which is then reflected in poor postural patterning. Alternatively, the cycle can start with poor postural positioning, which then leads to stress and depression. Someone with very poor posture will predictably be feeling some degree of depression. So which comes first: are they depressed because they slouch or do they slouch because they are depressed? The answer is that there is *no* answer. Our posture is the dense representation of our movement, thoughts, and emotional patterning and they all affect the other. The body, unlike thoughts and emotions, is something tangible that it can be seen and shaped. When breathing deeply and standing tall, it is very difficult to frown or feel depressed. In YogAlign, we have found that naturally-aligned posture helps heal the emotions and quiet a busy mind.

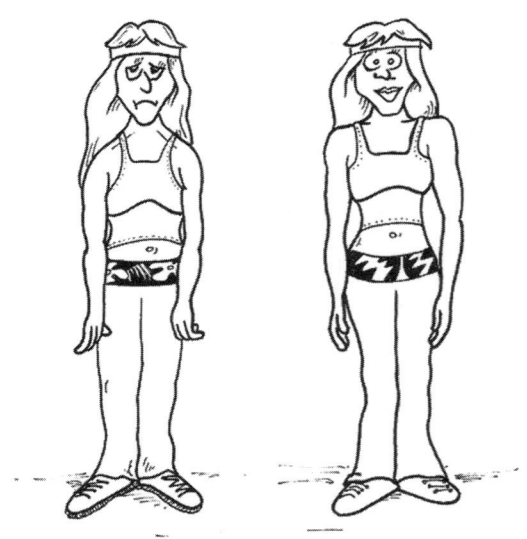

Whatever the situation, once you have chronic poor posture or emotional depression, you can start on a stress cycle that is hard to stop. Both depression and bad posture lead to fight-or-flight feelings of danger, shallow breathing, tense muscles, stress-related diseases such as digestion problems, chronic fatigue, and even more serious conditions like heart disease and arthritis. These health problems then cause more stress and create *more* fight-or-flight responses like high blood pressure, a faster pulse, and increased adrenalin, all leading back again to bad posture and depression. Breaking the cycle can feel impossible. On the other hand, with YogAlign change can happen very quickly as it did for Ross, a mountain climber and forest ranger, after only four days of doing YogAlign, (**Fig 5.4**).

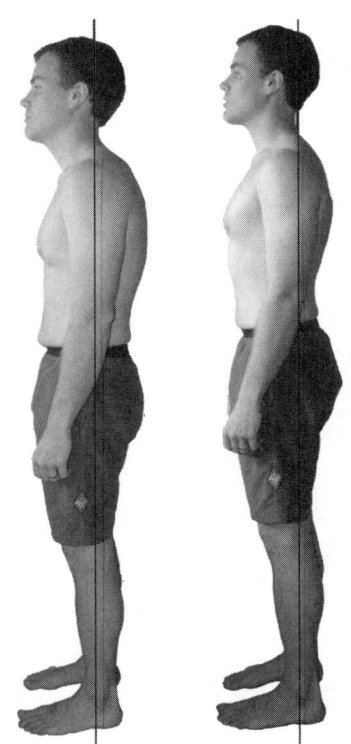

Fig. 5.4

We actually *can* break this cycle, by setting up beneficial nervous system patterning. In YogAlign we do this by practicing functional, natural spine alignment and conscious, relaxed deep-breathing. The nervous system responds to these practices by releasing tight muscles in the belly and pelvic floor providing relaxation and blood flow that facilitate beneficial encoding. This simple, natural approach is what makes YogAlign such a beneficial and powerful self-help tool.

EXPERIENTIAL EXERCISE #12

Posture Affects Nervous System Responses

Stand with a deliberate slouch in your body and exhale deeply. Just let the exhaling muscles contract strongly and notice what happens to your body. The contraction of the exhale will pull you forward, and compress your spine. Notice how this body position lends itself toward frowning and maybe even feeling a sense of agitation or tenseness. Try to smile and you may notice that it is difficult to smile or feel positive when your posture is poor.

Next, stand with your feet hip distance apart and pressed to the earth. Keep a slight bend in your knees and make sure they are not locked back in hyper-extension. Inhale with a deep Core SIP Breath feeling how the deep movements of breath create length and extension in your body. Keep the spinal extension that makes your waist and neck lengthen. Exhale softly out of the nose, and feel your belly contract while retaining the lift in your center. Relax and breathe through your nose and notice that by standing well, you feel a sense of relaxation. Try smiling and then frowning. Is it easier to smile and difficult (or almost impossible) to frown? A sense of ease in posture creates neuromuscular responses in the brain that help to elicit the relaxation response. Next time you feel a bit "blue" remember this exercise.

SELF-MASSAGE ENGAGES THE RELAXATION RESPONSE

Self-massage is a panacea for self-healing and longevity. It is surprising how few people massage themselves on a regular, daily basis. Massage is beneficial because it provides blood and lymph flow to areas of the body that are strained and oxygen-deprived. It is important to use self-massage on a daily basis to stimulate nerve centers in the skin, encourage the flow of *prana*, or *chi*, and also to increase our proprioceptive senses. Massage sends a signal throughout the nervous system that encourages the body to relax, helping to release endorphins. Massaging one area of the body affects the whole, so even just doing the hands or feet can profoundly affect the entire body through the fascia web and neural connections. In YogAlign, we try to massage the whole body, and we have devised innovative ways to do this massage while engaging the body in functional, comfortable yoga positions.

EXPERIENTIAL EXERCISE #13

Self-Massage

Standing with your feet hip-distance apart and keeping the knees soft, take a deep core SIP Breath. Keep the elongation and inner support that arises from the movement of the inhalation process (the gift of the lift). It is very important when doing any of these exercises that you pay attention to the body in its entirety. Stay aware of how you stand and support yourself. Notice if you lock your knees or jut your head forward and use the breathing process to align from your inner core.

Take your right hand and begin to massage your left hand with purpose and feeling. Press deeply on each fingernail and then roll each joint of every finger. Use your thumb to massage open your palm, sensing your entire body as you do it. Now let your arms hang down to your side and notice how differently not just your hand feels, but how your entire arm area, all the way to your shoulder, feels different as well. You may have a feeling of more space in the left shoulder compared to the right. Take your awareness to your hip and pelvic floor on the same side and you may notice that there is a sense of release and relaxation in those areas as well.

POOR MOVEMENT IS MORE THAN MUSCLE DEEP

Physio-emotional aspects of posture can hold a person in a state of tension. This may come from an acute trauma, or simply from a disposition that tends to hang on to mental anguish or suffering. Whether we have a physical accident or a broken heart, our muscles tense and our body goes into self-protective fight-or-flight, and can remain there long after the initial trauma has passed. Trauma and stress can cause a neural overload that shuts down the proprioceptive sense, and limits awareness of motor functions. This sensory "motor amnesia" causes loss of sensation in afflicted parts of the body, inhibiting movement, and leading to chronic pain. Frequently, an involuntary stretch reflex is activated, holding muscles in chronic contraction; this unconscious tightening makes muscles sore, depriving them of much-needed oxygen and cell nutrients. A lack of fluidity affects coordination and balance, and causes an overall energy drain. Habitual muscle contractions also cause postural problems, leading to poor weight distribution, herniated discs, back pain, migraines, vertigo, chronic fatigue, and arthritis.

This chronic congestion of energy and the tightness or numbness of muscles is called a "trauma reflex." When we have ongoing stress or a sudden accident, the trauma reflex emerges from the primitive part of the brain, and takes over our motor reflexes. The reflex manifests itself in a variety of bodily maladies, such as a back spasm that won't go away, jaw tightening, or neck tension. Muscle groups imbalanced from trauma reflexes do not permit joints to move well, and the over-contraction of tense muscles leads to thickened layers of fascia. We may find ourselves with pain that echoes an injury (or an insult) that happened years before.

This trauma reflex pattern remains deep in the nervous system, creating a semi-permanent fight-or-flight mode. Rest and drugs are the common prescription for relief from this "dis-ease." Some will try chiropractic, massage, acupuncture or other physical therapy techniques, but find that these methods provide only temporary relief, and a return to these practitioners is necessary in order to be "fixed" again.

Many of us are driving ourselves hard to *do* more, *make* more and *be* more; always pushing hard on the gas pedal, trying to drive to success. The nervous system gets stuck on "go," and although we may crave rest and relaxation, we are stuck in high gear with one foot on the gas and the other foot on the brake. Thomas Hanna in his book on somatics describes a condition he calls the "Green Light Reflex," a syndrome in which many of us are caught.

> **"**In our society, most people begin to "get old" early in life. Our technology lets us live a long life, but it also condemns us to live out those years in discomfort and fatigue. An industrial society is fueled by the energy of the Green Light reflex which is triggered incessantly. This relentless repetition guarantees that the muscular contraction of the reflex will be constant and habitual. The action response is so steady that, eventually, we cease to notice it. It becomes automatic, fading into oblivion. This is sensory–motor amnesia. All we feel is fatigue, soreness, and pain – in the back of our heads, in our necks, our shoulders, upper back, lower back, and buttocks.**"**

Hanna, *Somatics:
Reawakening the Mind's Control of Movement, Flexibility, and Health.*

All of our daily thoughts, habits, and experiences can then lead to a collusion of forces, causing us to experience sudden, sharp pain, seemingly out of nowhere.

How many times have you heard someone say, "I just bent over and suddenly, without warning, my back went out!"? In truth, the instability was preexisting. Chronic back problems result from the cumulative effects of trauma memories and/or poor posture and breathing habits. In this stressed state, chronic pain and injuries can occur simply from doing activities necessary for daily living. Unless a functional way of moving is encoded that releases the trauma patterns and allows one to move with less effort and force, a cycle of pain and stress reflexes will invade the entire body and mind, affecting quality of life. Many people are caught in a lifelong physio-emotional cycle of stress, tension, and pain. YogAlign provides individuals with powerful and pain-free ways to break the cycle, allowing them to become fit and functional. For back health, daily alignment and elongation exercises are better than money in the bank. When spinal muscles are toned but relaxed, they create more space between the vertebrae. Discs then decompress and can soak up fluid that nourishes, supports, and cushions the entire spine, protecting the fragile spinal nerve system.

Because of the tendency for our "issues" to wind up in our "tissues," we use a combination of techniques that support natural alignment using the emotional, physical, and spiritual elements of our entire being. It is very important when practicing YogAlign that one focuses on the fluid nature of our being, and the transitory nature of life itself. One must be willing, as well, to let go of old limiting beliefs and ideas that prohibit transformation. We can literally shape ourselves a new body by directing neuromuscular currents in the brain to recalibrate muscle tension, allowing ease in the body. This ease can bring us more fluid connective tissue, better circulation, and improved organ function, nerve strength, and joint health.

INTERNAL GUIDED IMAGERY

When we use proprioception to sense our body, we often think of the body metaphorically. Using self-guided imagery from the mind, we can help bring about changes in the physical. Called "Ideokinesis", this technique was incorporated into bodywork by Mabel Todd in the 1930s as a method for improving strength, flexibility, and balance.

One of the most important ways to use Ideokinesis is to practice sensing what might be called "the vibrational force of our being." All of our cells are vibrating with life force, and all life forms on the planet vibrate with this same energy. The yogis call the force *prana*, the Hawaiians *mana*, and the Chinese call it *chi*. No matter what you call it, this force is what we feel when we sense our being and our inner self.

EXPERIENTIAL EXERCISE #14

Feel Your Life Force

(Adapted from Erich Schiffman, yoga master and author of *Yoga, Moving Into Stillness*)

From a standing position with your feet hip-distance apart, spread the fingers on one hand as widely as possible. Bend your elbow and raise up your hand, gazing at your palm retaining the spread in your fingers. Close your eyes and visualize a sun radiating its energy in the palm of your hand. Visualize each finger as a ray of light and make the sun powerful, sending its energy from the center out to each finger tip. Now sense your hand in its entirety without thinking. Just feel the energy that is your hand. You now are not actually feeling the "hand;" instead, you are feeling the energy of the vibrational elements that make up your hand. The word "hand" becomes a concept, and feeling the energy that makes up your hand connects you to the vibration of our cells and of our life force.

Now visualize the sun in the center of your body. Stand and press your feet into the floor as you feel your trunk elongating. Visualize your entire body radiating with light and vibrations from the center. Practice sensing the flow of mana, or prana, in your body every day, whenever you can.

The quality of the food we eat, the amount of sleep we get, our relationships with others, and of course our posture and activities all affect how much life force is available to us on a daily basis. By focusing on increasing your life force, you will be helping to increase life force vibration in every cell of your body. By regularly focusing on the flow of life force in your being, you can start to imagine energy flowing to areas of the body in need. Not all functional problems that burden the body and encourage muscle compensation result from the physical. Some come from stress, or trauma, or even something as simple as breathing poorly. Whether from the physical or emotional realm, all of the issues in the tissues come from using the wrong muscles for the wrong jobs, wasting precious energy, and ingraining muscular patterning that is not efficient.

EXPERIENTIAL EXERCISE #15

Crimping the Hose

From a standing position, take a moment to massage your rib cage and diaphragm area, especially the muscles and cartilage between the ribs. After you massage there, begin to breathe in using the Core SIP Breath, noticing how your trunk lengthens with extension. Each time you breathe in, feel how your spine naturally elongates helping you to come into good standing alignment.

As you exhale, practice keeping this extension and lift. Notice how you can feel your invisible center holding and supporting you with very little effort.

As you continue in the exercise, hold this alignment pattern and be sure not to lock your knees, or pull your head or jaw forward. By using conscious awareness to stand well as you do the breathing exercise, your brain will start to memorize these codes for natural alignment and perfect body tuning.

Inhale, using the Core SIP Breath. Hold the breath for a moment. Increase the muscle action that occurs in the inhalation process for a few seconds and notice how inhalation creates extension in our body, increasing length in our trunks and spine. On the next exhale, keep the length of the waist and notice that the belly can pull in without losing the length created in the inhalation process. This is an eccentric contraction of the muscles of exhalation.

Do the SIP Breath again, holding for a moment and tightening. Now, exhale out of the mouth with an SSS sound through your teeth for a few seconds. Stop exhaling the air but hold the actions of the exhalation for a moment longer, accentuating the contraction of the exhalation muscles.

Still holding the contraction of your exhalation muscles, begin to breathe in again with the SIP breath. This will create a muscular resistance exercise between the forces that engage to inhale and the forces that engage to exhale.

Keep sipping without letting go of the actions of inhalation, and then release the contractions of the exhaling muscles all at once. You may feel your ribs pop open and experience a deep expansion of your chest and ribs. Try it a few times, as it may be difficult at first to keep the movements of inhalation happening when you are holding the forces of exhalation. A visualization that helps with this is to imagine that you are crimping a hose with your hand when you hold the muscular force of the exhale. When you begin to do the SIP inhale, imagine your breath as water trying to come through a crimped hose. The breathing muscles of inhalation get stronger as they try to contract against the resistance created by holding the muscles of exhalation. Let go of your belly and your exhalation muscles while you continue to use the Core SIP Breath technique. When you release the "crimp" in your breathing line, air rushes in and you will feel the expansiveness of inhalation that occurs when there is no excess holding or tension in the abdomen.

Many of us are imbalanced in the actions of our breathing muscles, and have muscular tension patterns that restrict the movements of inhalation. By using this PNF technique and accentuating the tightening of the exhalation muscles, you increase the performance of the inhaling muscles and the resting length of the exhaling muscles.

After your next Core SIP inhale, keep the lift and exhale deeply. Now tighten your pelvic floor muscles (as though trying not to pee).

Begin the Core SIP inhalation, holding the pelvic floor tightly for a moment. Keep trying to inhale at the same time, then release the contraction of the muscles in the pelvic floor area, which allows you to finish the inhalation. Sense how the relaxation of the muscles of the pelvic floor allows you to extend the inhalation beyond what was possible when your muscles were tightened. By engaging the inhale with the resistance from the muscles of exhalation, one can gain a deeper kinesthetic awareness of the connections between the rib and belly muscles and the pelvic floor.

Develop your proprioceptive sense by feeling these fascial and body/mind connections. You can now feel how a chronic tightening of the belly also causes the same tightening in the pelvic floor area. This unnecessary tension can greatly inhibit your movements, breathing, and bodily functions. After doing several sets of this exercise, notice how light you feel in your body. Walk around and imagine that your entire rib cage area is a helium balloon that effortlessly lifts you. Allow the weight of your head to be balanced on top of your spinal column, and imagine that your head almost floats. Imagine that you are so light now that you have to reach your feet towards the floor to keep from floating away. Feel how this lifted feeling frees your hips to swing naturally and lets your knees float below you and track without tension.

Notice how strong extension in the deep internal movements of breath releases congestion or compression in the hip socket, knees and feet.

Good posture happens when you have powerful breathing muscles. Deep breathing can help you rid yourself of chronic aches and pains in your body. It's like putting money in the healthy equity account everyday. This is your most important "bank account" of all.

By becoming aware and bringing your individual consciousness into your healing, you can also retrain your proprioceptive patterns and recode the brain to tell the body to move differently and with less effort.

In YogAlign, we call this concept "becoming sustainable and green in your own body." Obtaining and sustaining natural alignment will revitalize your overall health and longevity.

Remember This: When you practice PNF or "tightening the tightness," you can get flexible and strong quickly and painlessly. There will be no strain or pain in your joints, ligaments, or muscles.

The immediate benefits of using PNF active muscle contractions are the development of a strong flexible core, a graceful posture, and a pain-free body. Each session leaves you toned, energized, and relaxed, as if you just had a massage and a workout at the same time! Below are some important points to remember when practicing the YogAlign techniques.

YogAlign Neuromuscular Repatterning:

* Develops sensory awareness of the body

* Uses conscious breathing to go to the "Mother Board" of your body's computer

* Uses PNF exercises to reset resting muscle length for easy flexibility and muscle tone

* Practices positive imagery to pattern positive ideas about the body

* Maintains natural alignment by facilitating efficient breathing during exercise

Our posture affects every level of our being. By using tools like PNF, you can change your posture at the neuromuscular level to achieve natural alignment, becoming your own best healer and body worker. In the next chapter we will explore in-depth how to align your spine.

YogAlignMent Principle #8
Achieve sustainability in your own body by using PNF to calibrate your system, eradicating unnecessary effort in all of your postures and movements.

YogAlignMent Principle #9
Use imagery to align yourself with the fluid nature of your being, and to envision the posture that you want to have.

CHAPTER 6: ALIGN YOUR SPINE

ॐ **Bad Posture Is Everywhere**

ॐ **Spine Alignment Determines Our Overall Health**

ॐ **Alignment Based on the Body as a Tensegrity Model**

ॐ **Poor Alignment Is Exhausting**

ॐ **What Does Yogalign Natural Alignment Feel Like?**

ॐ **What Is Good Posture and How Do We Attain It?**

ॐ **Your Spine Is Not Supposed to Be Straight**

ॐ **We Aren't Designed for Chair Sitting**

ॐ **Become Aligned in Daily Life**

ॐ **The Body Is Designed to Move**

It is not what you do for exercise that is most important, but rather how you are aligned when you do it.

> **"**When a standing body is well aligned, gravity's vector travels through its central core.... Healthy posture is characterized by an easy grace, with movement flowing effortlessly between limbs and trunk. The movement of someone with unhealthy posture looks disconnected and labored.**"**
>
> – Bond, *The New Rules of Posture*

Being aligned with good posture is an essential element of a healthy life, and a key to longevity. Without proper alignment, our breath and movements are restricted, and our lives are infiltrated by pain, illness and limitation.

Bad Posture Is Everywhere

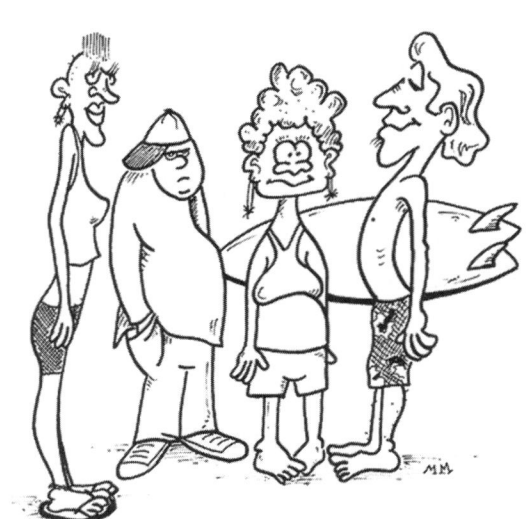

In the Western World, poor posture is a fact of life. People with rounded shoulders, hunched upper backs, and forward head carriage are everywhere. Young children sit poorly and spend more hours per day in a chair than any previous generation, and there is now evidence of arthritic spinal problems in some teens, with many more suffering from chronic back pain. Bad posture has become epidemic, and will cost us millions of dollars in treatment in the coming years.

We are fast becoming a nation that suffers from chronic back pain, and much of this pain is due to the excessive amount of time we spend sitting in chairs. Galen Cranz, in her book *The Chair*, addresses the root of back-pain troubles by saying that "the chair itself" is the problem. Upright, right-angled chair-sitting is bad for the body because it puts backward and downward force on the pelvis and sacrum. Because this causes us discomfort, we then slump or slouch into the backrest of the chair, weakening core muscles and spinal stability, and perpetuating pain. Poor and dysfunctional postural patterns resulting from this chair-sitting are so common that mannequins in the teen section of many department stores are made to look like "normal" teens, reflecting slouching, rounded shoulders, hyper-extended knees and a forward head position.

There has been much discussion about claims that students suffer from back pain because they carry about heavy books in backpacks. In truth, if these students had good alignment to begin with, and had ergonomic desks that encouraged strong back and postural muscles, the effects of the book weight on their backs would be minor. Alignment dysfunction and spinal weakness from prolonged sitting are both major contributing factors in student back pain; carrying a backpack is not the *cause* but rather the *symptom* of larger postural and pain issues. After all, humans have carried heavy loads for centuries and have not suffered from back pain and arthritis in the epidemic proportions that are common among our youth now.

Some schools in the U.S. have appropriated funds to provide two sets of schoolbooks to students—one set for school and one for home—in an effort to eliminate the need for students to carry heavy books at all. It would be far better if funds could be spent purchasing ergonomic chairs for the classroom that would engage postural muscles, foster natural spine alignment, and support better breathing habits. Schooling methods that allow children to move more and sit less would also help posture and strength, as well as mitigate serious health issues like obesity and attention deficit disorders. The human body is designed to move, and movement and posture should be core considerations in any educational approach. Yet sometimes it appears as if we're educating our children's minds at the horrible expense of wrecking their spines.

Because the body is a continuum, every movement we make reverberates throughout the entire body. Poor posture leads to weak breathing habits, which cause spinal compression, which in turn leads to chronic pain, accelerating aging in the body. According to health statistics like those outlined below, alignment and dysfunctional posture are directly responsible for the majority of chronic aches and pains in the body.

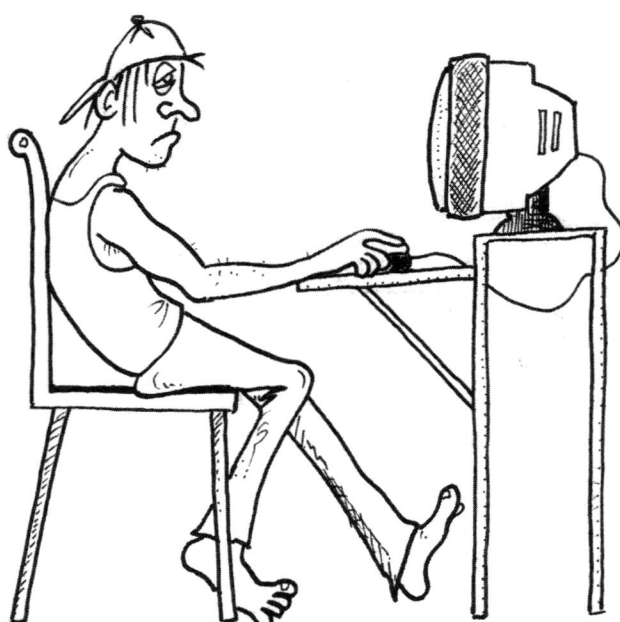

According to NIH: National Institute of Arthritis and Musculoskeletal and Skin Diseases, 8 out of 10 Americans will suffer from back pain at some point in their lives. Poor posture is a major factor in the epidemic of back pain, which-- after upper respiratory infections--is one of the most common reasons for seeking medical attention in the U.S. Poor posture creates not just back pain but also the following chronic conditions:

- Cervical kyphosis (straightening of the neck)

- Tension headaches—often misdiagnosed as migraine headaches

- Constant neck/shoulder strain

- Rounded shoulders

- Bicep/rotator cuff syndrome

- Degeneration of cervical (neck) and lumbar (low back) discs, usually caused by trauma or multiple micro-traumas

- Weak and stiff muscles

- Decreased range of motion (fascia thickening)

- Low back and neck pain

> **"***Despite a growing array of sophisticated drugs, diagnostics, physical therapies, and surgical techniques, the millions of Americans battling back pain may not be any closer to getting that quick relief than they were 20 years ago. Several recent studies indicate that even with the latest in high-tech medical intervention, effective treatments for back problems remain elusive.***"**
>
> *Newsweek Magazine*, Karen Springen, February 12, 2008

Postural-related pain is seriously affecting our health, and is one of the drivers of soaring health care costs. We shake our heads and blame government and health insurance companies for skyrocketing health care costs, but in truth large amounts of money are spent treating illnesses that are in the power of individuals to prevent. Most of what is "wrong" with us can be prevented if we take responsibility for our health through diet, exercise, and spinal care. The Western lifestyle does not promote good posture or encourage spinal health, and the consequence of these poor postural and breathing habits is increased health problems, which incur costs for medical insurance and treatment. Many healthcare professionals emphasize the importance of a good diet and exercise for overall health, but they rarely consider, much less know, how profoundly posture and breathing affect the body. In fact, exercise performed without good posture and spinal alignment could actually do more harm than good. By educating our children in good posture and breathing habits, we could make real headway in reducing back pain and other problems associated with alignment issues.

Focusing a child on wellness from childhood to adulthood encourages them to create their own preventative health care. People spend hours a day—sitting in chairs—planning financial moves and investments that will raise the equity levels in their bank accounts. In YogAlign, we practice paying into our daily health equity account by eliminating pain and tension, practicing good spinal alignment, and acquiring natural flexibility. Health equity dividends are priceless in their value because in the end, health is our most important asset.

Spine Alignment Determines Our Overall Health

Since spine alignment is a major determinant of our overall health and our quality of life, we need to support, engage, and encode habits that align the spine. This is why YogAlign emphasizes the tenet that all yoga poses need to simulate good posture and functional, real-life movement. Good health can be regained painlessly and quickly by addressing posture and breathing habits, in order to attain natural alignment during yoga, fitness, and life's daily movements.

When postural alignment is poor, evidence shows that over time joint problems such as arthritis or disc degeneration—as well as a host of other afflictions—can develop. Postural imbalance can also cause disorders such as bladder incontinence, which is a direct result of pelvic floor weakness and/ or tightness. Weakened breathing habits lead to sagging organs that compromise organ function, and spinal compression—whether induced by aging, bad posture, or chair-sitting—negatively affects the entire nervous system, as well as major organs.

Because fascial lines and ligaments are the wires that connect our inner structure to our outer structure, imbalance in these lines due to poor posture and tightened or weakened muscles can lead to crowding and displacement of the internal organs. Eric Franklin, creator of the *Franklin Method* of body awareness, teaches people how to use mental imagery to improve posture and alignment. In his book *Pelvic Power*, Franklin writes, *"In following down the line along the umbilical ligament to the bladder, I am amused by the thought that in the end the bladder hangs from the neck. For the bladder, this connection has value only if the body's posture is good."*

As Franklin points out, the body and the organs are not blocks stacked one upon another, but are rather suspended in space by balanced, tensile forces. Ligaments connect the pelvic floor and bladder to the navel, which connects to the liver. From the two lobes of the liver, ligaments connect to the diaphragm, which in turn is hung from the heart. The heart itself is suspended from the neck or cervical spine by ligaments. In this way, the inner organs of the body are strung together by ligaments that, as in Franklin's example, connect your bladder to your neck.

This connection is experienced by us in a number of ways. For instance, tight back muscles can inhibit healthy functioning of our kidneys, since these two filtering organs are literally held in place by the back muscles. The tone and tension of the diaphragm is connected fascially to the arches of the feet and the pelvic floor muscles. The tongue and the roof of the mouth are also in fascial communication with the diaphragm, and share the same tensile integrity. Because of this interconnectedness with the rest of the body, a weak diaphragm can affect everything from your internal organs, to your breathing process, to your extremities. Your alignment and breathing, which is dictated by diaphragm fitness, continually affects not only functional movements, but organ health and placement as well. It just makes sense to do exercises and yoga poses that support optimal movements of your diaphragm, since this organ affects your body in its entirety.

Fascia of the deep core line connects together the major organs of your inner body to your outer body (**Fig. 6.1**).

ALIGNMENT BASED ON THE BODY AS A TENSEGRITY MODEL

So what do we really know about alignment? There is rife misunderstanding of the nature of body alignment, and there are many conflicting methods, rules, and theories about how to attain it. In YogAlign, we view posture as the sum of the forces of dynamic tension (that control how we move), added to the somatic education of the nervous system (which is comprised of the neural patterns that direct movement). For example, when a person is naturally aligned, there is a feeling of fluidity and ease in movements. This is due to the balance of compressive and tensile forces in the body. According to Thomas Myers, a *Rolfer* and the developer of the *Anatomy Trains* system, natural alignment is not based on the Western model in which we are held up by bones that are stacked on top of each other like blocks. Instead, his approach is that alignment in the human body is based upon lines of pull, which are created by the fascia system as it connects and mitigates movement throughout the entire body. This approach is based on a movement continuum, in which all parts affect the whole.

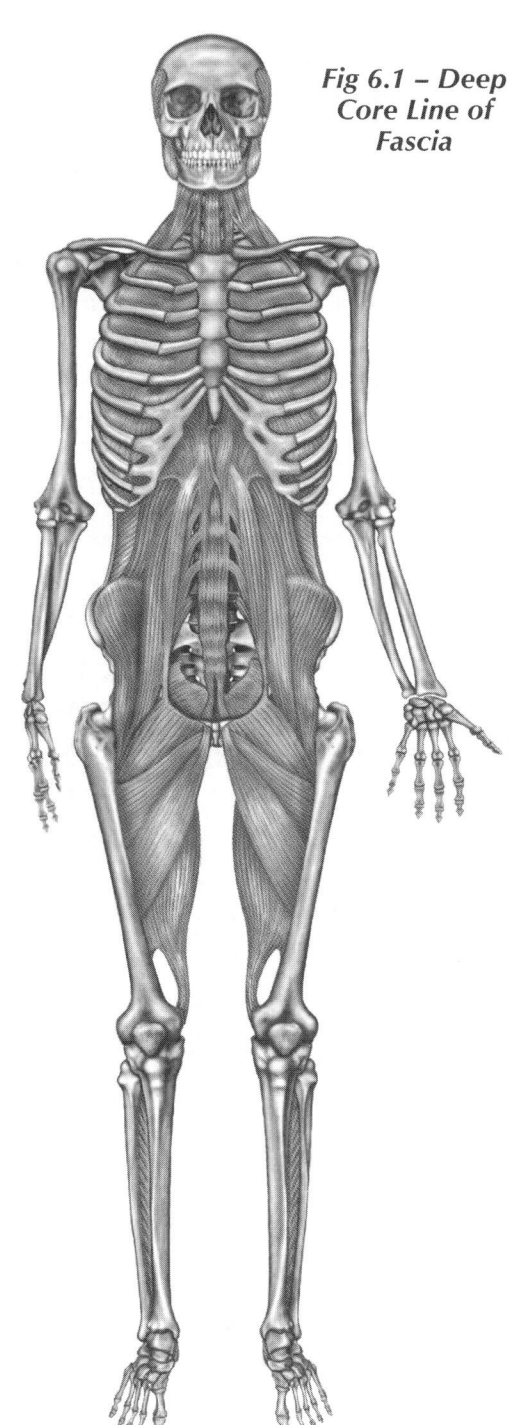

Fig 6.1 – Deep Core Line of Fascia

Redrawn from *Anatomy Trains* by Thomas Myers

According to Myers,

"Our commonly held and widely taught impression is that the skeleton is a continuous compression structure, like the brick wall. . . In this traditional mechanical model, forces are localized. If a tree falls on one corner of your average rectangular building, that corner will collapse, perhaps without damaging the rest of the structure. Most modern manipulative therapy works out from this idea: if a part is injured, it is because localized forces have overcome local tissues, and local relief and repair are necessary. . . A tensegrity model of the body paints an altogether different picture – forces are distributed, rather than localized. . . The compression members push outwards against the tension members that pull inwards. As long as the two sets of forces are balanced, the structure is stable."

The YogAlign Method uses the imagery of the tensegrity model (which was discussed at length in Chapter 2) in techniques that tune-up your posture with breathing and proper body position, allowing you to become your own body alignment specialist. Gradually, as you practice YogAlign, you attain the innate muscle memory that allows you to stay in natural alignment without thinking about it—moving gracefully and easily from the core center of your body—with a toned, flexible spine and strong, stabilized joint functions.

POOR ALIGNMENT IS EXHAUSTING

Almost everyone feels poorly after sitting in a chair for too long. This is because it's more tiring for our muscles to hold our body in a static sitting position than it is for it to engage and release muscles when moving. The poor body positions most people hold while sitting in a right-angled chair cause breathing to become labored and dysfunctional. This is because chair sitting creates a posture that reverses the spine's natural curves, causing the

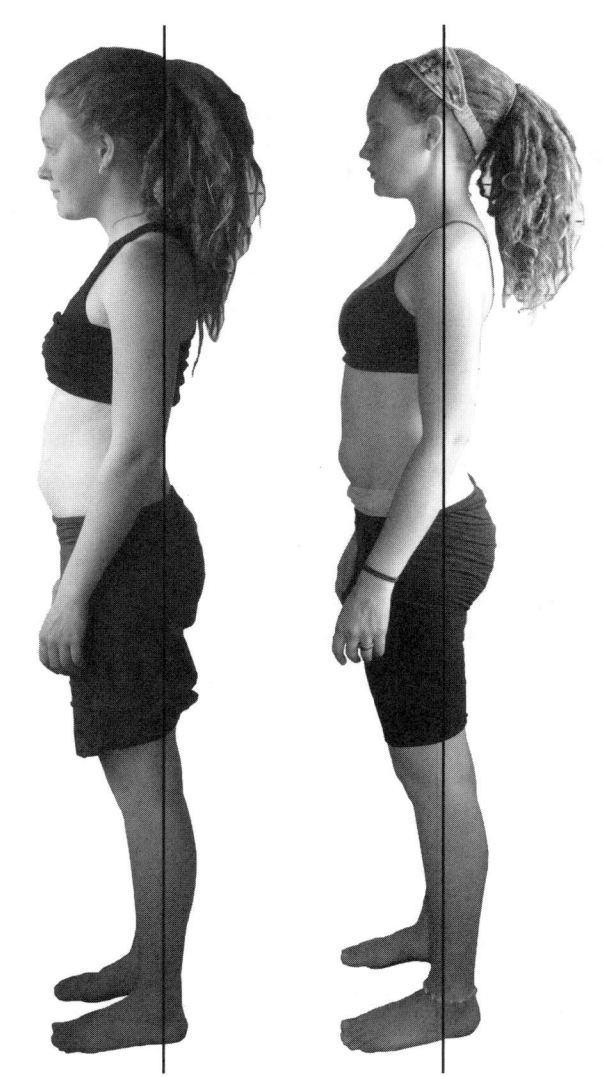

Fig. 6.2 – Athlete, counselor, and now YogAlign Instructor Cree, shown before and after 6 weeks of practicing YogAlign.

anterior spine to compress the discs and vertebrae. The head is then pushed too far forward, and the breastbone is dropped, causing the rib cage and diaphragm to be compressed and unable to move freely in the breathing process. And in many cases, sitting in chairs exacerbates—or originates—these postural problems.

The ligaments of the sacrum can become overstretched with excessive chair sitting. This leads to a condition I call the "S.S.S.", or the "Sagging Sacrum Syndrome." Normally, the sacrum should have a 30–degree angle to it and should never look flat or straight. When the ligaments connecting the sacrum to the hips become stretched out, the sacrum loses its naturally-tilted position and no longer provides shock absorption to the hips and knees. A loose and sagging sacrum is a health time bomb, and will lead to compression of the hip and knee joints during such mundane activities as walking and sitting. As a result, these overstretched ligaments can lead to arthritis, premature aging, and the oh-so-common hip and knee replacements.

Establishing natural spine alignment and sacral integrity is vital to becoming balanced and pain-free throughout your body. This alignment and integrity can be compromised by sitting or exercising—including doing yoga—with poor spinal alignment. Many people prematurely age their spines, hips, and sacrum by excessive sitting, or by doing exercises that keep the sacrum and lumbar spine flattened or reversed.

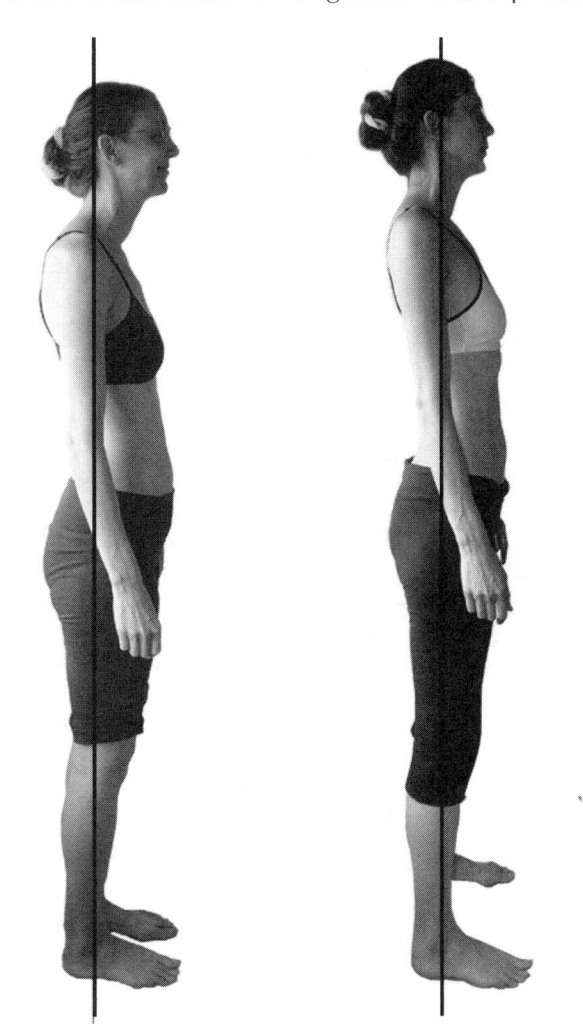

Fig. 6.3 – After only 4 days of YogAlign, Marjanne was able to stand taller with less effort.

In the latter case, these individuals are doing their bodies more harm than good, trying to stretch or move in positions that violate the natural form and function of the body. Using the fascia models put forth by Myers, YogAlign visualizes the body as a force rather than a structure, and emphasizes proper and natural posture and spine alignment in all of its poses.

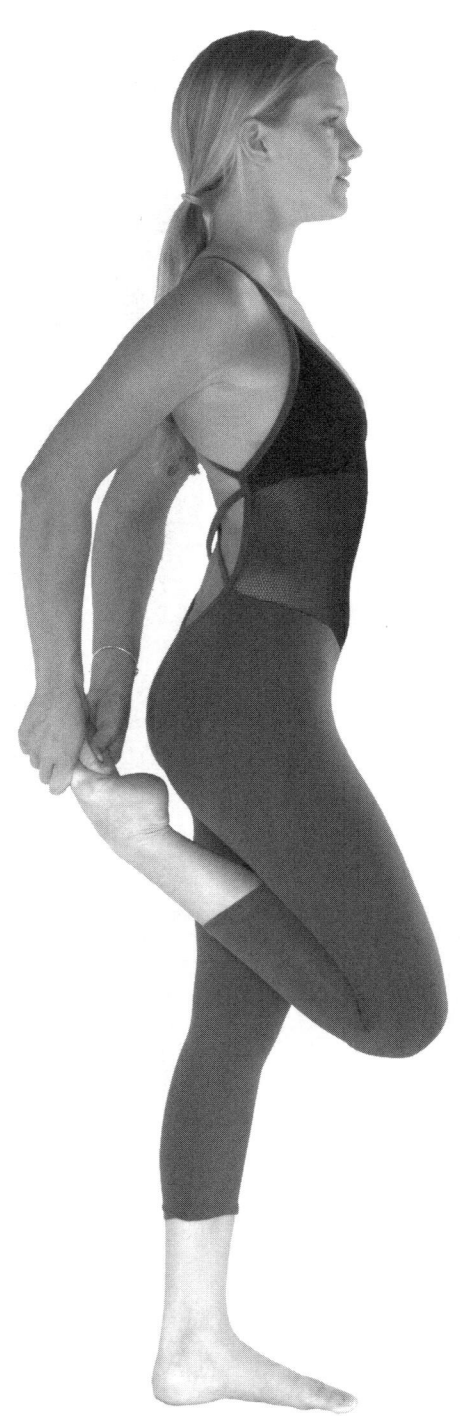

Fig. 6.4 Rayna does the YogAlign standing foot massage pose building strength, flexibility, balance, and massage; all in one maneuver.

What Does YogAlign Natural Alignment Feel Like?

Rather than thinking about stacking the body one part over the other in order to achieve good posture, YogAlign aligns us from the center, using the most core movement of all: the breathing process. By focusing on the muscle and fascia engagements that occur when we breathe, we gain the inner and outer support that arises from activating our inner core center. We use the inhale to extend the spine, engage core muscles, and align the body without peripheral control. This means one no longer has to lift up their shoulders, hold their belly, or use a lot of effort in the extremities to feel stable in their structure. There is a sense of economized movement, and a feeling of alignment that happens without effort. This is the way we felt as a child, and is the essence of the kid body.

Our body is like our car: when our car has front-end alignment problems, the tires and suspension system wear out. It is the same with the human body. Bad posture is responsible for a majority of chronic pain issues. It is essential to learn to tune your body's alignment by disposing of patterns and tensions that negatively affect your posture. The aligned spine you will achieve with the YogAlign method makes you feel like you're floating, as if the body has disappeared. We feel more life force when we are in alignment than when we are not, and the hips float and swing thanks to the empowered extension of the spine and the freed ribs and breathing process. We feel the movement of our legs beginning in the center of the body, where our psoas connect to our diaphragm. We feel our knees hinge easily, and our feet feel like springs that support us as we move from a place of no effort. Activities like hiking or running feel effortless when we are aligned, and all movement is balanced from the center.

Attainment of this natural alignment happens when you become sustainable within your own body. Sustainability means that you can live your life with relative ease in your body, freeing up your energy for activities that bring you joy. It also gives you the tools to fix aches and pains that may occur rather than always having to rely on someone else to fix what is "wrong" with you. There is no excess effort; the body moves with ease and simplicity. No huge amounts of stretching and toning are required, because there is no tension that needs to be stretched. Toning is achieved with each deep, unrestricted breath that massages and opens the inner body. One begins to become less a consumer of complex poses and more a radiant soul, reflecting out through a kid-like body.

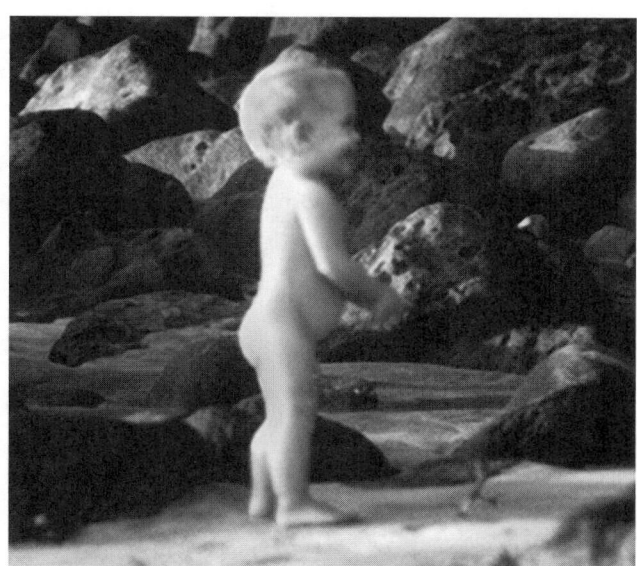

The kid body is joyous, seamless, and connected from the center.

❝*Tensions are our guests; we have invited them. Relaxation is our nature, we don't have to invite it. You don't have to relax; you have to just stop inviting tensions, and relaxation will start on its own accord. In your very being, in every fiber, in every cell of your being there will be relaxation. This relaxation is the beginning of meditation.*❞

Osho

WHAT IS GOOD POSTURE AND HOW DO WE ATTAIN IT?

If we learn to use our body consciously and economically, the weight of our body can be carried by a balance between the dynamic tensile forces of our muscles, bones, and fascia. Ideally, our head should be balanced on the top of our spinal column. Unfortunately, too many people walk around with muscle/fascia patterning that pulls the head forward of the rest of the spine, making natural alignment via tensile force impossible.

To correct posture, people often try to lift from the upper shoulder, neck or lower back, or pull in their navel to stay aligned during the day. Pulling in our belly or forcefully pulling back our shoulders are just band-aids, and don't address the underlying problem. Neither of these temporary solutions will produce a feeling of effortless movement or real freedom in our body. Instead, these movements waste valuable energy. Working on flexibility from positions that mimic bad posture or that encourage a compressed spine with no natural curves, is the opposite of how we ought to retrain our body into natural alignment.

YogAlign has special exercises that engage specific and conscious muscular actions to encourage natural spine alignment. When practiced with conscious breathing, these movements and poses help develop new alignment patterns from the inside out. You can use the breathing process to align your spine and overall posture, enlisting very little effort from the outside of the body. This is the way we are *supposed* to be supported, and in YogAlign, this is the way to achieve the "kid body," as the kid body is aligned, does not hurt, and always moves from the core.

> **"***People who never lose what they knew as babies are more apt to live comfortable, pain-free lives regardless of their age, culture, race, body type, or level of activity.***"**
>
> Porter, *Ageless Spine, Lasting Health*

YOUR SPINE IS NOT SUPPOSED TO BE STRAIGHT

Have you ever struggled in a yoga or exercise class after being told to flatten your back or to sit with a straight spine? Straightening the spine is actually anatomically impossible, and the effort to get into such positions can add copious amounts of tension to your body. Our spine is a flexible rod with natural curves, and is designed to act as a shock absorber as we move. There is no such thing as a straight spine, nor should there ever be an attempt to make one. More accurate terms for describing spinal positioning are "erect," "lifted," or "extended" rather than just the use of the word "straightened." When engaging and visualizing the spine, it is helpful to have words that convey spinal integrity and extension.

Seen in **Fig. 6.4**, there are four shock-absorbing curves in your spine: two *lordotic* (concave) curves and two *kyphotic* (convex) curves. Twenty-four vertebrae make up the vertebral column, and the sacrum and tailbone are each composed of fused vertebrae. There are seven vertebrae in the *cervical* (neck) curve, twelve in the *thoracic* (mid-back) curve, and five vertebrae plus the sacrum in the *lumbar* (lower-back) curve. The *coccyx* (tailbone) alone comprises the fourth curve. The neck and lower back spine including the sacrum have a lordotic curve or secondary curve. The mid back or

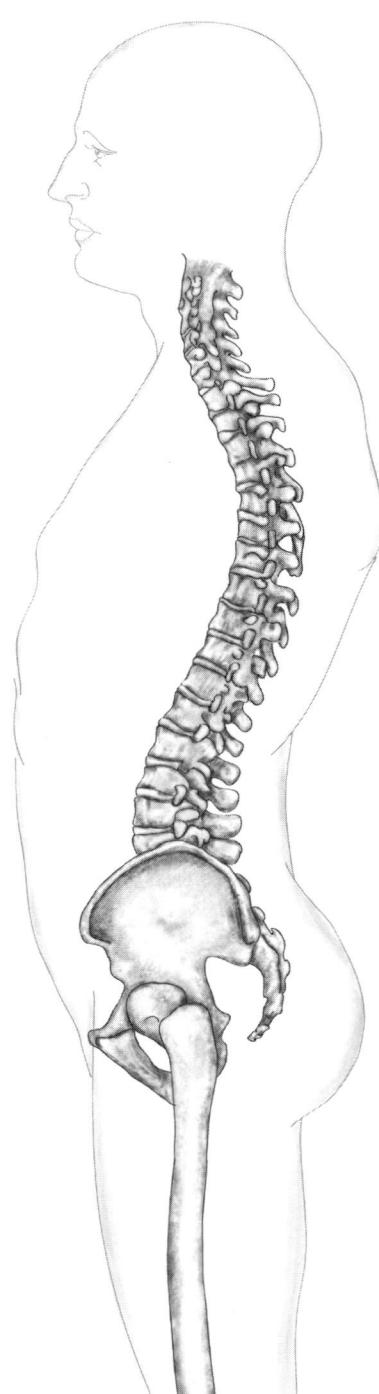

Fig. 6.4 – Natural spine alignment supports the four curves.

thoracic part of the spine and tailbone (coccyx) have a primary or kyphotic curve.

The sacrum is positioned between the hip bones, connecting the spine and the two sides of the hips. Sacral integrity is a major determinant of having a healthy and a pain-free body. When positioned optimally, the sacrum has a 30-degree angle that acts as a vaulted bridge at the base of the spine, providing important shock absorption. Proper tilt of the sacrum helps protect the skull, the vertebral column from neck to tailbone, the hips and the lower extremities from shock and compression. The front of the sacrum is considered the anatomical center of the body and is sometimes referred to as the "sacred bone."

Aging people and the "young and misaligned" often have a "flat"' sacrum, with loose and overstretched sacral ligaments and nerves resulting from sitting and exercising with the posterior pelvis flattened and pulled under. If the sacrum is flat, it is overstretched, and if the sacrum is sagging, the breastbone will do the same. In this case, the spine cannot extend properly and, over time, body weight will compress the hip socket and knee joints.

For these reasons, the sacrum should not be flattened or tucked under when practicing yoga poses or performing fitness exercises. Many people treat the sacrum and tailbone as one structure, and when attempting to draw the tailbone down they flatten the sacral curve. One of the most common causes of overstretching the sacrum occurs when folding into a forward bend with both legs straightened. YogAlign's directive is to *always* maintain the tilt and lift of the sacrum in all active positions.

Deep breathing facilitates a subtle internal descending movement of the tail bone, which allows the supportive lift and curve of the sacrum to remain active. On inhalation, there is also a descending of the tip of the breast bone at the xyphoid process. The sternal part of the breast bone lifts and spreads as the fascial connection from the xyphoid to the descending diaphragm keeps our ribs aligned with our hips and knees. In this way, we can pull our ribs back over our hips simply with the internal movements of deep breathing (as seen in **Fig. 6.5**), rather than by using belly muscles to hold in the rib cage.

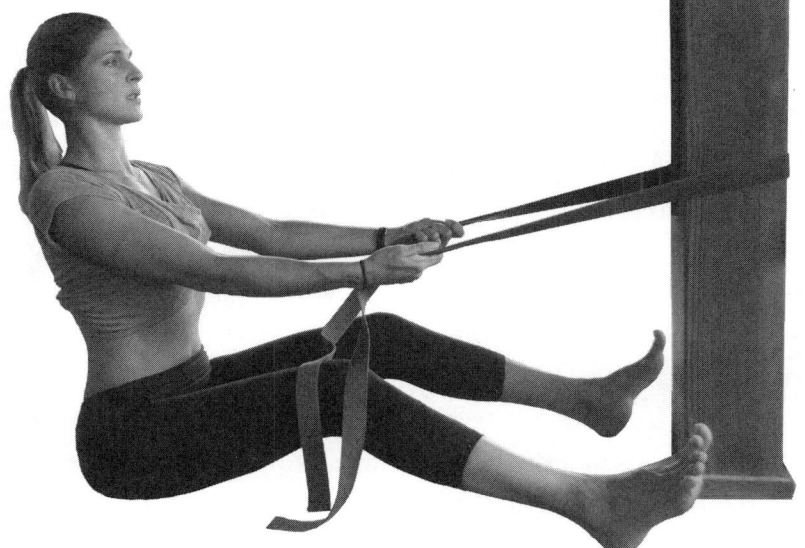

Fig. 6.5, Gabrielle "Gabby" Reese tuning her whole body with deep breathing while in the YogAlign "Spine Aligner" pose.

The health of our spine and our nervous system is also increased through the movements of deep breathing combined with functional body positioning that simulates ideal posture. The daily stress of a sedentary lifestyle weaken the forces of extension in our body, leading to poor postural habits that can cause arthritis, bone spurs and compression in the 24 vertebrae in our spinal column. Our spine contains all of the nerves that radiate from our brain out to our body, and the quality of our spinal health is crucial to our overall functioning and well-being. The vertebrae themselves are separated by discs which cushion the spine and provide shock absorption and space for proper functioning of the nerve tissues that exit from the spine. The discs themselves make up one-fourth of the length of the entire spine. Each disc is like a radial tire with a tough outer core composed of collagen fibers and a gel-like center that is not connected to the vascular system. Because there is no fluid supply, each disc must absorb fluid from the surrounding tissue in order to keep its shape. We are taller in the morning since the discs soak up fluid during a good night's sleep, while the body is positioned horizontally. During the day our upright position, combined with gravity and tension, compresses the discs, and we lose length in the spine.

❝*During non weight-bearing rest, the discs expand as they soak up fluid, increasing the length of the spine by as much as one inch over night. In weight-bearing activity, this fluid is squeezed back into the adjacent soft tissues and vertebrae, to be replaced by fresh fluid during the next rest period. If these normal healing mechanisms are inhibited by poor posture and loss of flexibility, the discs become thin, brittle, and easily injured. This condition, called degenerative disc disease, can lead to bulging or herniated discs.*❞

Schatz, *Back Care Basics*

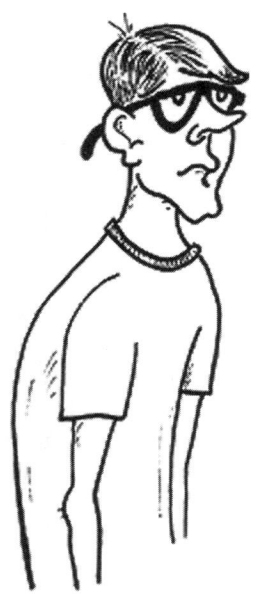

As children, our discs are more watery in substance, but the discs thicken with age and poor posture, leading to less mobility and stiffness of the spine. This thickening is a result of how our fascia system works: where there is tension or compression, the body will produce an excess of collagen fibers, thickening the discs. As the disc thickens, the gel-like nucleus loses water and compresses, leading to spinal nerve impingement and stiffness. We can assist our disc physiology by practicing good alignment and doing therapeutic exercises that increase spinal extension. Avoiding caffeine, cigarettes, and alcohol can help disc hydration, since these substances act as diuretics. Practicing yoga that optimizes engagement of the natural spinal curves can be like getting an extra eight hours of sleep, helping your discs and vertebrae to remain youthful and supple.

"The integrity of our structure is not only crucial to our being comfortable and pain-free, it contributes to many aspects of our overall health and well-being. The natural placement of our bones in any activity and movement determines whether vital energy—the very pulse of life itself—flows freely through our bodies or is blocked and stagnant. The former leads to vibrant health; the latter, to pain and disorder."

Porter, *Ageless Spine, Lasting Health*

Sitting well is an essential tool for surviving the modern lifestyle which revolves around us sitting in chairs. Learning to correct poor breathing habits and aligning the spine can fix much of what is hurting in the body. In a world where humans live primitively, people do not sit in straight-back chairs or try to sit or bend over from standing with straight legs. These are simply unnatural positions that are encouraged by the trappings of our modern lifestyle.

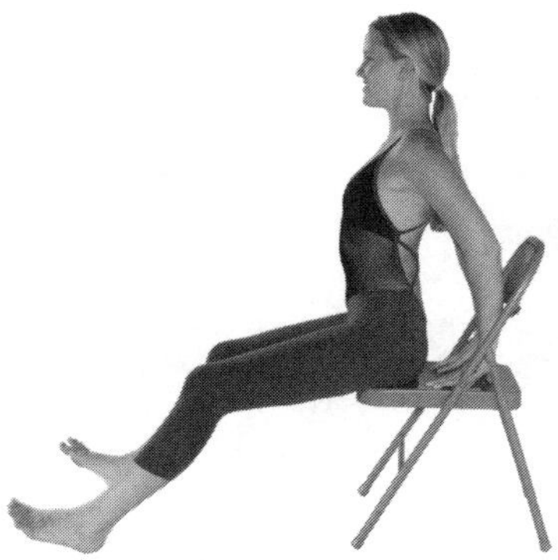

WE AREN'T DESIGNED FOR CHAIR SITTING

Sitting is first among modern practices that have resulted in abundant breathing and structural dysfunction. If we had never used a chair, we would all be quite flexible and agile into old age.

Fig. 6.6 – Rayna in the supported Spine Aligner is learning to sit in a chair with core support created by the internal movements of breathing.

If we had never used a chair, we would also have more natural breathing and postural habits, and beneficial movement and sensory patterns. Sitting in a chair, forcing our muscles to hold the body upright without moving, is actually harder work than walking.

Chairs put our trunk and legs into a right-angle position that causes our sacrum to sag and our spine to compress. While sitting in a chair, our core muscles weaken because the back of the chair does the work of holding up the spine. The butt, pelvic floor, and hamstring muscles can become chronically engaged, and are left tight and shortened from sitting in chairs.

We also move from place to place sitting in cars, and many of us must sit when we work, unless we have outside occupations such as construction or landscaping. Since the modern world demands that most of us must sit, it is vitally important to develop beneficial sitting habits and to take moments to relax and release the muscles that hold us in a sitting position. Frequent breaks and seated yoga twists or deep breathing can help alleviate muscle tension from lack of movement. Sitting on a ball or having one in your office is a reminder to stretch out your front when you have spent a few hours in a chair.

EXPERIENTIAL EXERCISE #16

The Full Body Stretch

Lie down on your back with your legs straight and toes pointed. Reach your arms up over your head, shoulder-width apart, with the arms straight, if possible. Engage yourself in a full body stretch—as though you are just awakening from a good night's sleep **(Figs. 6.7 A&B).** As you reach overhead, spread your fingers wide with your palms facing the ceiling. Your hands and toes do not need to be touching the floor. While reaching, pull your shoulder blades down while drawing your arm bone in towards the shoulder socket, keeping your elbows straight, if possible. Feel the musculature and fascial energy of your arms connecting back to the center. Practice drawing in with your limbs as you radiate out in a stretch from your core center.

Take a deep breath while tuning into your whole being. Point your toes like a dancer as you contract and squeeze your muscles tightly towards your bones. Feel and accentuate the muscle energy in your arms, legs, and trunk. Use the SIP Breath, the core breathing technique for inhaling, drawing the breath slowly through your pursed lips.

Retain your next inhale and tighten all of your muscles, making fists with your hands to add more contraction to the muscles that are already engaged. Tighten your pelvic floor muscles. Hold and squeeze, noticing the feeling of your muscles as they contract. When you need to exhale, release the extra tension you added but stay in the stretch.

Open your fingers, toes, and mouth as widely as you can. Fully extend your tongue like a yawning cat and release the breath with a firm inward squeeze of the rib and belly muscles. Release the muscles of exhalation and let your breathing happen naturally now, without any conscious control. As you witness the breathing happening automatically, imagine all of the tension in your body flowing out of you. Visualize your body like water, as though you are a liquid pool of energy.

Rub your scalp muscles briskly. Take another deep breath and then exhale with your mouth wide open, and your tongue extended long for a few seconds. Bring your arms back down to your sides, feeling your body as though it has melted into the floor. Flow like water and notice the length, openness, and alignment of your being.

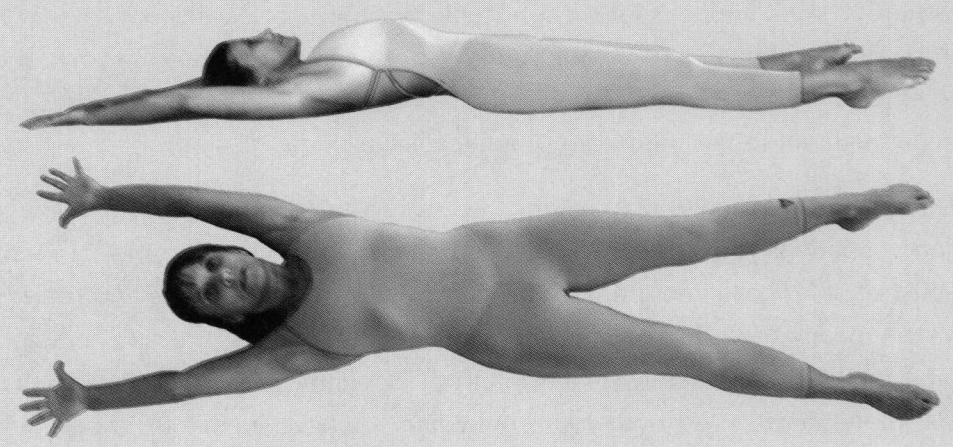

Fig. 6.7A & B – The "Full Body Stretch" always puts you in natural alignment.

Your Office Chair is Killing You

"What fascinates me is that humans evolved over 1.5 million years entirely on the ability to walk and move. And literally 150 years ago, 90% of human endeavor was still agricultural. In a tiny speck of time we've become chair-sentenced." – James A. Levine, obesity specialist, Mayo Clinic, *Science Magazine*, issue 28, January 2005: 584-586.

"Sitting too much is not the same as exercising too little. They do completely different things to the body... If you're standing around and puttering, you recruit specialized muscles designed for postural support that never tire. They're unique in that the nervous system recruits them for low-intensity activity and they're very rich in enzymes.

"One enzyme, lipoprotein lipase, grabs fat and cholesterol from the blood, burning the fat into energy while shifting the cholesterol from LDL (the bad kind) to HDL (the healthy kind). When you sit, the muscles are relaxed, and enzyme activity drops by 90% to 95%, leaving fat to camp out in the bloodstream. Within a couple hours of sitting, healthy cholesterol plummets by 20%." – Marc Hamilton, microbiologist, University of Missouri, *"Your Office Chair Is Killing You"*, by Arianne Cohen, Bloomberg Business Week, April 29, 2010.

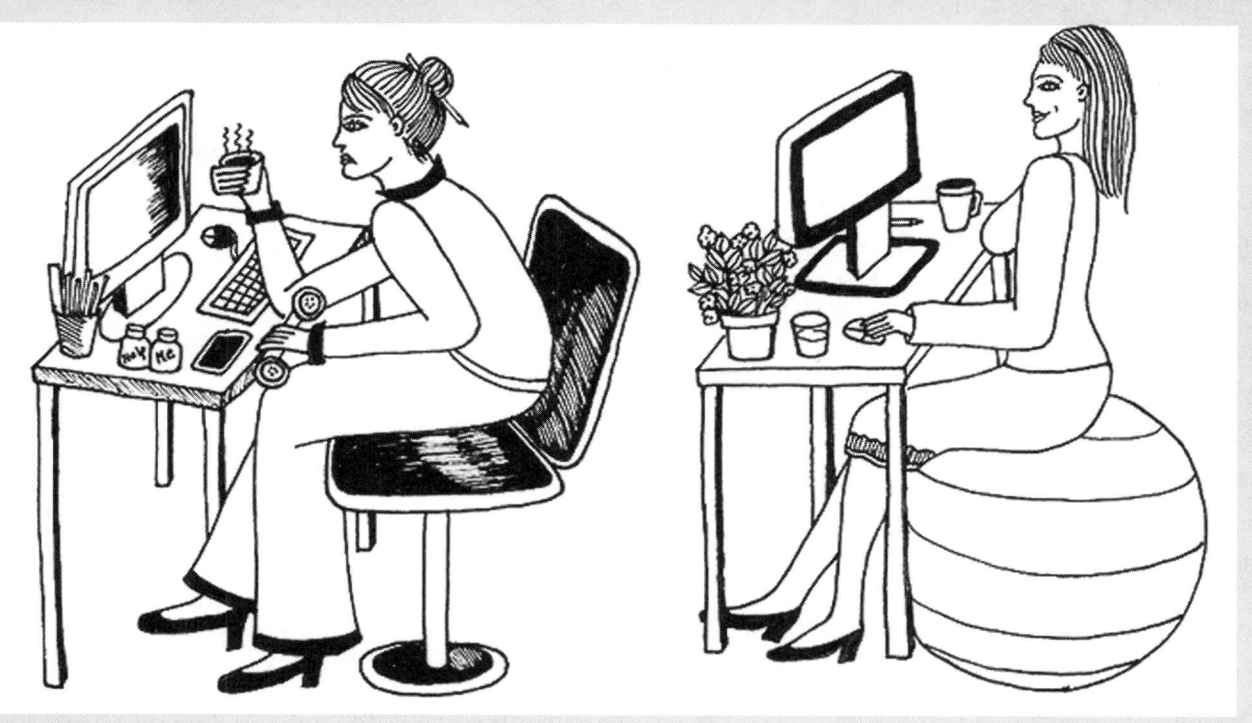

Poor sitting posture can also affect productivity and mood. Chair-sitting also shifts the way in which your body burns fat, and too much time spent in a chair can lead to weight gain and high levels of LDL, the "bad cholesterol." Because of the way our fascia lines pull, sitting in a chair creates fascia tension on the sacrum and lower back, and can even cause tension all the way up the back fascia line attaching to the neck and skull. Sitting at a right-angle is an aberration of natural body positioning, because it forces the sacrum out of its natural tilting position, the ligaments get overstretched, and the discs get compressed, severely impeding our ability to maintain natural, beneficial alignment.

"*Our chair habit was created, modified and nurtured, reformed and democratized in response to social—not genetic, anatomical, or even physiological—forces.***"**

Cranz, *The Chair.*

BECOME ALIGNED IN DAILY LIFE

The human body is designed to squat, not to sit in a chair. Cultures without modern furniture or that have avoided modern right-angled chair-sitting boast a population with stable and erect posture. Such cultures can squat easily at any age and do not require pills, adjustments, and surgeries to keep going. Modern life, unfortunately, often requires that we sit to do paperwork, schoolwork, and duties for our jobs, so chair sitting has become a fact of life.

So what can be done to mitigate the potential dangers of chair sitting? Finding a desk that supports your body by having the computer at eye level and your knees lower than your hips is a good place to start. There is a list in the back of this book of where you can purchase chairs that support good alignment. Many people are even starting to work while standing up and walking on a treadmill. This is especially good for folks who spend all day typing or on the phone.

While not as dangerous as sitting, standing in place can create difficulties too, as many people do not have balanced posture or the elongated, strong trunk muscles needed to protect their hips and knees when standing. Occupations such as hairstyling and dentistry have epidemic amounts of pain and posture dysfunction. Many people stand with their knees hyper-extended and their heads jutting forward. Learning YogAlign techniques and recruiting the breathing process to align and tone the spine and posture has been very helpful to people with jobs that require long periods of standing. The primary goal is to be aligned in your daily life, no matter if you are at work or play.

Many people pride themselves on running or cycling to stay in shape with cardiovascular exercise. While it is important to get the heart rate up, it is equally important to be aligned in the process. YogAlign trains the body into postures that engage the body in optimal natural alignment and which support all of the systems of the body with an economy of movement. As you practice optimal posture, your brain begins to memorize the codes to keep you there, and better posture begins to happen naturally, without conscious effort.

THE BODY IS DESIGNED TO MOVE

Sitting shortens and tightens our muscle patterning because the body works harder when maintaining a static position. Doing exercises and yoga poses that support ongoing patterning of beneficial alignment will help you in all that you do. Natural alignment serves as a warranty against injury, preventing aging and cultivating vitality. Consciously maintain a natural balanced alignment in whatever you are doing, whether it be when working, doing yoga, riding a bike or riding a horse (**Figs. 6.8A & 6.8B**). When you look at these two photos, the naturally-aligned posture looks young and agile, and the misaligned posture appears old and stiff.

Natural Alignment Characteristics:

· Standing feels easy and stable. No peripheral support is needed to stay in position.

· Breathing feels effortless and ribs are free to move and expand in all directions.

· Leg bones are aligned and centered under the pelvis. The pelvis is aligned with the rib cage.

· All weight-bearing joints—shoulder, neck, knee, spine, hip and ankle—are aligned along a central axis.

· Spine and trunk are engaged in extended stabilization, providing support and space to the internal organs, which are themselves positioned comfortably with no compression forces.

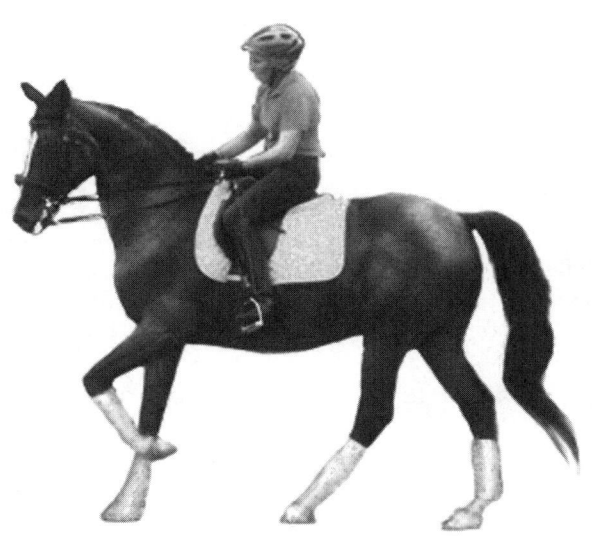

Fig.6.8A – Equestrienne's alignment before YogAlign breathing and posture exercises. Notice the flat lower back curve and forward head carriage.

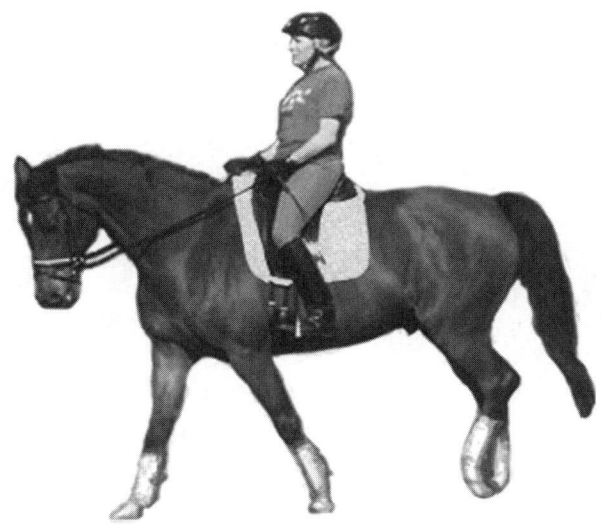

Fig. 6.8B – Equestrienne's alignment after one month of YogAlign. This talented equestrian is 70 years young!

- Effort to stand comes from a dynamic balance of tension, compression, and inner core-strength.

- Fascia lines are in balance with each other, so there is no force or pull on the skeleton.

- There is no pain or tension anywhere in the body, and a sensation of floating, ease, and a relaxed nervous system is evident.

Misalignment Characteristics:

- Standing takes a great deal of effort and peripheral support is needed to stay in position.

- Breathing feels labored and ribs are not free to move and expand in all directions.

- Leg bones are not aligned and centered under the pelvis. The rib cage is not aligned over the hips.

- All weight–bearing joints—shoulder, neck, knee, spine, hip and ankle—are not aligned along a central axis.

- Spine and trunk are engaged primarily in flexion, providing no support and space to internal organs, which in turn are compressed and displaced.

- Effort to stand comes from the outer body and is a dysfunctional combination of either collapse and locking out, or peripheral stabilization efforts such as pulling in the navel, holding up the shoulders, tensing the jaw or tucking under the tail bone.

- Fascia lines are thick and ropey and not in balance with each other. There is great force and pull on the major joints and spine, affecting the organs, joints, and the entire skeleton.

How YogAlign works to create and maintain beneficial postural and breath patterning:

- YogAlign can add longevity to your life by providing a fascial template that will keep you vital, relaxed, and highly mobile well into old age.

- YogAlign emphasizes maintaining the neuromuscular programming of natural body positioning.

- YogAlign engages focused deep-breathing, training the muscles of your trunk to engage primarily as extended stabilizers rather than shortened flexors.

YogAlign has only a few rules for every position. It is important to engage in the following dialogue with yourself while you practice, and to develop discernment that will empower you to use your body intelligently. When you do a pose or a position, ask yourself some important questions:

- Can I take a full deep breath here?

• Do my spine and sacrum maintain their curves and integrity?

• Does this pose or position simulate functional movement, allowing me to feel comfortable and stable?

The importance of practicing exercises or poses that support the physiology of natural alignment cannot be overemphasized. Such exercises will benefit us for our entire lifetime. Remember: it is not what you do that counts, as much as how you are aligned while you do it.

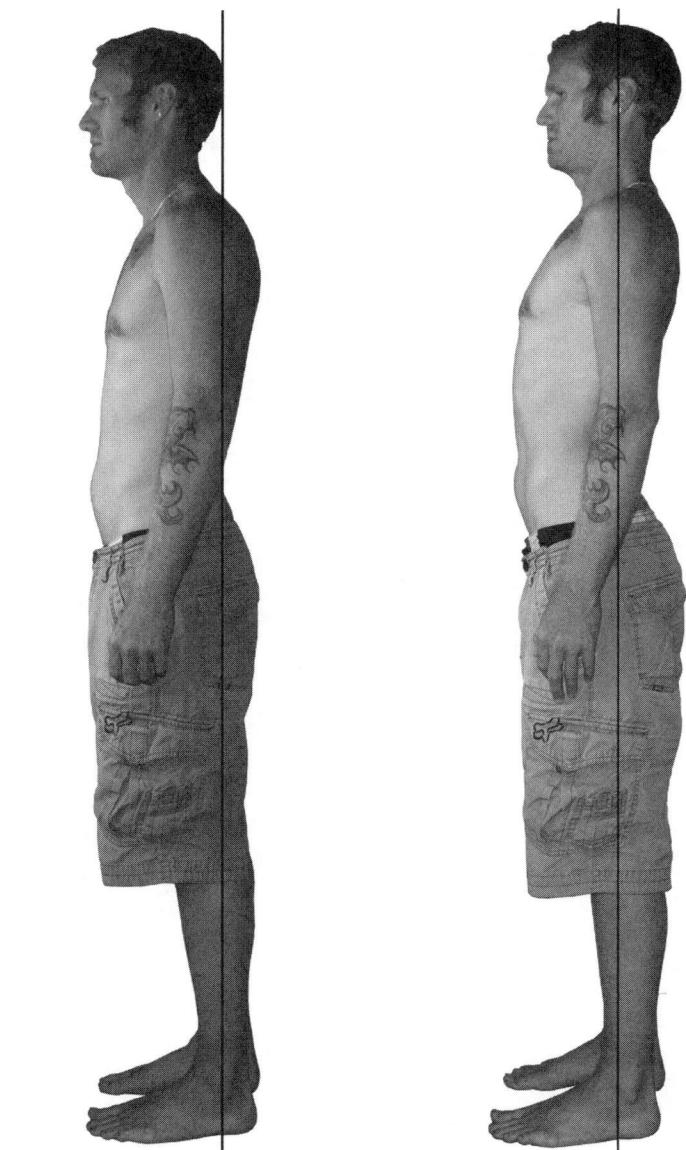

Andrew's alignment made a huge shift after just one two-hour session of YogAlign with Michaelle!

YogAlignMent Principle #10

All poses should engage muscle actions that facilitate the natural curves of your spine, and the shock-absorbing angle of your sacrum.

CHAPTER 7: STABILIZE YOUR CORE

A toned but relaxed belly keeps us healthy, aligned, and pain–free.

Chapter 7
Stabilize Your Core

"By strengthening your muscles around a compressed infrastructure, you close your body more, solidifying your body's imbalances."

Bond, *The New Rules of Posture*

What really gives us a strong core? People often think it requires getting a tight, hard six-pack that gives a washboard look in the front of the body. Getting hard and tight abs will give you a good core, at least according to fitness magazines, and so a flat and tight stomach is what many people aspire to. In reality, it is hard to pinpoint exactly where and what the core is, so it is vital to educate yourself about how the abdominal and trunk muscles are wired together in form and function. Our body is a continuum and every movement we make affects the whole, so understanding what it takes to achieve a strong fluid core can help you lay the foundation for strength, flexibility and balance throughout your entire body.

A Tight Belly Can Create a Sore Back

Some people strengthen their abs in order to acquire a beautiful waist or an impressive six-pack that is void of fat. Many also use ab exercises to tighten or flatten the outer belly in an effort to stabilize sore back muscles. That this is a proper remedy for back problems is a common fitness misconception, and is one of the biggest blind spots in the yoga and fitness industry. Many people—even yoga and fitness instructors—erroneously believe that a strong core means having a tight belly; however, it is a *toned and relaxed belly* that will keep us flexible, aligned, and powerful in the long run. Back pain is caused not just by weakness but also by excessive tightness in the core; thus over-contracting the core is not a panacea for back pain, but rather a trigger for it. Exercising the abs to make them tight causes a chain reaction affecting the entire body, inhibiting breathing, feeling, movement, sexual energy, and even digestion and elimination. The poor advice that suggests tightening the front-body to strengthen the core is worsened by traditional back-stretching exercises that urge practitioners to contract their abs and lean forward, particularly in movements such as seated or standing forward-bends. These exercises are not beneficial to a sore or tight back; in fact, they may simply exacerbate the problem and can actually be detrimental.

Millions of people routinely exercise themselves into a muscular vice-grip trying to "tighten" their outer core. A tight six-pack in the abdominal muscles can be dangerous to the health of the spine, nerves, organs, and even emotions. Individuals with a six-pack may appear to be athletic and seem to be very fit, but they may not actually be *functionally* fit. Common flexion exercises, like abdominal crunches, elbow-to-knee type sit-ups, and straight-leg forward bends continually contract the entire front of the body, leading to a shortening of the front fascial connections that run from head to toe. Trunk muscles then become habituated to a shortened and contracted state, rather than engaging in the more important task of stabilization. This constant contraction of the forces in the front of the body puts pressure on the discs in the spinal column, and can compress the nerves exiting the spine. This contraction creates a muscular train of tension that pulls the sternum or breastbone towards the pubic bone, creating shortness and restriction of movement all over the body.

As we have discussed throughout this book, the way to becoming pain-free begins with moving and breathing from the center of your body, and letting go of abdominal exercises and belly tensions that restrict your ability to breathe deeply. Yet social culture has dictated that a tight, sucked-in belly is beneficial and sexy. Rarely does the idea of toning the belly take into consideration how this emphasis on the *exterior* affects our *interior* functions. One of the simplest ways to ascertain if a pose or exercise is beneficial to your internal well-being is simply to see if, while performing the pose or exercise, you can take a deep SIP breath that allows free movement of both the diaphragm and the muscles that expand and contract the rib cage. When one is not aligned well, or is doing a pose that engages the periphery to control the interior, breathing will be inhibited and restricted. When exercising or practicing yoga, it is important to inquire within and use breathing to determine if a pose is serving your body's needs.

How one breathes when doing exercises that focus on contractions of the abs—such as sit-ups—will determine the exercise's overall benefits, as breathing is the primary determinant of the quality of our movements. For example, most people do strong exhalations as they come into a sit-up, curl, crunch

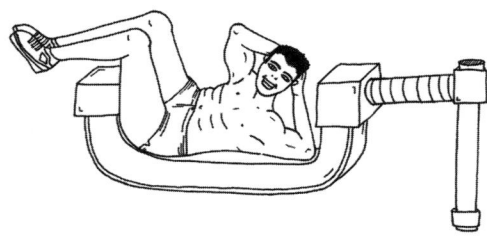

or forward bend. Exhaling as you do ab-strengthening movements further contracts the front body, which reinforces shortening of not just the ab muscles, but also the entirety of the superficial front fascial lines that run from head to toe. In addition, when muscular actions that flex the spine are combined with the movements of exhalation, immense pressure is put upon the anterior discs of the spine, which can detrimentally affect spinal health.

Many fitness and yoga classes stress the importance of keeping the navel pulled in tight to keep core strength. When practiced consistently, these tightening signals eventually get wired into a chronic, tense nerve-patterning that restricts rib and diaphragm movement, and affects organ functioning. This "muscular vice-grip" created by strong, tight abs is a recipe for back pain and dysfunctional breathing, and is the reason why fit people are often in pain and are frequently injured. The body can be strong yet wired incorrectly, and it needs to be recalibrated at the nervous system level to remove unconsciously-held muscle tension. YogAlign focuses on creating neuro-muscular signaling that directs core muscles to act primarily as stabilizers that elongate your spine, increasing length through the neck and torso.

How we breathe defines our structure, and any tension that inhibits breathing can sap precious energy resources. In YogAlign, we emphasize that it is not what you are doing, but how you breathe while you are doing it that defines the quality of your movements and brings you to true center.

CASE HISTORY

Bruno Ewald came in complaining of chronic low-grade back pain and a more serious severe shoulder pain. He attributed the shoulder pain to an injury in his anterior bicep tendon where it attaches to the coracoid process. He was in no way weak or disabled, nor was he even the average weekend athlete:

he was, in fact, the 2006 World Jiu–Jitsu Champion in the masters division, and the 2010 reigning Hawaii champion in all age groups.

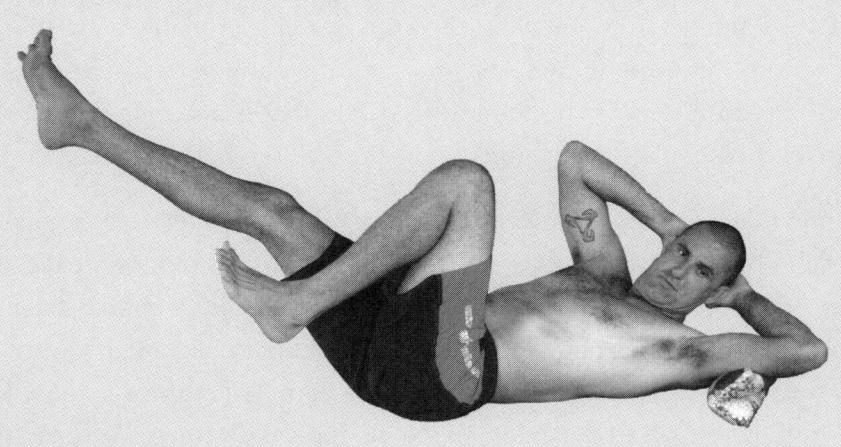

Bruno had some of the strongest abdominal muscles I have ever seen, and when I palpated them, they felt like iron. However strong his abs, he still suffered from back and shoulder pain due to the contractions of his strong

Bruno practicing the "Bicycle SIP-Up" exercise.

abdominals, which were pulling his breastbone towards his pubic bone and his arms forward of neutral. I was able to show him that by changing the way he breathed when he was training his abs, he could acquire strength that would release the tension patterns that were actually migrating from the abs out into his entire body.

The amazing solution was simply to use the Core SIP Breath as he practiced contracting his abs, allowing them to function more as stabilizers. I also showed him how to do PNF exercises that opened his chest and arm lines while at the same time engaging his back to increase extension forces. In particular, I focused on helping him strengthen his mid-back and lower shoulder blade area, as he was very "top" heavy in the large trapezius muscle. Having natural spine alignment in all exercises enabled him to breathe more effectively and I advised him to stop focusing on exercises that compressed and flexed his spine, and to focus more on exercises that create optimal posture and spinal balancing. He was able to experientially feel the fascial connection between the six-pack, the chest, and front of the shoulders as well as the lower connections to the pelvic floor and knees. He has spread the word to his students and is now approaching fitness in a whole new way, with more awareness of how training the entire body using breath can create a more flexible functional structure.

Fluid Movement of the Ribs Creates a Powerful Core

In YogAlign, how we breathe in a pose becomes our most important focus, because how we breathe significantly affects the quality of our movements. Strong muscles of inhalation create length and strengthen the forces of extension in our structure, providing us with a warranty against pain and the effects of aging. In contrast, the movements of exhalation create flexion of the spine, pulling the body forward and reversing the lumbar curve of the lower back, unless one learns to focus on keeping the trunk area extended while the abs contract. This will enlist the core muscles primarily as stabilizers rather than flexors of the spine. Because of time spent in chairs, most of us already have an overall shortness in our front body which is a good reason to avoid abdominal exercises that exacerbate this shortening. What is of vital importance is to learn to engage the actions of the core with a balance between the forces of extension and flexion.

To find that balance and to get to the core, we must to learn to engage the functional use of the intercostal muscles between the ribs, as discussed in Chapter 4. In our rib cage, inhaling requires engagement of the outer intercostal muscles, and exhaling requires the inner intercostal muscles. Balancing the forces of these muscles is an important factor in becoming naturally aligned. If any muscle that attaches to the ribs is over-contracted or weak, this can affect the movement of our ribs and our breathing process. People who over-strengthen the forces of flexion above the forces of extension create muscular patterning that inhibits fluid movements of the rib cage, which prevents the functional breathing that is key to functional alignment.

In YogAlign we spend time recalibrating the signals that cause muscles to over-contract and restrict the free movements of each rib when we breathe. In order to be pain-free and aligned, one must have all ribs free to move. The movement of our diaphragm is greatly assisted by a flexible rib cage, as well as by body positions that engage the psoas and the QL as muscular foundations to the diaphragm's descent during breathing. Breathing that initiates from the shoulders or from sticking out the belly overrides the natural movement that should be occurring at a deeper level, where the movement of the breath begins with an equal expansion of the rib cage. Basically "the beginning creates the ending," so if you try to breathe from your periphery, the quality of your breath will be shallow, inefficient, and superficial.

More Harm than Good

Back-pain sufferers in America cost this country more than $100 billion annually in medical bills, disability insurance, and lost productivity at work. Eighty percent of Americans will deal with back pain at some point in their lives, making it the second most likely reason for doctor visits, after coughs and other respiratory infections.

Doctors commonly recommend surgery, drugs or physical therapy to relieve their patient's pain. Besides these "remedies", many people also try holistic therapies like massage, chiropractic therapy or stomach-strengthening exercises. Massage and chiropractic therapy can definitely help us feel better and give temporary relief, but oftentimes they are only "quick fixes" and the pain soon returns.

The TV and Internet are full of products, pills, and gadgets to strengthen the core, fix your aching back, or give you a flat and sexy belly. Stretching and yoga are often prescribed, despite the possible dangers of yoga and the alarming increase in yoga and fitness injuries. Most people try to tighten their abs in order to combat back pain and increase support in their trunk; adding to the problem is the fact that these same people may sit for hours in positions that compress the spine and diaphragm, overriding any possible benefits of working out. In many cases the desire to exercise hard creates a muscular barricade against pain which begins a vicious cycle of ab shortness that actually *increases* back pain, compression, strain, and tension instead of relieving it. To treat this epidemic of pain, we need to begin by addressing the deeper structural imbalances that are the true root causes of back pain. While the body can be pushed and pulled back into alignment, without active, conscious engagement by the individual, the new patterns cannot hold.

To stop pain in the back, we must go to the root source, which, in many cases, stems from weak breathing muscles combined with short and weakened (or overengaged) abdominal and pelvic floor muscles. These issues can be allayed by stretching open the front, and strengthening the back extensors; this is accomplished by initiating all movement from the core center with deep, unrestricted breathing. When we engage the deep center, the periphery releases incorrect holding patterns, allowing the front and back lines to become balanced in tensile forces (**Fig 7.1**). Once beneficial breathing patterns are engaged to activate the core, we can then develop aligned posture naturally from the inside out, and balance our lines of fascia, which in turn can correct the postural issues that perpetuate chronic back pain.

Many people hold strong beliefs about fitness and yoga that can cause some serious injuries in both the long and short term. When we push the body into poses that compress the spine and restrict breathing, we are training our body to restrict free, fluid movements. In many cases what we "think" is good for us winds

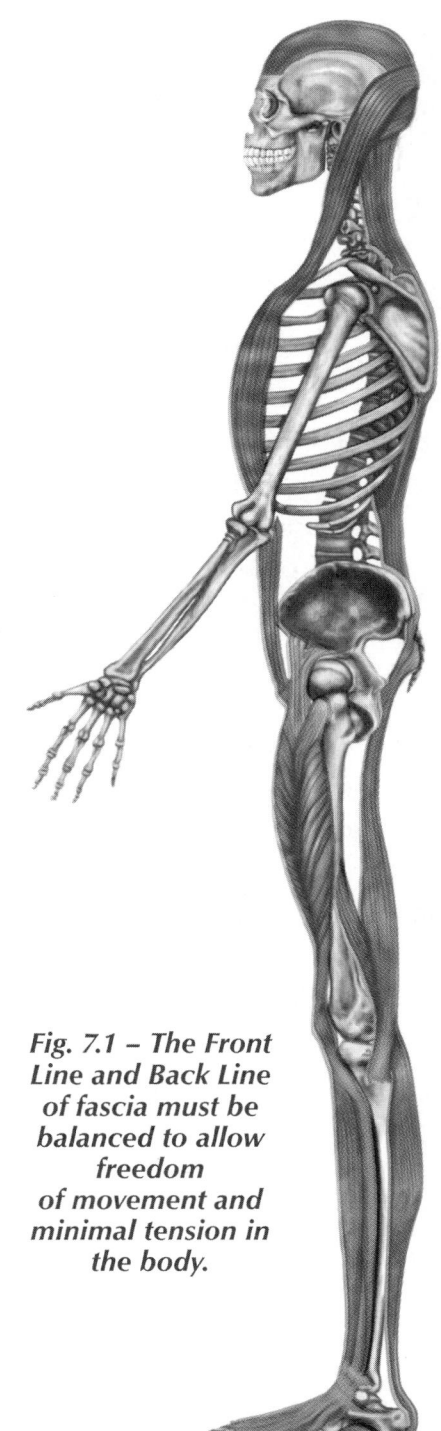

Fig. 7.1 – The Front Line and Back Line of fascia must be balanced to allow freedom of movement and minimal tension in the body.

Redrawn from *Anatomy Trains* by Thomas Myers

up becoming a contributor to our problem; despite this, it can be very difficult to let go of our usual practices even though they may actually be hurting us. Oftentimes people are uncomfortable in a pose, but they breathe through it or persist because of the common belief that we have to "experience pain" in order to get flexible or stronger. Such beliefs are part of the blind-spot that is a major contributor to the increase in yoga- and fitness-related injuries. Yoga and fitness instructors, practitioners and theorists have a responsibility when teaching routine practices to accommodate natural human design and the body's anatomical reality.

One of the ancient Yoga Sutras of Patanjali says:

> **"***anityasuciduhkhanatmasu nityasucisukhatmakhyatiravidya***"**
>
> *(Misapprehension leads to errors in comprehension of the character, origin, and effects of the objects perceived. What at one time feels good or appears to be of help, can turn out to be a problem; what we consider to be useful may in time prove to be harmful.)*

From *Heart of Yoga* by Desikichar

GETTING OUT OF PAIN IS JUST A BREATH AWAY

Oftentimes people do outer core ab work and multiple sit-ups, only to feel their back pain getting worse, or to find that they have developed a potbelly. "Ab Crunch" is a fitting name for a compressive movement that literally "crunches" your spine. Any exercise that focuses on enlisting the periphery—as opposed to the core—to support our center can only be counterproductive to natural breathing and alignment. Keeping the navel pulled in towards the spine occurs naturally during the breathing process, yet fitness and yoga instructors sometimes encourage students to keep the navel *artificially* pulled in as much as possible. Keeping the navel chronically pulled in makes no anatomical sense when you consider how it sabotages spine alignment and breathing function.

> **"***Our cultural obsession with having firm abdominals binds up the diaphragm and creates stress for our entire system. The sympathetic fight-or-flight response is turned on in a low-grade, chronic state. Chances are we don't even recognize that this is happening since our regular state of tension has become our norm and we no longer know what it feels like to be fully and naturally relaxed.***"**

Porter, *Ageless Spine, Lasting Health*

Strengthening the outer abdominals overrides the spine stabilizing action of important core muscles like the psoas. When outer peripheral abdominal muscles are over-contracted and shortened—as is the case in many athletes—the ribs are being pulled down, squeezing the organs and keeping the diaphragm compressed, and the psoas are unable to function as stabilizers of the spine. By over-contracting the abs to shorten our front body, we may be inadvertently giving ourselves more back, neck, or hip pain in the process. A combination of overly strong abs and a weak or tight psoas group (**Fig. 7.2**) compresses the lumbar spine, affecting the vertebral discs and nerves throughout the body.

Experiential Exercise #17

Exhalation Creates Shortness (Spinal Flexion), Inhalation Creates Length (Spinal Extension)

Lie on your back with your knees bent. Inhale, and then cough or exhale, focusing on how muscles engage to make the exhalation happen. Hold the exhale out while accentuating the feeling of the contraction of the exhalation muscles. Stop pushing air out but continue to hold the actions of the exhalation muscles tightly for a count of 5–10 seconds. Release the exhaling muscular actions and just relax for a moment before you start to inhale with the Core SIP breathing technique. While inhaling, notice how your spine lengthens or extends with the inhalation process.

Now exhale and again, keep your exhaling muscles engaged for 5–10 seconds without taking a breath. As you do this, can you feel how your spine compresses to the floor and the lumbar curve is reversed? Notice how even your neck is pressed flat to the floor. This movement does not take you into natural spine alignment, nor does it engage muscles in beneficial patterning, but you *can* learn to exhale while retaining length and extension in the spine.

Now stand up and cough or exhale strongly, holding the action of the muscles that engage. Still holding the exhaling muscles, take a few steps around and notice how constricted the body feels. Try to lift your arms. Can you feel how a chronically tight belly is not an ideal to strive for? Breathe in now, and feel how the muscles that help you inhale bring extension and lift to the spine.

This time as you exhale try to stay extended by keeping the length of your waist area. Notice how little effort it takes to stay lifted and aligned from the inner core.

Inhale again with the Core SIP Breath, noticing extension of your spine and how the space between your ribs and hips and your shoulders and head is now greater. Practice maintaining this space and keeping the length in your entire torso area as you exhale. This requires a conscious effort to engage your belly muscles as stabilizers rather than flexors. Focus on maintaining the extension of your spine during the exhalation. This is the essence of YogAlign— keeping "the gift of the lift" that comes with focused inhalation and exhalation.

Tight abs are overrated and will not "fix" a sore back. Superficial tone in the abs leads to poor posture, organ compression, rib cage inflexibility, shoulder instability, and inhibition of movement.

When engaging abdominal muscles primarily as flexors, it is very important that you inhale into the movement. The inhalation process creates an extension in the spine and lengthens your trunk muscles as they contract. If instead you *exhale* when you do the popular "Ab Crunch," the movement of exhalation will accentuate the pull of the chest towards the pubic bone, the flattening of the lower back curve, the rounding of the upper back, the tucking under of the tail bone, and the moving forward of the head on the spine—all of the hallmarks of poor alignment. Exhaling while flexing the trunk and pulling the knees toward the head creates a super-tight outer core that sets you up for injuries and pain that will migrate all over your body. When the trunk muscles get trained to act primarily as shortened flexors in this manner, the back line of the body must compensate for the shortness in the front line. The back muscles become lax and overstretched and/or tight and go into spasm. This over-contraction leads to restricted blood flow and chronic tension. Discs become dysfunctional and nerves can get impinged, leading to pain in the back, hips and knees as well as conditions like sciatica, IT band inflammation, sacroiliac pain, and inflexibility.

Not many people realize that superficial (outer) core strength also creates a tight pelvic floor, since the contracting of the ab muscles causes a commensurate contraction in the pelvic floor muscles. If you have abs that are wired in chronic tightness, you will have the same tightness in your pelvic floor area, because both areas are basically parts of the same structure. Chronically contracted pelvic floor muscles can play a role in the cycle of back pain and inflexibility, affecting the hips and pelvic angle. When we keep our belly chronically tight, the breastbone pulls toward the pubic bone, creating tension in the muscles of the pelvic floor while also pulling the head forward. This creates a state of tension that affects the whole body, and in particular sends painful contractions to

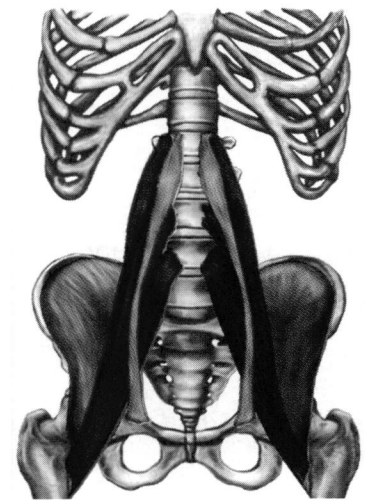

Fig. 7.2 – The Psoas Muscles. Depending upon pelvic tilt, tight psoas can either shorten the spinal curve causing "sway back" (lordosis), or flatten the sacrum and lower back, impinging spinal nerves that innervate the leg from hip to foot.

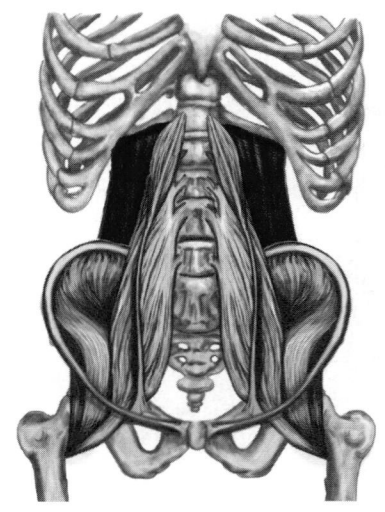

Fig. 7.3 – The Psoas and the Quadratus Lumborum (QL) work in synergy with the abdominal muscles and the erector spinae muscles in the back, providing whole body core support.

the lumbar spine that affect the nerves and discs of the lower back. The nervous system proceeds to encode this repetitive tightening movement, and hard wires the muscular action of the outer core muscles primarily as flexors. These holding patterns then override our natural ability to breathe and move with ease. In this way, a chronically-tightened belly inhibits free movement and diminishes general well-being. Six-pack abs chronically contracted can also cause the entire body to shrink in appearance, which can be a primary cause of many of the characteristics of aging.

CREATE SYNERGY BETWEEN THE SIX-PACK AND THE PSOAS

The deepest layer of abdominals, below the *rectus abdominus* or six-pack, is the *transverse abdominus* (TA) (**Fig. 7.4**) which connects to the diaphragm and rib cage. The second deepest abdominals, the *internal obliques*, work alongside the transverse abdominus, the QL, and the psoas to stabilize the spine.

Deep intrinsic muscles attaching to the vertebrae called the *rotators* and the *multifidus* are other strong forces in spine extension and stabilization. Without a functioning psoas and QL group, the back extensors, paraspinal muscles and even the neck muscles become hardwired in an exhausting state of chronic tension. By requiring the nervous system to enlist the psoas and QL group in stabilization, the deeper muscles of the spine engage and support the body from the inside out, relieving the excess energy use and chronic tightness brought about by over-reliance on the tightened muscles of the belly.

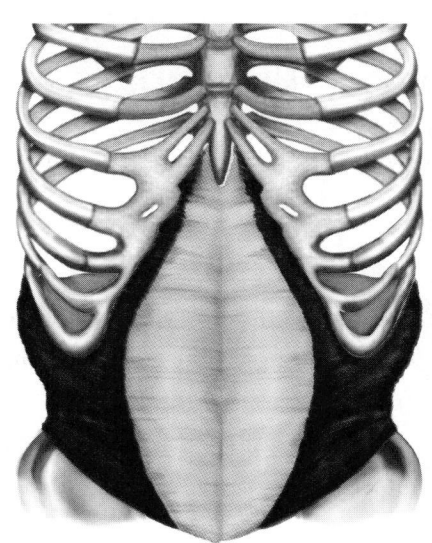

Fig. 7.4 – The Transverse Abdominus muscle provides an inner ring of core support, toned and lengthened by regular practice of the YogAlign SIP Breath.

Abdominal muscles acting predominantly as flexors override the spine-stabilizing function of the inner core muscles. The stabilizing muscles are multi-functional and are a combination of slow- and fast-twitch muscle fibers, meaning they function for quick bursts as well as for slow, stabilizing contractions. Normally considered an abdominal compressor, the TA is affected by the movements of inhalation created by the SIP breath, lengthening even as it contracts. The unique SIP breath creates a ring of support for your spine while giving you a toned and extended waistline. In YogAlign we strengthen the surface abdominals, or outer core, as stabilizers working in synergy with—not in place of— the inner core. We tone and activate the breathing muscles of the rib cage and diaphragm with the psoas, quadratus lumborum (QL), the erector spinae muscles and the other abdominal muscles (**Fig. 7.3**). As a result, neck and back muscles alone are not required to take over the job of stabilizing the spine, holding up the head, or keeping the ribs above the hips.

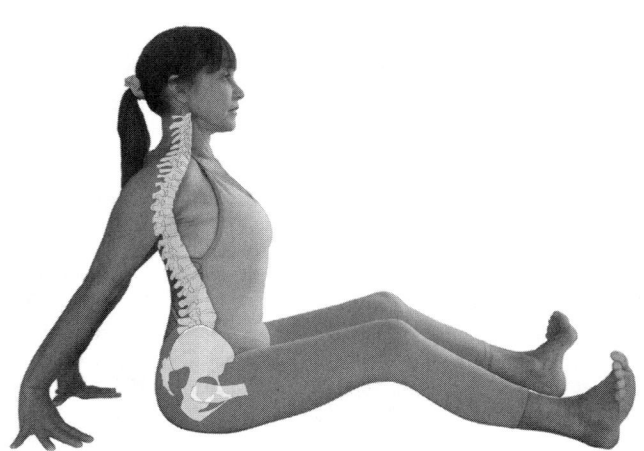

Fig. 7.5 – The "Spine Aligner" activates the deep core line, creating internal support of the four curves of the spinal column.

The "Spine Aligner" (**Fig. 7.5**) is a panacea for back pain relief because of the SIP breathing techniques used throughout the pose's movements, including the contraction of the abs in concert with the lifting of the trunk. These movements (in combination with the breathing technique) create abdominals that work in synergy with the diaphragm, psoas and muscles of the pelvic floor to stabilize and elongate the torso. The "Spine Aligner" is also a "posture reorganizer" that balances all of the fascia lines in the body at once. In particular, it helps to release tension in the muscles of the neck and upper trapezius by creating a template for natural alignment. This pose also relaxes the lower back muscles, balances inner and outer rotation in the hips, tones the core in stabilization, and re-establishes beneficial neuromuscular codes for natural posture. Notice how the knees are bent to simulate real life movement in the body, and all four curves of the spine are engaged. Efficient movement patterning is attained when we learn to activate the deepest core muscles that stabilize the spine while using only necessary effort in the neck and shoulder area.

It takes so little effort to be sustainable in the body. When a pose is balanced in YogAlign, it will feel effortless, like you are floating. You are simply a "force of energy" and feel no density in your physical being.

YogAlign's SIP breath techniques, in combination with functional body positions, engage the core trunk muscles primarily as stabilizers instead of flexors. It is not necessary or particularly healthy to develop a super-tight six-pack in order to be fit. Remember, even the process of simple, daily, focused exhalation is enough to keep your six-pack and your abdominal compressors toned. Becoming stable from the inner core involves learning the essential core breathing techniques of YogAlign and orchestrating the deepest core muscles of the rib cage, spine, and diaphragm. When we put the body in a natural position and breathe, these stabilizing muscles awaken like the sun coming out after a rainy day.

EXERCISING THE ABS WITHOUT THE CRUNCH

So if outer-core-strengthening Ab Crunches don't relieve back pain, create more tightness, and fail to increase mobility, how, then, should we go about strengthening our abs?

Balancing the abdominals starts with activation of the deepest core muscles of the body. This activation happens through focused breathing combined with stabilizing muscular actions around a neutral, naturally-aligned spine. In this focused breathing, inhalation enlists muscular/fascia actions that extend and lengthen the trunk and spine, and exhalation is combined with a conscious effort to maintain this extension. It may seem backwards at first, but when you take the stabilizing roles of the involved muscles into account, it makes more sense to inhale when you do any front-compressing exercise.

Most people have compression of the diaphragm and ribs, due to excessive time spent sitting in a chair. There is already a poor, ingrained breathing habit in many of us because of this, and many of us use the upper shoulders and back to initiate the breathing process. Using deep breathing to engage the abdominal muscles in synergy with the psoas muscles and deeper spinal muscles—as opposed to depending upon the extremities—is an essential element of the YogAlign system. Abdominal muscles and the psoas group need to be strong, flexible, and stable in order to keep the spine out of compression, to promote effective breathing, and to facilitate kid-like freedom of movement.

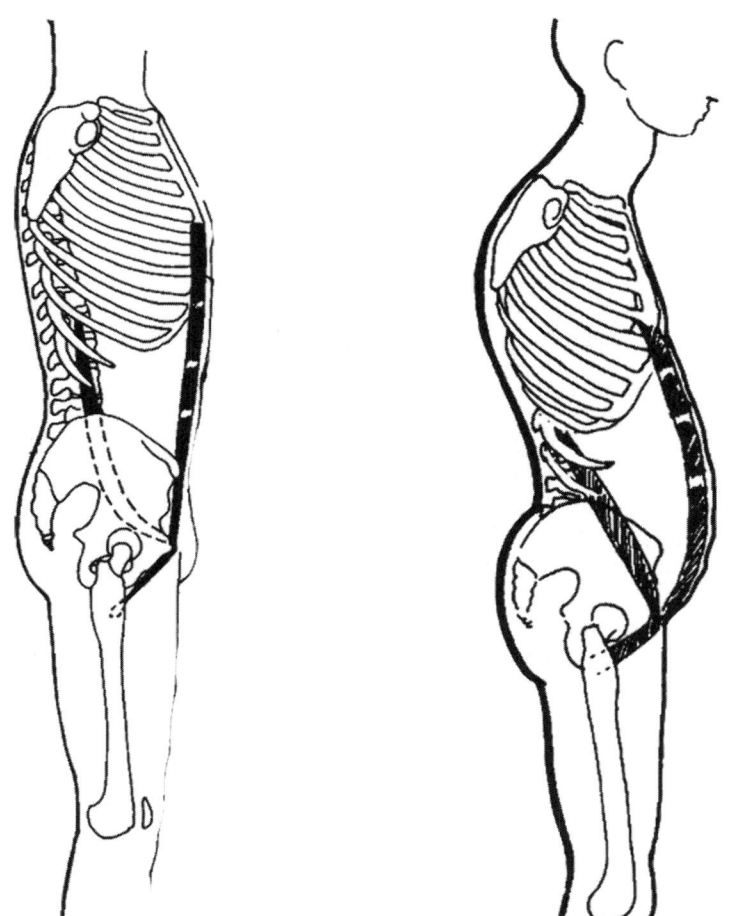

A chronically short psoas group can pull the pelvis forward, leading to a drop in the chest. This causes a loss of tone in the six-pack or rectus abdominus. The result, as shown in **Fig. 7.8**, is no tone in the belly muscles, which leads to a pot belly and swayback posture; this is a recipe for chronic back pain. In YogAlign, we use the movements of inhalation to protect the spine from disc or nerve compression while at the same time engaging and strengthening the body's core stabilizing muscle groups. Inhaling as you contract your abdominal region creates stabilizing muscle actions that lengthen as they engage.

Fig. 7.8 – A tight psoas (left) can cause swayback and a pot belly.

EXPERIENTIAL EXERCISE #18

SIP-Up and SIP-Up Twist

Lie on your back, knees bent, feet placed hip distance apart. Interlace your fingers behind the back of your head and press your elbows towards the floor with your shoulder blades pulling down towards your hips and in towards your heart (**Fig. 7.6**). Focus on breathing with rib movement and keep the fingers softly woven together without over-engaging your neck muscles. Begin to practice the Core SIP Breath. As you inhale, lift your upper body, including your head and shoulder girdle, off of the floor. Keep the elbows wide. Do not lift by pulling on your neck spine.

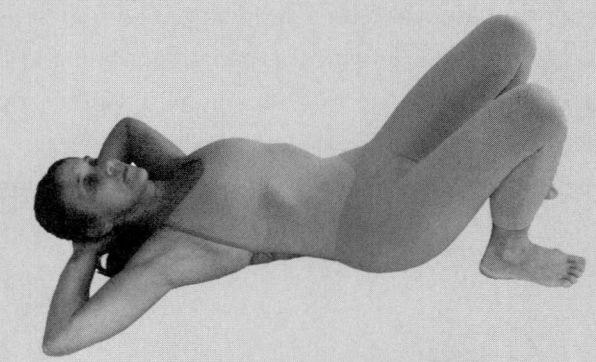

Fig. 7.6 – SIP-Up

You are lifting the entire body by engaging the core through breathing. Always focus on initiating movement from the effort of the SIP breathing technique.

Breathe as deeply as you can, expanding your rib cage deeply on the inhale and drawing it in on the exhale as you lower to the floor. You may exhale through your nose or mouth but do not push your lower back into the floor as you exhale. Simply pull the inner rib cage muscles together, drawing the belly in towards the spine without losing the length and curves in your lower back. Repeat this exercise, beginning your movement first with a few seconds of inhalation and then lifting your shoulders and head off the floor. Keep the movement of your rib cage active and lift straight-up, rather than trying to curl your body up towards your knees.

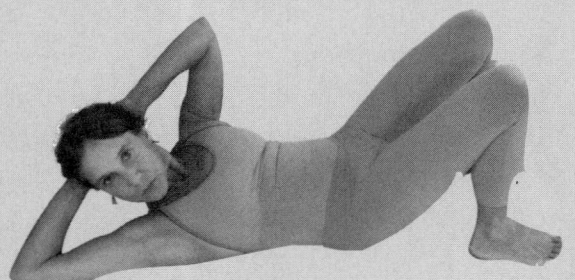

Fig. 7.7 – SIP-Up Twist

To use more of the lateral trunk muscles, add a twist to the right side as you inhale up, and slowly lower yourself to the floor as you exhale (**Fig. 7.7**). Repeat on the other side, twisting to the left, making sure to initiate your lifting movements with the SIP breath. Breathe slowly and deeply, making your rib cage expand deeply in the breathing process. Start with five Sip-Ups on each side, then go one step further. On

> **EXPERIENTIAL EXERCISE #18 (CONT.)**
>
> your next inhale, twist to one side as before, and then, stay up while exhaling slowly through your mouth making a "ssss" sound like a snake through your teeth. Inhale again slowly using the Core SIP breath. Intensify the twist, and then lower yourself back to the floor as you slowly exhale through your nose. Continue to the left side and try to stay up for a round or two of inhales and exhales. Finish with a full body stretch, then massage the upper psoas-diaphragm area located just below the breastbone.

By using the inhalation-into-flexion process, the nervous system encodes the action of the core muscles as stabilizers. These actions support the spine and free your extremities from trying to support and stabilize your structure. When the belly is relaxed, all of your ribs are free to move when you inhale, and breath happens deeply, with little effort. Remember that most of the time our breathing process is unconscious, so we must reprogram the nervous system using our breathing muscles so that strong, efficient breathing will happen unconsciously. Once we do this, optimized breathing and natural alignment is intrinsic and automatic. All postures and movements in YogAlign involve using the movements of the inhalation process to bring the body into natural alignment.

> **"***Our relationship with our bodies is ruled by myths that take us ever further away from our body's natural design. Prominent among these myths is the as-yet unchallenged belief that strong rectus abdominus muscles, or 'abs', are not only necessary in order to support our backs but that they must be firm in order for us to be attractive, the definition of which is regulated by a culturally accepted standard. This standard says we must conform to an ideal appearance that may have little to do with what is natural or healthy for any particular individual. Millions of people in our society are dedicating themselves to a quest for "killer abs" when actually, back support comes from relaxed rectus abdominus muscles. These free the bones of the pelvis, sacrum, and spine to align in a natural relationship to one another and allow the deeper transverse abdominus or "corset" muscle, to provide the necessary elastic support.***"**
>
> Porter, *Ageless Spine, Lasting Health*

As we have discovered, the long-term solution for tight back muscles lies in empowering the psoas, QL, transverse abdominus, and all of the core trunk muscles in a synergistic fashion. When these muscles activate in synergy, the spinal curves are naturally aligned, and the external back and belly muscles are

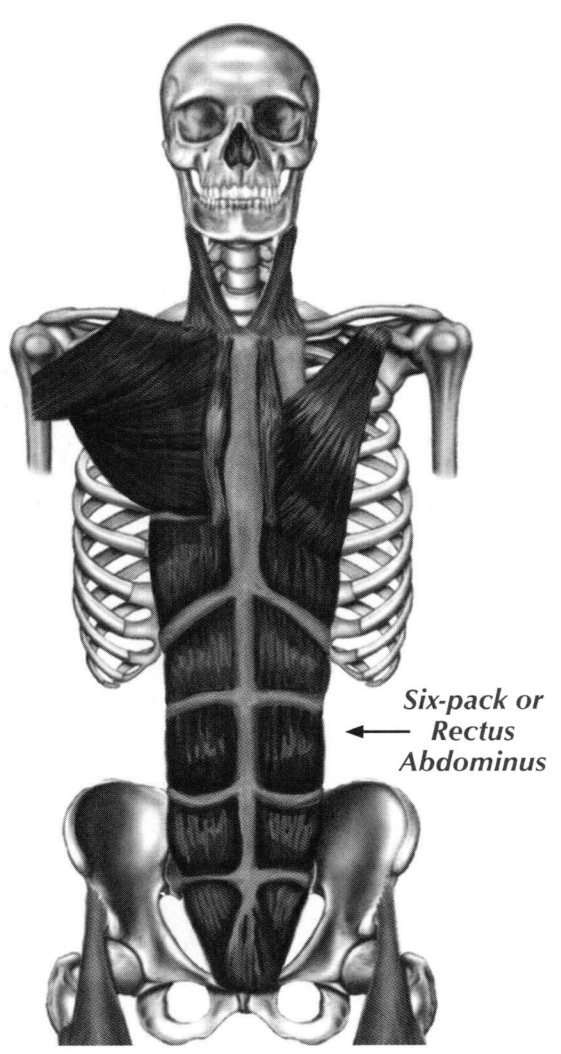

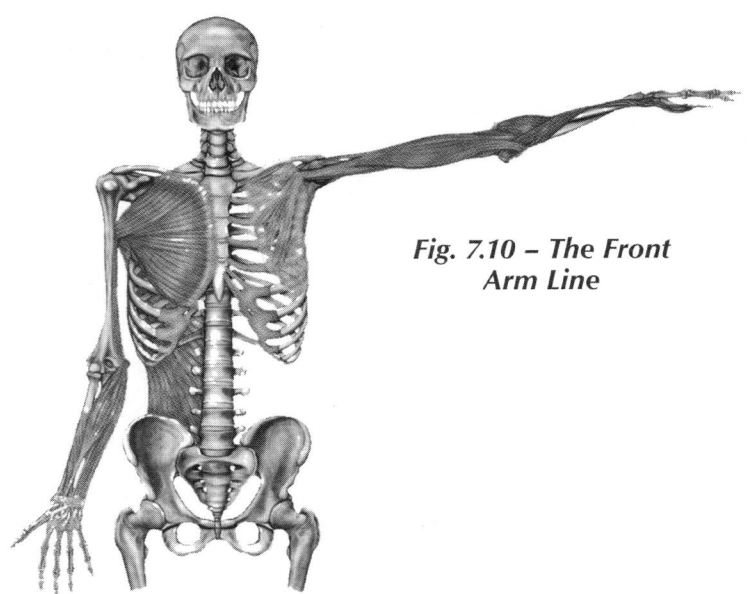

Fig. 7.10 – The Front Arm Line

Redrawn from *Anatomy Trains* by Thomas Myers

Six-pack or Rectus Abdominus

Fig. 7.9 – Muscle tension in the abdomen directly influences the alignment and functions of the arm and shoulder joint. The ab muscle's most important function is to stabilize, not flex, the spinal column.

toned but not tight or tense. The body then feels light, and moves effortlessly, especially in the lower back and in the neck muscles. So many people with strained and exhausted back muscles could be pain-free if they simply learned how to actively relax the back and belly muscles and how to stabilize, lengthen, and strengthen the psoas via deep breathing and functional movement poses. Deep core breathing—not contracting the outer core into shortness—must be practiced to functionally awaken our trunk muscles as stabilizers.

Core Synergy Connections

Since we have now learned that over-tightened outer-abdominals inhibit breathing, it is important to review how this affects the body as whole, due to the interconnected nature of the human structure. The breathing function is connected to the upper chest and pectorals, and helps to align our shoulders and arms. Tight abdominals, therefore, through their effect upon the breathing process, can restrict movements of the body all the way up to the shoulders and into the arms. **Fig. 7.9** shows the abdominals and their connection to the arm lines in **Fig. 7.10**. Upon examining these illustrations, you can clearly see how tight and short abdominals will affect the arm lines and pull the arm forward in the shoulder socket. The tension of the abdominals migrates to the arm and can restrict the shoulder joint, create a forward head-carriage and possibly invoke an indirect fight-or-flight nervous system reaction.

Tension and over-contraction in the outer trunk muscles can also seriously inhibit endurance, wasting precious energy and resources. Recall that the muscles in our arms, legs, and outer belly are called phasic or "fast-twitch" muscles. They are designed to fire and release, propelling us forward, and they are primarily fed by glycogen. When we are hiking and start to get hungry, it is the arms and legs which begin to fatigue, as opposed to the deeper core and spinal muscles. This is because the deep posture muscles of the back and spine are "slow-twitch" muscles designed to stay contracted for long periods, supporting our upright position throughout the day. These muscles are primarily fueled by oxygen, which is why breathing is so important to them, and why sedentary chair sitting weakens them by replacing them (with the backrest) in their main task of structural and postural support.

Recall also that some muscles in the trunk area can engage as fast- *and* slow-twitch muscles in combination. The transverse abdominus and the internal and external obliques can be abdominal compressors with fast contractions as well as slow sustaining stabilizers. The transverse abdominus acts like a corset wrapping the trunk when we exhale, but we can also feel it engaging as a stabilizing ring of support from the inside when we inhale using the SIP breathing technique.

Issues in the Tissues

In addition to the six-pack and lower back, the pelvic floor is uniquely connected to movements of breathing. In order to be truly fluid and connected in our movements, we need to be in touch with the muscle tension in the pelvic floor region. Ideally the pelvic floor is relaxed during the movements of inhalation and it naturally contracts with the six-pack, TA, and the internal intercostal muscles on exhalation. The six-pack is the most superficial muscle of the abs at the ribs, but below the navel this muscle group actually dives below the other abdominal muscles and connects at the pubic bone, becoming the deepest abdominal muscle. The tension in the six-pack is, in this way, wired to the pelvic floor region. As a result, chronic tightening in the six-pack is a significant cause of unnecessary holding and tension in the pelvic floor area, causing tightness in the hips and legs.

Emotions can also be affected by over-tightening in the belly area. Feelings that are held back can cause one to hold excess muscle tensions that become the "issues in the tissues" and the pelvic area (by virtue of its connection to the belly) is one of the main areas of the body where people can become locked up, both physically and psychologically. This is because the pelvic floor, belly, and hip regions are zones that hold unreleased emotion, memories, and sexual repression. "Stuck feelings" are often exacerbated by a weakened or tight psoas group, and by the excessive strengthening of trunk muscles through forced abdominal exercises. The constant tensing of the abdominals and pelvic region (as well as the repression of feelings that is common in many people) can inhibit breathing and, ultimately, movement. Almost anyone can benefit from using PNF exercises to find and unravel the unconscious tension areas that sap our energy and lead to restrictions.

This next Experiential Exercise shows how to reset muscle tension in the pelvic floor region. Use of the PNF technique exaggerates tension, which on the release resets the resting length of the core breathing muscles, increasing the tone and fluid balance of the core.

EXPERIENTIAL EXERCISE #19

Pelvic Floor Tuning

From a standing position with feet hip-distance apart and arms to the sides, contract and pull up on your pelvic floor muscles by acting as though you are trying not to urinate. Notice how your navel pulls in at the same time.

Exhale and pull the navel in even more. As you exhale, feel how the pelvic floor and the belly muscles engage together. Try to let go of the belly without letting go of the pelvic floor area. It is difficult to do this because they are connected in their actions and fascia reinforcements. Any contraction of the outer belly automatically causes a tightening in the pelvic floor area, and also the muscles of the inner rib cage that work in the exhalation movement.

Now tighten the pelvic floor more and try to walk. Can you see how difficult this is? Imagine how even the slightest amount of unnecessary tension in the pelvic floor and abdomen can inhibit movement, creating a feeling of inflexibility. Tighten your pelvic floor ("stopping the pee" action) as well as your belly, then lift your arms up alongside your ears. Notice how movements feel with these areas contracted. Now do it again without the added tension and feel the difference. This difference arises because the arms are ultimately connected to the belly area; there are no separate parts in the bodily continuum. Tension that is unnecessary affects not just the area that is tight, but the entire body as a whole. Tight abs and a tight pelvic floor cause pain, injuries and restrictions that can show up in the shoulder and arm area. Focus for a moment on allowing the expansion and stretching of the pelvic floor on the inhale, and feel how it naturally contracts in the exhaling process. Your body is connected as a whole and the body cannot lie.

CASE HISTORY

A BBC cameraman in his late 30's came from Europe to see me after visiting my website and learning about the work I do with the psoas and chronic pain. He had severe chronic back pain and psoas problems, and was hopeful that I could provide him with some relief.

His story was intense and he most definitely held some traumatic memories that were affecting his ability to release the excess tension patterns in his abs, psoas, and pelvic floor muscles. He was reticent about his history, but he did tell me he had spent 17 years filming the horrors of war and the tragedies of natural disaster, plague, and famine all over the planet. He had learned how to suppress his emotions in order to get the job done, but these feelings were stuck in the neuromuscular patterning of his inner core, especially in his navel area, psoas, diaphragm, and pelvic floor. He had been doing power yoga and primarily ashtanga yoga for years, but had never felt any relief from his persistent back pain. He had also tried massage, physical therapy, and acupuncture with no success. He found YogAlign after being told by a therapist that he had "psoas issues."

The idea of doing yoga that did not require painful positions and that focused on ideal posture and body stabilization from the inside-out intrigued him. He came to Kauai and spent a few weeks learning YogAlign in private and group sessions. He did specific PNF exercises (including the core synergy exercises), with me assisting him in the process. He was able to gain an experiential awareness of the tension patterns he carried in his abs and pelvic floor that were leading to his chronic pain. As his psoas released and assumed proper functioning, tension in his pelvic floor relaxed, and he became more fluid and calm in both his physical and emotional body. The chronic back pain that had plagued him for years disappeared. During one session, he had a spontaneous release of internalized sadness and deep emotion which was very helpful in the overall process, and showed he was able to "let go and feel" once he relaxed the chronic armoring in his belly and pelvis. It was through this inner work of engaging and releasing deep core structures—and in particular, the trauma reflex in his psoas and pelvic floor patterning—that he was able to release himself from the emotional and physical pain-prison that inhibited his structure and expressed itself as chronic pain.

Like this cameraman, while practicing YogAlign, some may feel a release of deep emotions that are the "issues stuck in the tissues." In a sense, the physical body is a dense representation of our experiences, memories, belief systems, and thought processes. Ignoring the body's pain signals, holding our emotions, and making ourselves do positions that go against our natural design just masks the real issues and drives dysfunction deeper into the body. Gradually this peripheral armoring, whether caused by a conscious effort to tighten the belly or brought on by emotional guarding or traumas, can cause serious harm and hasten the aging process. In YogAlign, we acquire the tools and awareness to unlock the rivers of tension that can impede the uninhibited flow and spirit of our naturally joyous state of being.

STABILIZATION IS THE ANSWER

Beyond movement restriction or chronic pain, keeping the belly tight has very serious consequences for our overall health and well-being. Tension or over-contraction of the outer trunk muscles seriously inhibits breathing, sending a person into the cycle of restricted movement, chronic pain, and emotional holding. Exercises and yoga poses that teach us to control our inner body by tightening the navel can lead to chronic imbalances that seriously affect the quality of our lives. By using the movements of breath to align and stabilize our core area, we can cultivate a body-wide balance of effort that arises from our inner body. Having this inner support allows us to drop the unnatural tensing that armors and impedes our breath, feeling and movements. Using only the effort that is needed becomes a welcome feeling that leads to the fluidity of a kid-like body that is freed of unnecessary effort, tension, and strain.

YogAlign Essentials That Develop a Pain-Free and Sustainable Body:

- **Breath:** Deep, conscious, full functional-breathing at the psoas/diaphragm level.

- **Fascia:** Balancing all the fascia lines by aligning with our core through the breathing process.

- **Alignment:** Poses in natural alignment for balanced strength and natural flexibility and suppleness, always strengthening and stretching from functional movement positions.

- **Proprioception:** Sensing the whole body, and connecting with the feeling-sense using conscious breathing and PNF exercises, functional and balanced positions, and self-massage.

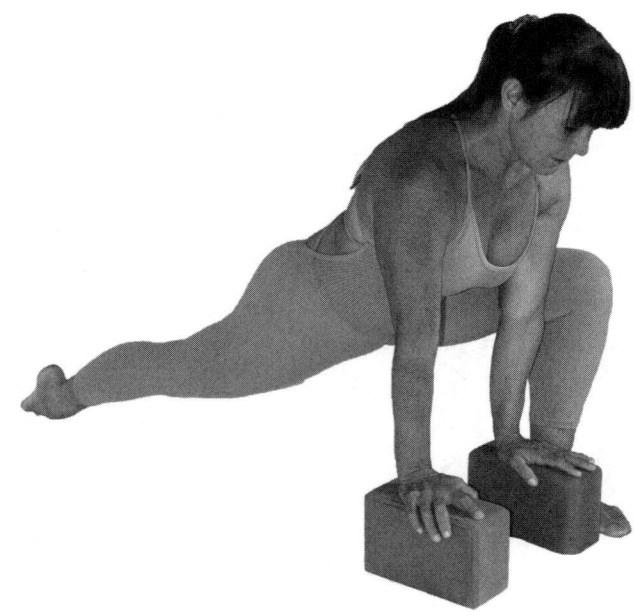

Fig. 7.11 – This deep lunge tones the "femoral triangle," sometimes also called the "armpit of the groin."

YogAlignment Principle #11
Abdominal muscles can be programmed to lengthen while contracting
creating a fluid, toned core and a longer waist.

CHAPTER 8: YOGA DOESN'T HAVE TO HURT

ॐ **Gain without the Pain**

ॐ **Right-Angle Poses Do Not Follow Nature's Design**

ॐ **Flexibility Can Be a Liability**

ॐ **Don't Be Inflexible in Your Belief about Your Own Flexibility**

ॐ **YogAlign Perfects Your Posture**

ॐ **Downward Dog Misconceptions**

ॐ **YogAlign High Dog**

ॐ **The Straight-Leg Forward Bend**

ॐ **Beneficial? Or Dangerous?**

ॐ **Arm Extension from Your Inner Core**

ॐ **Conclusion**

The hidden reason why yoga can hurt
and cause injuries is that
many commonly practiced yoga poses
require one to use the body
in a way that makes no
biomechanical sense and there
is no "correct" way to do them.

"Sthira sukham asanam"

(That which is stable, that which is comfortable. That is asana.)

"Heyam Duhkham Anagatam"

(Pain in any form must be anticipated and avoided.)

From Patanjali's *Yoga Sutras*, an oral tradition estimated to be 5000- 6000 years old, transcribed to the written word approximately 2400 years ago.

GAIN WITHOUT THE PAIN

The Yoga Sutras are ancient yogic teachings that outline the art and science of Yoga meditation, with the goal of reaching Self-Realization. The ancient sutras or "threads of wisdom" explain the process of systematically encountering, examining, and transcending each of the various gross and subtle levels of false identity of the mind, until the true self is revealed. The teachings in the sutras are predominately focused upon the mind and meditation. The above sutras suggest that our body should be stable and comfortable and pain is to be avoided when in a pose or *asana*. This could be interpreted as working through discomfort to find ease and comfort, but it will never mean keeping the body in sustained uncomfortable, contorted, or painful positions, as practiced by some. Pain is a message from the body telling your conscious mind that you need to change position, or that something you are doing is causing tension, which is leading to pain. Experiencing pain will not bring gain. Instead, pain can actually signal the body's autonomic nervous system into the fight-or-flight response, bringing unconscious nervous system reactions like higher blood pressure, rapid pulse, and the tightening of muscles and connective tissue bands.

In my years of teaching yoga, I have frequently heard people say that they can't practice yoga or stretching because it hurts. Many people don't feel comfortable while performing poses or exercises, and decide that they will never be "good" at yoga. Others persevere despite their pain, and hold out a hope that at some time in the future they will indeed be flexible if they keep practicing, however painful that practice may or may not be. For those who are naturally flexible, yoga may seem easy in the beginning, but in a long-term practice, many experience joint de-stabilization from the repetition of moves and poses that are anatomically questionable.

Most of us don't look like the glamorous folks in magazines or the yoga stars in the front row of class. Many more ignore the fact that in the course of their yoga classes they seem to be feeling more pain than enlightenment; some people even suffer injuries. It is estimated by some physiotherapists that 30-40 percent of people in yoga classes are getting hurt. Yoga injuries are in the news and on the rise. Why? Many experts believe that most injuries are a result of inexperienced teachers or students that are pushing too hard. There is no doubt that these *are* major factors. YogAlign practices, however, suggest that many injuries are more accurately the result of positions and poses that cause injury because they conflict with the physical realities of the human body's design.

In YogAlign, we actively seek out positioning, alignment and movement that reflects how we move in daily life. We avoid uncomfortable, unnatural, and compressive positions that restrict deep breathing or that cause spinal compression. When we are aligned with the spine in its natural curves, the body connects naturally as a continuum and we feel relaxed, balanced, secure and peaceful. We attain a comfortable and natural state of being, connected to our true essence. We keep our practice simple, focusing on attaining naturally-balanced posture, instead of being excessive "consumers" of yoga poses or asanas.

A recent quote in a yoga magazine by Adhil Palkhivala, a renowned Iyengar-style yoga teacher, boldly suggests that "90% of yoga asana is a waste of time," – interview with Adhil Palkhivala by Andrea Kowalski, Yoga Journal , May 2009 page 140. Poses aligned with human biomechanics create no discomfort. When we do yoga asanas that oppose the body's natural design, we create an internal and external struggle that spawns tension in our mind, body, and emotions. This state of tension is the *antithesis* of the ideal Yogic state of alert attention. Poses that allow the body to engage naturally in breath and movement do not inflict pain, rather they allow us to move into a deep, yogic state of full-body awareness with a clear mind and an open heart.

If you were a rock climber, you would study route maps ahead of a climb to understand where you were going, and to determine the best route to take you there. You would also ensure that your body was fit and that your climbing equipment was sound. You would certainly make sure that the lead climber was experienced, educated about the area, and trustworthy. The practice of yoga requires the same amount of preparation and inquiry, and a crucial part of this is determining if a teacher is qualified, and learning whether the poses you will be doing are safe and comfortable for the design of your own body. Many people go to yoga classes and put themselves, usually unknowingly, in a very dangerous position, allowing other people to lead them into places that do not serve their highest good. It is important to have a map of where you are going and make sure that you take care of yourself in any kind of yoga class or fitness exercise. Individual injuries and chronic pain issues should always be communicated and discussed with a teacher qualified to guide you into poses that will foster natural alignment and heal imbalances and obstructions. A yoga practice designed to optimize postural patterns has more benefit than a repetitive, pose-based practice that ignores current discomfort for the sake of a possible gain in the future.

In YogAlign, we always maintain a dialogue with our body about what feels comfortable and beneficial. Students are encouraged to develop individual discernment based upon a foundation of questioning and knowledge, rather than following a "rote" yoga program that requires one to follow the pack. Students should feel free to adapt poses to their own level of comfort, and to practice in a calm state of presence that retains awareness and keeps inquiring, evaluating, and learning in each moment.

We begin by exploring the anatomical roadmaps of our own bodies, which teach us about our body's natural design, and our optimum state of being. In practice, we use a combination of breathing, self-massage, fascia-balancing, and PNF techniques to re-establish or strengthen natural alignment and movement patterning. Our students learn to honor the body, warming-up, and preparing ahead of time before undertaking a challenging practice. Having a deep understanding of the anatomy of the human structure, the nervous system, and the biomechanics of movement helps one to gravitate toward poses that assist in joint stabilization and real life functionality.

Right-Angle Poses Do Not Follow Nature's Design

We spend untold hours performing mental tasks while sitting in positions that distort our spine into a C-shape. Most of us sit with poor posture, compressing our spine and restricting the movements of our diaphragm. As our muscles work hard to hold our body in unnatural positions, these dysfunctional posture patterns eventually become normalized. The nervous system then encodes these patterns, the fascia thickens, and the resultant habituation encourages shallow breathing and chronic misalignment. This process is unconscious and entirely involuntary. The first we may notice of the implications of this ingrained dysfunction may be back pain, muscle tightness, or joint strain. As these pain signals start telling us we need to do something different, some people will try massage, while some will try chiropractors or prescription medications. Others embark on exercise programs in which certain poses are suggested for the stretching of the specific sore or painful area, without regard for the structure as a whole.

As we have learned, yoga poses best serve us when they help us reverse the detrimental effects of sitting. Yet many yoga practices *insist* that we must repeatedly practice forward-bends with straight legs—or that we must sit with a straight back—the very postural positioning created by sitting that is causing our discomfort in the first place. There are no straight lines in nature; all of creation is formed of, and exists in, round and spiraling shapes. Where is the sense in going against nature's design and performing poses that have more to do with *sitting* and less to do with our natural movement patterning?

In the effort to address back pain, many positions are suggested that try to alleviate that pain through toe-touching exercises, done in a seated or standing forward-bend with the legs held straight. Unfortunately, stretching out tight back muscles by sitting with straight legs and leaning forward can wind up causing more damage to a sore back; anytime we keep both legs straight and position our trunk at a right angle to our legs, we are jeopardizing the health of our spine and hindering our chances of healing. The back is sore in the first place because the front of the body is either weak and shortened or strong and shortened. In either case, bending forward to stretch out the back is like robbing Peter to pay Paul: as you bend over to stretch out the back, you are in fact further shortening the front line, which leads you right back to the same back pain you are seeking to eliminate. Spine alignment that is functional will prevent back pain and heal injuries. In YogAlign we seek the same alignment principles in every pose, which create muscular forces of extension through our breathing that align our spine into optimal posture. These conscious actions serve as a warranty against injury and lead to posture that is functional and fluid, and that happens without us having to think about it. Whether you are standing, sitting or reclining, poses that compress the spine and reverse the spine's natural curves jeopardize the longevity and vitality of the body's structure. We need to keep a neutral spine in all yoga poses, training our brain to direct our body into natural alignment, no matter our activity or body position.

The "Plow Pose" is another example of an anatomically-questionable body position, much like straight-legged seated or forward bending positions. The "Plow Pose" puts the neck and lower-back spine in dangerous compression by reversing the angle of the spine's natural curves, all the while engaging muscular actions to hold the spine in that compromised position. The "Plow Pose" also places body weight upon a fragile neck area that is bent at a right angle, and that is not designed to support the weight of the lower body. This pose not only looks uncomfortable, it is extremely dangerous, as it can cause compression fractures and/or herniation of the discs along the neck as well as along the entire spine. Another infrequently mentioned danger is the overstretching of the nerves and ligaments of the spine, which can lead to deep structural imbalances that disable the forces that hold us together.

> **❝**One of the few exercises known to modern man where you can injure your neck and back while sustaining a stroke, all in one maneuver, is the yoga plow. The plow puts inordinate stretch and stress on the blood vessels to the brain and the upper spinal cord, and as a result, strokes have occurred because the circulation to the brain or spinal cord was cut off.**❞**
>
> Dominquez and Gajda, *Total Body Training.*

Many people practice poses like the yoga "Plow" or the "Shoulder Stand" placing the entire weight of the body on the neck or cervical spine. These poses are considered by many to be safe when assisted with yoga props, however this is still anatomically questionable, according to biomechanical experts. I personally consider these poses to be so dangerous that I will not demonstrate them— nor will I allow others in my class or teacher trainings to do so—thus when assembling this book I chose to illustrate these poses using drawings instead of photos. The anatomical reality is that the neck spine is simply not designed to be placed at a right angle while holding the weight of the entirety of the body that exists below the neck. The physical danger and obvious liability issues stemming from these unsafe poses are the major reasons that some health clubs and yoga studios do not permit "Plow" and "Shoulder Stand" to be taught. However, many teachers continue to instruct students to do the "Plow" and the "Shoulder Stand", believing that the possible benefits (such as stimulating the thyroid) outweigh the risks involved.

There is no question that inverting the body is beneficial but not if it is done at the expense of the health and stability of the spinal structure. Many doctors and sports medicine therapists have been warning people for years about the dangers of these types of poses. Yet many people continue to believe that these poses are safe, because they have been told that the poses are ancient practices that have stood the test of time. A recent book, however, refutes the assertion that modern asana is based on ancient practices, and the information this researcher found may spur a re-evaluation of the assumed sanctity and safety of some popular yoga poses.

The book, entitled *Yoga Body*, was written by historian and yoga practitioner Mark Singleton, who received a grant from the University of Cambridge to research the origins of modern postural yoga poses. According to the research in *Yoga Body*, instead of being the fruit of thousands of years of spiritual tradition, yoga poses were actually hugely influenced by contortionists, British Army calisthenics, and women's stretching and gymnastic exercises of the late-Nineteenth and early-Twentieth centuries.

Contrary to popular belief, Singleton found no evidence that proves that the way in which yoga poses are commonly practiced dates back thousands of years, or that this method of practice even stems directly from the ancient teachings of the Yoga Sutras. In fact, yoga postures as practiced today actually emerged from a variety of disciplines and movements which swept across Europe in the wake of the Industrial Revolution. With mechanization creating less physical activity for the masses, people began to worry about the demise of the physical and moral fitness of men, and many set out to create religiously-oriented physical exercises that would elevate the spiritual and bodily steadfastness of their practitioners, even as the world around them was experiencing fundamental change.

For this reason, many societies of the late 1800's saw religion being combined with exercise, spawning fitness movements such as "spiritual calisthenics" and "muscular Christianity." It was in this time period that the famous YMCA was founded, which sought to combine physical fitness and religion through an ideology of the union of "body, mind and spirit." At the same time that these movements were sweeping across Europe, India's yogis were also being influenced by these disciplines, which were incorporated into the nascent Indian Nationalist movements that called upon individuals to be fit and powerful, readying themselves to be part of the possible uprising against British Rule. The Yoga poses and sun salutations that have developed during

the last 50 to 100 years are, in actuality, a combination of ancient yoga philosophy and this modern physical culture.

There is much evidence that the yogis of yesterday and today are able to control heartbeat and to achieve almost superhuman feats of strength and flexibility, and often display mental powers beyond ordinary waking consciousness such as precognition and lucid dreaming. Yogis have achieved fame for being able to go without food and water for long periods of time, in order to gain control over the body and the senses, freeing themselves into trance-like states in which they can access higher realms of consciousness. In their view, the body is simply a shell that is cast off when we leave this world, and there are claims that many yogis can and do leave their body at will.

In some sects of yoga, the body and its needs became something to conquer. Prolonged fasting, austere diets and even sexual abstinence have been used by yogis for centuries to try to get beyond the physical and make a connection with divine consciousness. There are many accounts of Yogis who sit for hours in deep meditative states, denying the needs of the body and the psyche, and not interacting with the outer world. There is the standard example of the yogi lying on a bed of nails or living naked in a cold cave in the Himalayas, relying on developing internally-produced body heat to keep warm. Another one of the ways the yogis tried to express their domination over the body was through the practice of poses that were extremely difficult, such as putting their feet behind their heads, or standing just on their head without any assistance from their arms. Strikingly similar to contortionism, many yogis sought to overpower the body by making it do positions that seemed impossible.

Just because yogis have done or are doing these poses does not mean they are safe or that they are biomechanically correct for the human body. I regret to say that I have spent a great deal of time in my life doing yoga poses that did not feel comfortable, and yet I persisted because I believed that the pain was some kind of weakness and the pose would make my body more open. As a result of my former practices, I have spent countless hours healing myself (and others) from yoga injuries, all the while trying to figure out why we were getting hurt. With millions in the world practicing yoga, it is crucial that people use discernment and get educated about both the history and mechanics of yoga poses, to make sure that they engage only in body positions that are safe and functional. With yoga injuries happening in epidemic numbers, it is important to evaluate and be informed about what is safe for your body. For these reasons, I have spent the last 20 years developing a hatha yoga style that would be effective, safe, and comfortable. There are others now sharing their stories about their yoga injuries and the dangers of poses like the king of asanas—the headstand.

Yoga teacher Patricia Sullivan wrote an account of the neck damage that she suffered from the long-time practice of headstands. Her article, which was published in the Nov. 2010 issue of *Yoga Journal*, talks about the nerve damage she incurred by practicing "Headstand" for 10 minutes a day, ignoring all of the pain and the signals from her body that the pose was not beneficial. At last Patricia had a doctor examine her and they found "extensive damage, including a reversed cervical curve, disk degeneration, and bony deposits that were partially blocking nerve outlets." By her own admission, "my longing to excel both in my asana practice and as an asana teacher had led me to ignore my body's signals and cries for relief."

I commend Patricia for speaking the truth and for alerting people to the hidden dangers of prolonged headstand practice. It just makes sense to avoid inverted poses that position the weight of the lower body above the skull and neck area. To be safe, in a YogAlign practice, we suggest using yoga wall ropes, a hip swing or inversion table when you want to invert the entire body. Doing a downward dog or a bent-knee forward-bend can also give you a great inversion of the trunk and traction of the neck area, without the risk of more aggressive inverted poses. You can also use a headstand lift if you want to go upside-down.

Many people enjoy the headstand and may be surprised to learn of Patricia's injury, which occurred as a cumulative result of years of practice. Others would not dream of even *trying* a headstand. But what about the poses that are not so obviously dangerous? What about those poses that don't feel very comfortable, but which we do anyway, harboring a belief that there will be some benefit that will occur later on?

In the same way that chair sitting compresses our spines, many yoga poses are built upon sitting in right-angled positions that strain the integrity of our spine and pelvis. Many commonly-practiced yoga positions can create serious injuries to nerves, tendons, discs and vertebrae in this way. The long-term serious (but less apparent) effects of these positions include increased tension in our body, and the joint destabilization

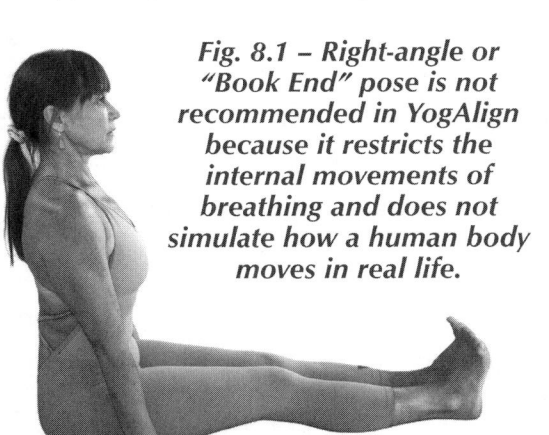

Fig. 8.1 – Right-angle or "Book End" pose is not recommended in YogAlign because it restricts the internal movements of breathing and does not simulate how a human body moves in real life.

that can occur with repeated practice. If a pose makes your spine lose its naturally good posture, the pose can be causing the same problems created by slouching; the pose may even engage the fight-or-flight response in your nervous system, particularly if the belly is artificially held-in in order to execute the position.

Our bodies are designed to move, and we never move without having to bend at least one knee; yet many yoga and flexibility exercises direct us to try and bend over while keeping our knees straight. Keeping both knees straight goes against the natural function and design of our body, which is constructed for engaging movement through voluntary contraction of muscles that create a bend in our knees for ambulation. Even though we have this built-in design feature, about 35 percent of yoga poses use what I call the "bookend" or "driving with the parking brake on" template, shown in **Fig. 8.1**. When we do these types of poses, our anterior spine compresses and our sacrum ligaments are overstretched, leading to a gradual weakening of the natural sacral platform that is needed to provide shock absorption for the spine. Similarly, sitting poses that require the toes to be extended toward the shin while keeping both knees straight actually contract not just the foot muscles but the whole superficial front line of the body, from the top of the feet to the jaw-area of the skull. When the forces in the front body are chronically contracted, the back line responds by engaging a line of pull to counterbalance the shortness in the front. The fulcrum point of tension in this body position is the lower back and sacral area. Another frequent by-product of this type of compartmentalized stretching is compression of the lumbar discs and sacrum and/or overstretching of the ligaments, undermining the complex structural support provided by the spine, sacrum, hips and pelvic floor. When one is hyper-mobile and easily flexible, years of practice in these poses can lead to hip and knee replacement surgeries. In "tighter" folks, there may be persistent discomfort — and in the long run the possibility of disc herniation or nerve compression — leading to sciatica and hip pain.

Here is an important point to remember: Sitting on the floor with our legs straight, or trying to bend over from standing with the knees locked, has the potential to weaken and compress the spine, as well as reinforce the postural and breathing dysfunctions perpetuated by time spent sitting in a chair.

FLEXIBILITY CAN BE A LIABILITY

When we straighten both legs with our trunk bending over at a right angle to the legs, the discs in the front of the spine are compressed, the sacrum ligaments are stretched, and the sacral stabilization platform is flattened. If you are really flexible and the pose seems easy, you may be unaware that you are overstretching your sacral ligaments, causing eventual instability to the sacrum, which is the human body's important shock-absorbing structure. When the sacral platform is destabilized, there is no tone in the buttocks, the spine loses its shock-absorbing, youth-perpetuating curves, and the tailbone is tucked under in what I call the "wounded puppy" position.

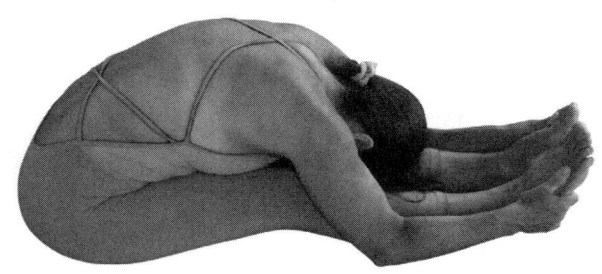

Fig. 8.2 – Seated forward bends overstretch the ligaments of the spine and sacrum while compressing the anterior portion of the spinal column.

When the highly-flexible person repeatedly performs straight-legged forward-bends, **(Fig. 8.2)**, the sacral ligaments get over-stretched. There is hidden danger here for "bendy" people because there may be no pain to sound a warning that ligament-stretching is causing harm. Over time, performing these poses may cause a sagging of the sacrum, and the eventual destabilization of the entire sacral platform.

However, for those following the YogAlign method, there is an obvious warning signal in this pose: the practitioner will not be able to take a full, deep breath because of contracting forces created by the body position of spinal flexion. This contraction—created when bending forward—restricts the inhalation or extension movements of the diaphragm and rib cage, and essentially creates a muscular fascia pattern that compresses our deep infrastructures and the inner forces of breath. In this way, through this pose we wind up emphasizing the contraction of the front body, instead of the extension of the entire body as a whole.

> **❝***The function of the sacral ligaments, like all other ligaments in the body, is to provide support for joints. It is especially important that the sacroiliac ligaments are not overstretched in the practice of asana.*❞
>
> Lasater, *Yoga Body: Anatomy, Kinesiology, and Asana*

In **Fig. 8.2**, notice how the natural curves of the lumbar spine are flattened when the legs are straight and the pelvis is tilted in a posterior fashion. This pose compresses the spine and the discs, pulls the sternum towards the pubic bone, tightens the hips and pelvic floor, and destabilizes the sacrum. The sacral angle is affected by how the legs are positioned because the fascia lines connect the entire back body from the bottom of the feet to the top of the legs, then all the way up the back and over the head to the eyebrows. When we extend our toes back towards the shin while sitting with straight legs, the entire front of the body is shortened from head to toe. This puts strain on the back line to balance the shortening of the front. You cannot stretch your legs in this manner without it adversely affecting your entire body.

Leaning over with a rounded spine to stretch out your back is like digging a hole in the sand. The more you stretch forward without the natural spinal curves intact, the more insistently you are wiring your muscles to pull you into poor posture. You may feel a temporary release of tension in the back after doing this pose, but the pain soon returns, much like sand sliding back into and filling the hole. Remember that the back is sore because the muscular forces in the front body are either weak and tight or strong and tight, and the sore back is a byproduct of the body's attempt to counterbalance this tugging upon the fascial pulleys in the superficial front line. The answer to relieving back pain lies in creating a strong breathing process that is achieved through the activation of the forces of the deep core line. Once you have cultivated this strong breathing process, you no longer crave stretching or have back pain, because the forces of extension in your body which are linked to the movements of breath become your central support system. You no longer have tense back or neck muscles, because your body has developed internal forces that naturally support fluid movement and natural spine alignment.

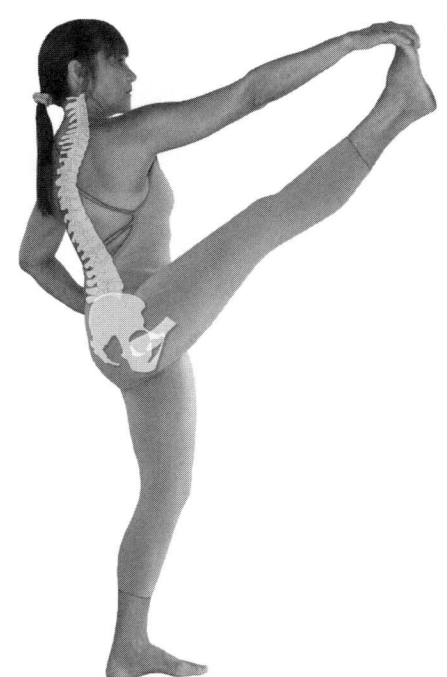

Fig. 8.3A

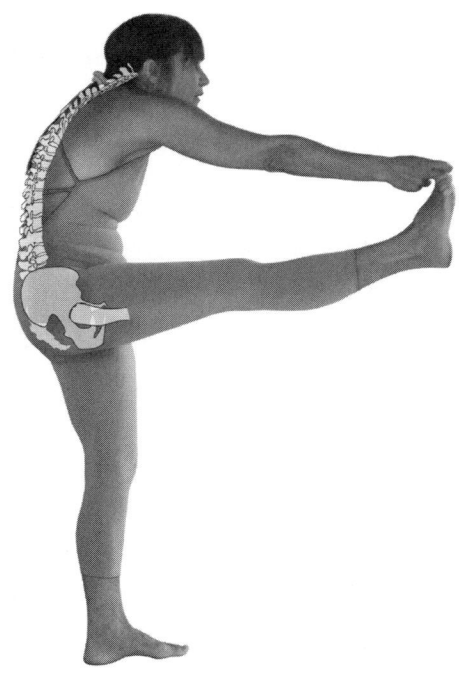

Fig. 8.3B

DON'T BE INFLEXIBLE IN YOUR BELIEFS ABOUT YOUR OWN FLEXIBILITY

Many people think they are not flexible if they cannot lean over and touch the floor while keeping their legs straight. We don't walk, run or swim with straight legs, so why do we think we aren't flexible if we can't keep our knees straight when bending over? Our body is designed to move, and we move with bent knees. It is much more biomechanically advantageous to exercise with bent knees, and to engage movement from the center of the body for power and extension.

In YogAlign, we avoid poses that position us out of naturally-aligned good posture and instead focus on basic functional movement positions that maintain the balanced tensegrity of all fascial lines, in support of the structure as we use it in the movements of daily life. There is really only one pose in YogAlign, and that is the pose of good posture; it is the template for all standing, sitting, inverting, reclining, lunging or twisting poses. **Figure 8.3A** shows balanced front and back fascia lines, running from head to toe. We seek to have fascial balance and natural alignment in every pose using good posture, utilizing the least amount of effort to keep the inner body fluid.

In yoga and exercise classes, we are sometimes told to pull in our navel, tuck under our tailbones, and straighten our spines. In many cases these outside adjustments waste a lot of energy, and compress the very infrastructure we are trying to engage. It makes no sense to attempt yoga or fitness poses that cause us to lose the curvature of our natural spinal design, as in **Fig. 8.3B**. A healthy spine has curves that provide support for posture, movement, and shock absorption. Pressing the lower back to the floor or rounding the upper back to make it possible to grab your toe is what many people do to get more flexible. It may seem like a way to stretch the pain out of your aching back, but that move in and of itself recreates the very position that is causing the pain in the first place.

According to Roger Cole, a well-known yoga teacher specializing in yoga anatomy and in the prevention of yoga injuries, one of the most common injuries in yoga is to the sacrum. My work has shown that this is primarily due to the right-angle positions that permeate so much of modern yoga asana. In order to be comfortable in the body and to increase authentic flexibility, we need to move and position the body in ways that imitate real life function and alignment, and which are based on stabilization principles that protect the integrity of our joints and ligaments.

> **"**Asana variations help us achieve maximum gain and minimum effort by intelligently addressing our physical needs.**"**
>
> Desikachar, *Heart of Yoga*

In this quote, Desikachar is reminding us to ask ourselves an important question in Yoga asana: Are we intelligently addressing our individual body needs? Does it make sense to assume uncomfortable positions in the hopes that we will somehow, someday be comfortable? If we are not comfortable right now, we are not going to be comfortable later. In order to be "comfortable," yoga poses must imitate how we move in daily life, and *no one* can walk around with both knees straight and get very far, as it is akin to driving with the parking brake on.

If you are still unsure about the sensibility of keeping the knees straight in yoga poses, stand up and keep your knees from bending as you try to walk around the room. Sense how your entire body feels when you do this. Where does the compression go? Do you feel how the tension and compression affects the alignment of the sacrum? Does this really feel like an intelligent use of the human body?

Take a moment to consider the pose shown in **Fig. 8.4A.**

Although he may be trying to do so, Zack will never get flexible by sitting with both of his legs straight. Instead, he is compressing his anterior spinal discs, while increasing the front line muscle/fascia shortness that overtaxes the muscles along the back line and holds them in a chronic state of tension. Notice how the curves of Zack's spine are reversed. **Figure 8.4B** shows this seated posture photo rotated to standing, revealing that no matter how you do it, bending forward with straight legs compresses the spinal curves. Seated or standing, Zack's spine is compressed and he clearly

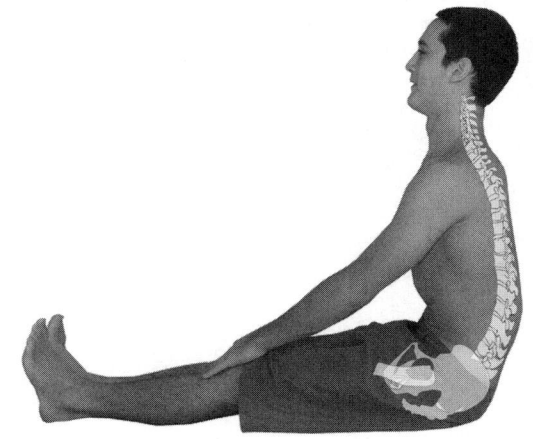

Fig. 8.4A – Zack is not comfortable here and his spine is definitely compressed and in an unstable position.

has bad posture. It's in opposition to the health of our spine to sit on the floor in a straight-leg pose because we are not designed for this; we are designed to squat, walk, and run and in these, as in all of our movements, bent knees are a vital part of the alignment equation. Whether we are exercising or working, we are doing damage to our spines if we are not properly engaging our four spinal curves.

YOGALIGN PERFECTS YOUR POSTURE

YogAlign practice encourages ease and economy in our movement, with poses designed around naturally-aligned positions that engage our muscles from the core and stabilize our joints. In YogAlign, the entire body is engaged, with all fascia lines in balance, so that every pose feels effortless. The nervous system and body then memorize this engagement, and the result is an aligned, extended, and balanced posture that becomes intrinsic and automatic.

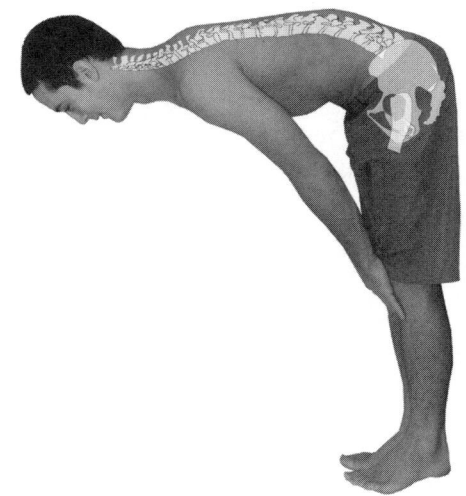

Fig. 8.4B – Seated posture from Fig. 8.4A turned to standing reveals another familiar yoga pose in the book end position that is so unnatural for the human spine.

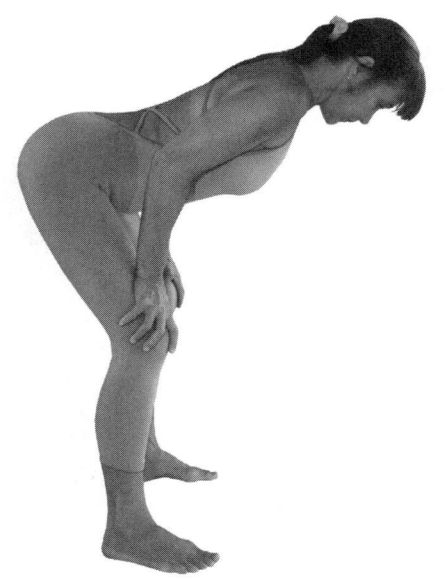

Fig. 8.4C - "Half-Forward Bend" YogAlign style has knees bent and spinal curves in neutral.

"An aligned and balanced body has no need for either extreme strength or flexibility yet has more than enough of each to function in all activities of daily living. This natural strength and flexibility can be maintained with little effort well into old age. Real flexibility comes about through the capacity of bones to inter–relate by way of mobile joints that are moved by elastic muscles in a natural way. This does not come about by indiscriminate stretching of specific muscles at the expense of the integrity of the spine."

Porter, *Ageless Spine, Lasting Health*

EXPERIENTIAL EXERCISE #18

Right-Angle vs. "The Spine Aligner"

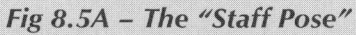

Lie on the floor on your back, knees bent. Begin by exhaling slowly. Deeply inhale using a Core SIP Breath. Take a long, deep breath and AS you breathe in, pay attention to how long you can engage in the inhalation process. Come up and sit on the floor with your legs straight out in front of you as in the "Staff Pose" shown in **Fig 8.5A**. Pull your toes towards your shins, reaching through your heels and try to keep upright with your spine and trunk.

Once again, inhale with the SIP Breath and notice how long your inhalation lasts. Notice how the contraction of the muscles in the top of your feet creates a tightness that travels to the belly area, immobilizing the ribs and diaphragm and inhibiting your ability to take a full, deep, and easy breath.

Fig 8.5A – The "Staff Pose"

From the same floor-seated position, place your feet hip-distance apart and bend your knees as in Spine Aligner, **Fig. 8.5B**. Spread your toes and press through the ball of each foot as though you are pushing on gas pedals. Place your hands behind your back as shown in **Fig. 8.5B**, and once again take a full, and deep Core SIP Breath. Notice how much longer you can inhale and how much easier it is to breathe when your feet and knees are in positions that simulate how you engage them in real life movement.

You may find it difficult to hold the "Spine Aligner" very long at first, but don't let yourself fall into poor posture trying to hold yourself up. If you have difficulty, you can also do this pose while sitting on the edge of a chair instead of the floor. Engage the position in short intervals until you have built adequate core strength. You can also support yourself in this position by holding a strap attached to a wall, pole or doorknob in front of you.

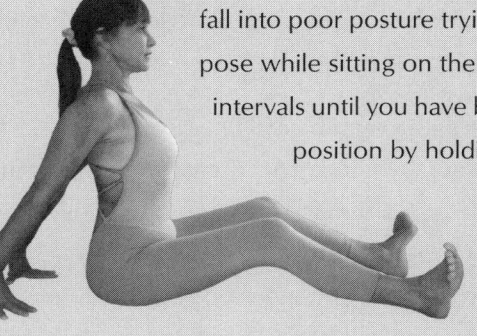

Fig. 8.5B – "Spine Aligner" pose simulates how the body moves in real life allowing the movements of inhalation to happen with ease.

Remember to do the core breathing technique–The Core Sip Breath to align your spine from the inside out, especially if the pose feels strained. Keep in mind that what you do is not as important as how you are aligned and how well you can breathe when you do it. You should always be able to take a full, deep breath without a feeling of restriction in the movements of the rib cage or diaphragm area.

So what did we learn from comparing the standard straight-legged yoga position with YogAlign's "Spine Aligner" position? As you experienced, the simple acts of straightening your legs and extending your toes toward your shins impeded not only your ability to maintain natural alignment, but also your fundamental ability to breathe in a deep and natural way.

Because we are designed to move—walk, run, and dance—we must bend our knees to ambulate anywhere; therefore we must also bend our knees for our exercise to be functional. In YogAlign, we keep our knees bent and focus on engaging our core muscles as stabilizers, instead of making the abs "tight" or contracting the pelvic floor in order to achieve what *we have been led to believe* is our core strength. Learning to activate the core muscles as stabilizers is *the most important skill we can learn* when it comes to protecting our spine and functionally activating our core.

The spine should always have its natural curves engaged in all yoga and exercise poses, especially if you are tightening or contracting muscles around the spinal column. Compression of the spine while exercising causes serious injuries and engages support from the extremities, leading to structural and neuromuscular imbalances. The "Spine Aligner" (**Fig. 8.5B**) maintains the natural curves of the spine, while at the same time encouraging core muscle stabilization, fascial opening and functional balanced strength. Freeing the spine and allowing the natural curves encourages deep breathing and fundamental stability that does not stretch ligaments or compress discs. The exercise is effective, beneficial, and comfortable.

Remember: You will not get comfortable by being uncomfortable. In YogAlign we teach that if you are not comfortable now, you are certainly not going to be comfortable later, so it is vitally important to listen to and honor your body's signals.

DOWNWARD DOG MISCONCEPTIONS

The traditional yoga pose "Downward Dog" is in reality just another right-angled pose, which can be uncomfortable and dangerous unless the heels are lifted, and the knees are kept softened or bent.

"Downward Dogs" can be **bad dogs.** The heels-down-knees-straight version of "Downward Dog" (**Figs. 8.6 A , B & C**) shows spinal compression through the lumbar-sacral region, and creates pressure on the neck and cervical spine by pushing the face towards the thighs. This position is also known to cause injuries to the wrists, shoulders and low back area. This is because the tendency in this pose is to stretch into the back of the knees or hang from the shoulder ligaments, rather than to engage from the core and keep the natural spinal curves. This "bad dog" version contributes to forward head carriage; weakening and overstretching of the shoulder, wrist, and knee joints; and compression of the lumbar spine and sacrum. Rotating these poorly aligned versions of "downward dog," 45-degrees, shows the body in essentially the same position as the seated right angle that compresses body function and movement.

Bad posture is hard work, and the ongoing strain of poor posture causes chronically-tense muscles,

"The Bad Dogs"

Each "bad dog" seen at left is shown rotated to a sitting position on the right. The rotated photos reveal the inherent poor postural alignment in these poses. Practicing the "bad dogs"-- with legs straight, and joints in lock-down--encourages joint overstretching, de-stabilization, and spinal compression.

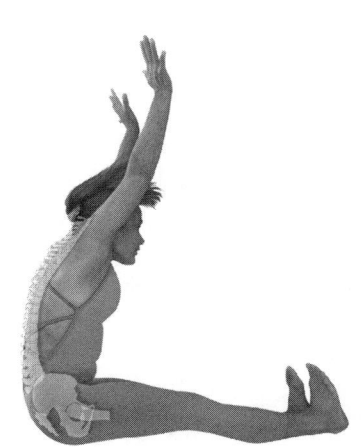

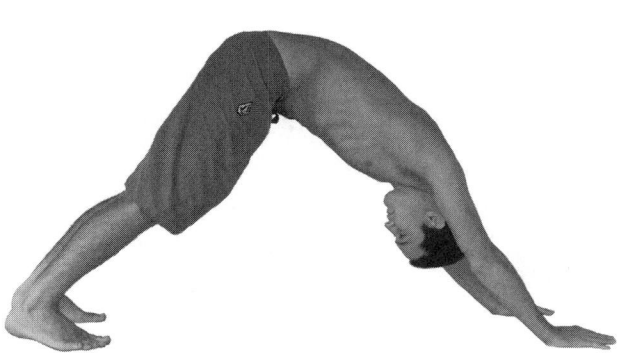

Fig. 8.6A – The "Shrugging Dog"

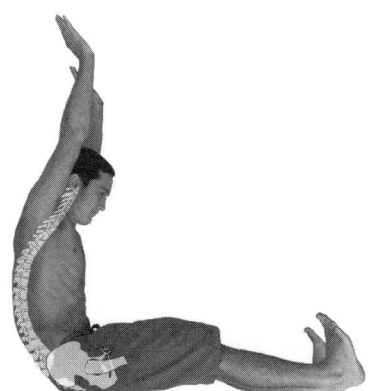

Fig. 8.6B – The "Spinal Compression Dog"

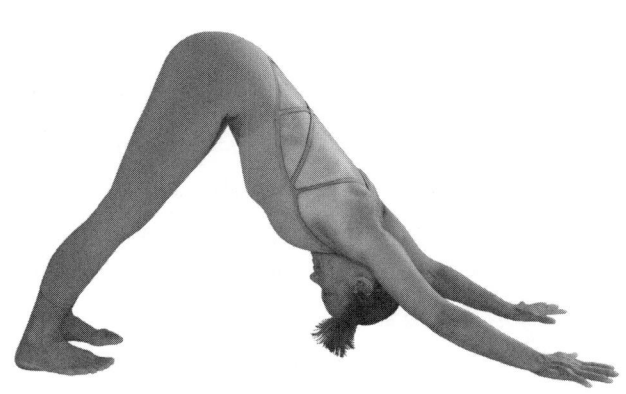

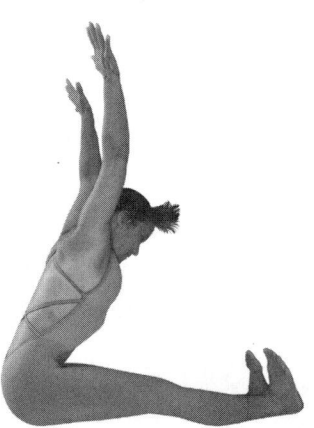

Fig. 8.6C – Shoulder hyper-extension thanks to the "Hanging from the Ligaments Dog"

thickened fascia tissue, and even feelings of depression and despair. When we have misalignment and tense muscles, we may constantly feel a need to stretch. If we stretch in a way that doesn't respect our body's natural movements, we can exacerbate our original bad posture, and we then get caught in a cycle of pain and stress. When the body is in alignment, there is very little tension in the body, and a pose can actually feel effortless. We then stretch because it feels good, rather than because we *need* to due to feelings of stiffness and tension.

YogAlign High Dog

The YogAlign version of "Downward Dog" is called "High Dog." In this version, the heels stay lifted as highly as possible, while continually pressing through the ball of the foot, spreading the toes, and engaging the arches (**Fig 8.7A**). The focus of the pose is concentrated on keeping the extension of the spine in its natural curves. (Those with backs that cannot retain the spine's natural curves in this position should keep their knees bent.) The sacrum stays naturally tilted in and up, with no pulling or pressure in the sacral ligaments. The head and neck are extended from the core, maintaining the same alignment that one would have if they were standing well with good posture. The upper arm-bone stays lifted, aligned, and in the socket, while the head is free to turn.

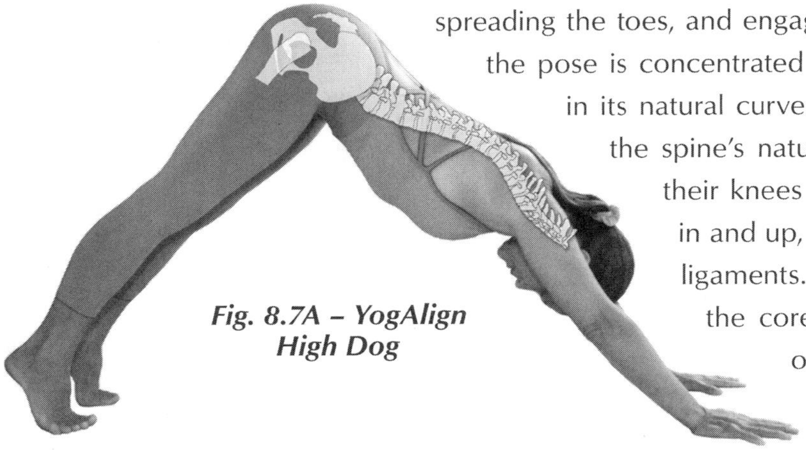

Fig. 8.7A – YogAlign High Dog

One should never push the face forward or drop the belly, chest, or shoulders down towards the floor or back towards the thighs. Many folks over stretch the shoulder ligaments in this pose causing a dangerous pattern of joint destabilization. Keeping the knees bent as in **Fig. 8.7B** helps to take pressure off of the spine and sacrum.

In YogAlign, we also practice a one-legged version of the classic "Down Dog" called "Core Dog." In this pose we keep the lifted-leg straightened and the standing leg bent (**Fig. 8.8A**). This activates the core trunk muscles and stabilizes natural spine alignment. Notice how the rotated photo of the "Core Dog" is essentially a sprinting or skating position, showing how this pose imitates real life movement.

With "Core Dog" rotated you can also see how this pose is essentially the same position as Part Three

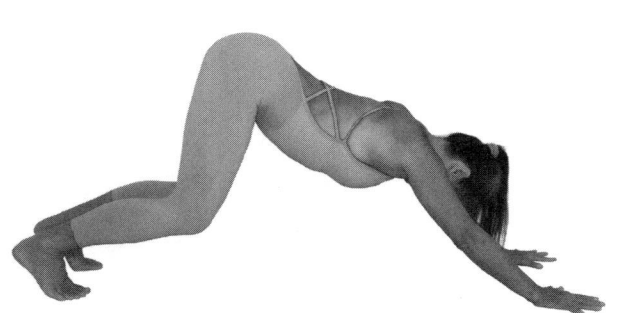

Fig. 8.7B – YogAlign Traction Dog

of the "Warrior Dance" series (shown in the Methods section of this book), in that both are standing, one-legged balancing poses. In each pose, the hips and sacrum are level, the foot is pointed, the standing leg is bent, and the fingers are wide open. The head is always in a neutral position relative to the rest of the spine, simulating how one would stand with good posture.

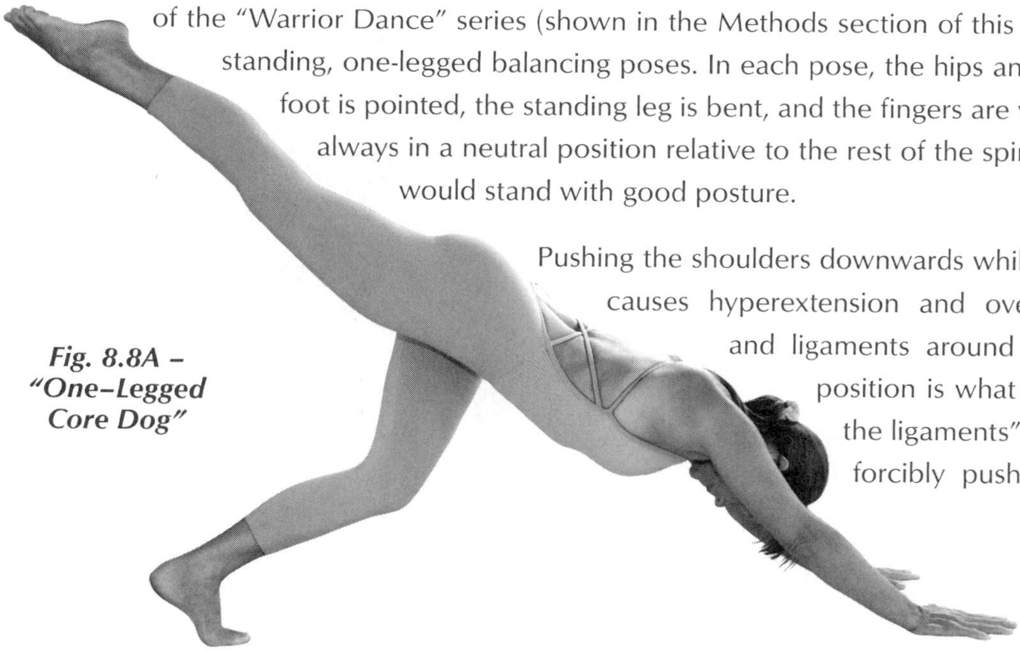

Fig. 8.8A – "One–Legged Core Dog"

Pushing the shoulders downwards while in "Downward Dog" causes hyperextension and overstretching of nerves and ligaments around the rotator cuff. This position is what we call "hanging from the ligaments" and the overly-flexible forcibly push the chest and heels down, utilizing very little core muscular effort. In daily movements, standing with the knees locked back and the chest thrust forward is considered postural dysfunction, but somehow, in "Downward Dog", it has become good form.

In many cases, relying upon the extremities to support the body—such as when "Downward Dog" is done with a rounded upper-back and lifted shoulders—is a result of poor breathing habits that keep the body in misalignment. These habits include lifting the shoulders on inhalation, or breathing in and protruding out with the belly, rather than letting the movement of the ribs lead the breathing process. Poor posture and breathing habits executed in exercise positions like these (or in the course of our daily lives) waste energy, and create structural imbalances that set us up for injuries, chronic pain and eventual joint deterioration.

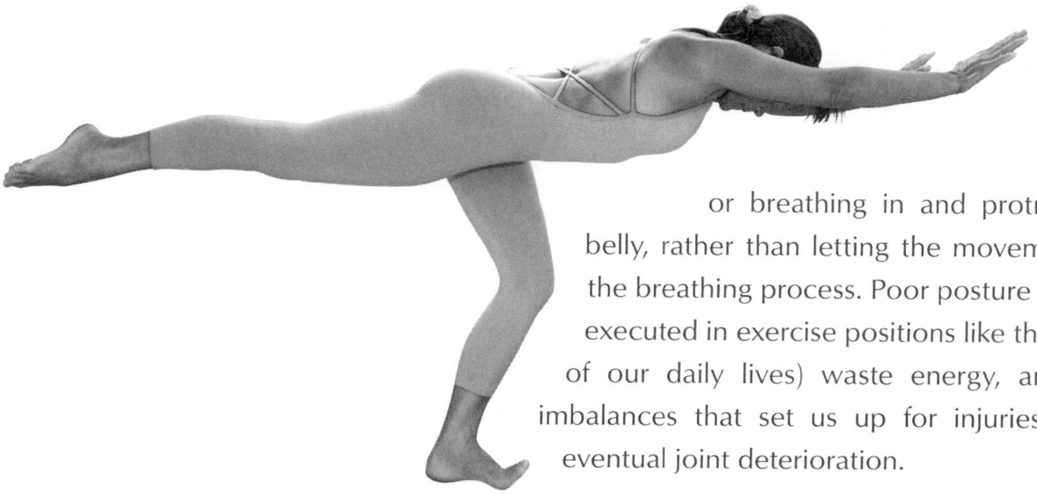

Fig. 8.8B – "One–Legged Core Dog," photo rotated.

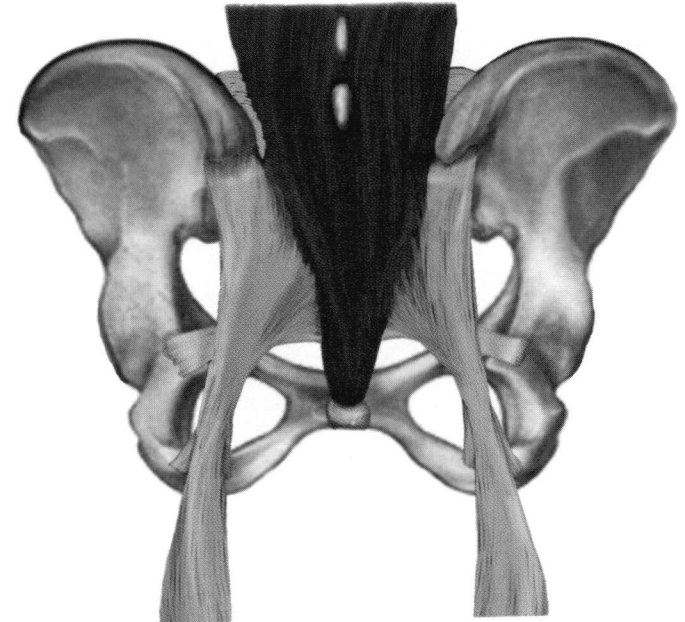

Fig. 8.9A – Sacrotuberous Ligament

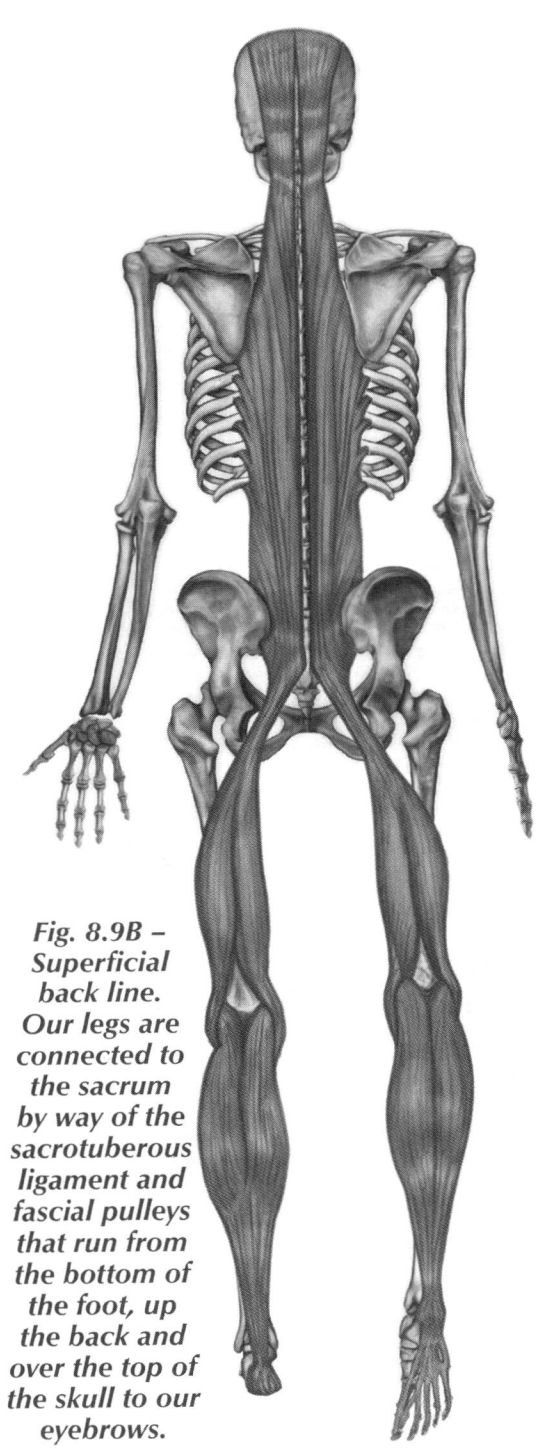

Fig. 8.9B – Superficial back line. Our legs are connected to the sacrum by way of the sacrotuberous ligament and fascial pulleys that run from the bottom of the foot, up the back and over the top of the skull to our eyebrows.

Redrawn from *Anatomy Trains* by Thomas Myers

Poor postural patterning and exercise programs that aggravate—and contribute to—a flat, compressed sacrum are dangerous to our sacral ligaments and spinal nerves. **Figure 8.9A** shows the sacrotuberous ligament connecting the spine and the legs. Exercises that stretch out sacral ligaments and nerves do more harm than good, as overstretching the sciatic nerve is actually a major cause of sciatica pain.

Many popular poses and exercises emphasize stretching out areas that are sore, rather than addressing the true source of the soreness, namely, poor breathing and postural habits, and overly-tense or weak spinal muscles. True healing of a sore back involves engaging the breathing process to direct internal core support, and developing alignment that respects the natural curves of the spine. Because our modern lifestyle involves so much sitting, most people are placing their bodies in right-angle-type poses all day long in their chairs, before they even get to yoga class.

THE STRAIGHT-LEG FORWARD BEND

As we have discovered, sitting with straight legs (**Fig. 8.10A**) while bending forward causes a fascial pull from head to toe that can lead to an overstretching of the pelvic and sacral ligaments needed for long term stability in our structure. These positions also shorten the muscles and fascia of the superficial front body. The core fascia line, which enables us to breathe efficiently, is not engaged functionally in the right-angle body position. What, then, is the benefit of poses that cut off the breathing process and compress the spine and internal organs in order to stretch the legs and back? Movements like these cannot change the underlying structural and postural deficiencies that allow these conditions to exist (**Fig. 8.10 A&B**). Instead, these poses exacerbate alignment and pain issues that are already present. They are an inefficient and compartmentalized attempt to gain flexibility that not only falls short, but can also cause harm or injury.

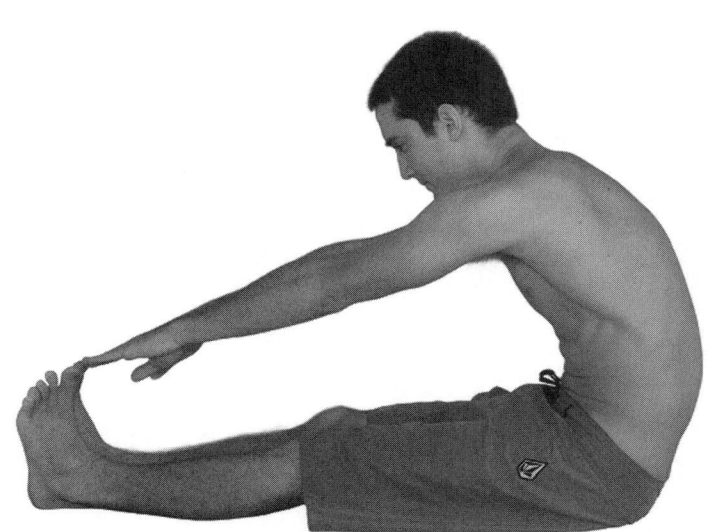

*Fig. 8.10A – Forward Bend.
It simply makes no sense
to shorten the front in order to stretch the back.*

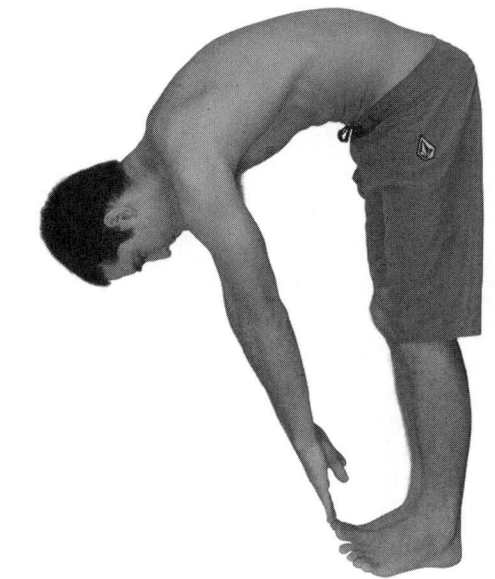

Fig. 8.10B – Rotating the same photo shows how poor the posture is whether we're sitting or standing.

Fig. 8.11B shows a pose called the "Common Forward Bend" in yoga and "Toe-Touching" in fitness classes. Done in a traditional manner, this maneuver eliminates the four natural curves of the spine and puts enormous strain on all of the structures in the lower back, stressing ligaments beyond their normal limits. The muscles of the back cannot give any support when you are toe-touching; you are actually stretching on—and hanging by—your ligaments. Toe-touching also puts a great deal of stress on the discs, and can cause ruptured discs in an adult who has an underlying disc problem.

However, this can be a safe and beneficial pose when it is done with the knees bent and the front spine extended (**Fig. 8.11A**). By inhaling as you lean over, the breathing muscles will naturally keep the spine in extension. Keeping length to the front spine facilitates full rib-cage breathing, and prevents compression of the discs in the lower back.

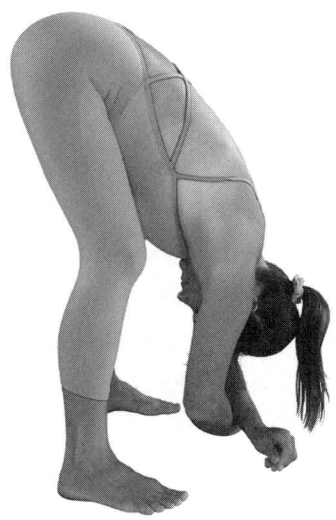

Fig. 8.11A– CORRECT:
YogAlign "Forward Bend"

Only when we recognize the realities of our anatomical design structure, and the power of natural alignment, can we engage in yoga and fitness in ways that will be truly beneficial, and never harmful.

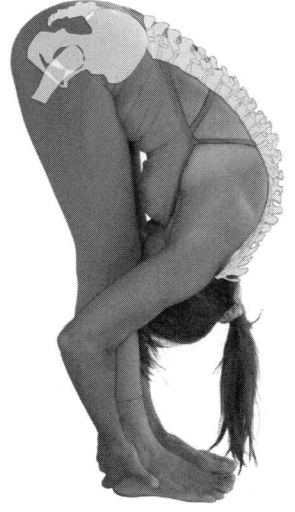

Fig. 8.11B – INCORRECT:
"Common Forward Bend"

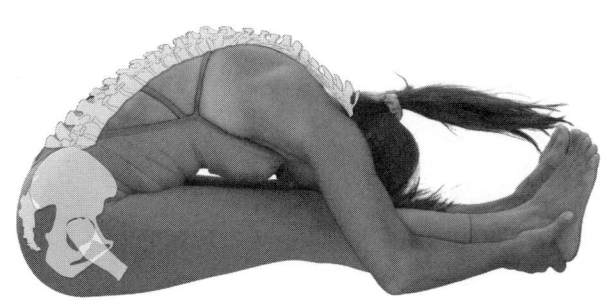

Fig 8.11C – INCORRECT:
"Forward Bend," photo rotated.
Straight-leg forward bends will compress the spine
and restrict the movement of your diaphragm,
whatever the position of your body.

> **❝***Toe-touching has been thought of as a good exercise to 'relax' or 'stretch' a tight back, but it does just the opposite. It will make your back muscles even tighter because of the strain.... You will get no benefit from this exercise, only pain – and you also risk serious injury in the process.***❞**

Dominquez and Gajda, *Total Body Training*

The YogAlign "Forward Bend" is executed with a strong inhale, knees bent, and the feet placed hip-width apart. In executing this pose, we bend over carefully, letting the internal movements of inhalation create extension in the spine. This protects the spinal discs from the excess pressure that can be generated by the action of bending forward, as both exhaling and leaning over cause a shortening of the anterior spine. We seek to provide an internal support for the spine through the focused movements of breathing. When bending over, the knees are always kept bent to protect the important ligament-stabilizing structures in the body. If one attempts to accomplish this pose with straightened knees, the "driving with the parking brake" action is invoked. This action creates body tension that inhibits breathing, and creates a fascial-tension that destabilizes the sacral platform and lumbar vertebrae. This is particularly dangerous when practiced across the span of many years, because ligament structures can slowly loosen, causing a loss of shock absorption mechanisms, which can lead to the compression of the hip socket and bursa of the knees. People with strong, tight hamstrings should keep their elbows on their thighs and avoid leaning all the way down without using their arms when they do this pose; this is *especially* important if there is a history of previous back injuries or surgery.

In the forward bend shown in **Fig. 8.11A**, pressure is relieved by keeping more weight on the inner edge of the feet, and not rolling into the outside of the heel. Rolling to the outside edge of your feet can cause fascial pulling that goes from the outer foot to the outer hip, contracting external rotators and pulling on the sacroiliac joint. Practicing a pose for an extended period without attention to proper foot alignment can cause chronic pain and destabilization of the sacrum and other distal parts of the body.

Life force, or "mana" as the Hawaiians call it, flows freely to the crown of the head in the YogAlign "Forward Bend." The curves of the neck are maintained in neutral and natural alignment. This alignment affords ease of breath, core engagement, and presence to the posture.

BENEFICIAL? OR DANGEROUS?

Throughout this book we have explored the paradox of how many yoga and fitness positions and poses seek to heal and strengthen, yet they consistently reverse the spine's natural curves, and place a huge amount of compression on the ligaments and joints. It is not true that "you need to feel pain to gain", or that "the pose begins when you want to come out of it." Pain is your body's way of telling you that the position is not natural. Use discernment and listen to your body.

With yoga injuries on the rise, it is imperative that we take a look at the biomechanics and common sense of what we are doing with our body. For instance, when we stretch ligaments in our sacrum, knees, and shoulders, we lose the necessary tension to hold our joints together. Stretching these ligaments can permanently destabilize a joint and cause compression in the hips and knees. As they age, many yoga practitioners who have overstretched their ligaments are now having hip and knee replacement surgeries. The years, hours and minutes spent overstretching ligaments in

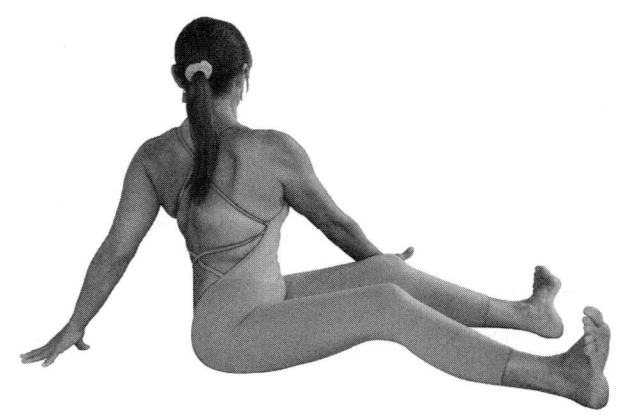

Fig. 8.12A – CORRECT:
The YogAlign "Spine Aligner Twist"

poses that reverse the spine and its natural curves are largely to blame. The sad part is that yogis are for the most part unaware of the potential dangers of stretching ligaments, and many still continue to teach others the very poses that have led them to pain, injuries and—in some cases—replacement surgeries. What is important is to practice the art of discernment, using both the brain and the body to make serious inquiries about the basic elements of yoga poses. In YogAlign we stress the importance of examining the risks, and adding modifications to poses to keep the body safe and naturally aligned.

Some people believe **Fig. 8.12B** is a beneficial twist, but look again. Engaging the body in this pose causes shortness of the superficial front line of fascia and locks in the back line, compressing the vertebral column. Straightening the leg causes the entire back line of fascia and muscle to contract. Even flexing the foot and reaching with the heel will shorten the front body, causing further locking in the back. This twist is cumulatively dangerous and leads to compression of the lumbar discs and overstretching of the ligaments connecting the sacrum from the spine to the hips. For these anatomical reasons, YogAlign seated twists are never practiced with one or both legs straightened.

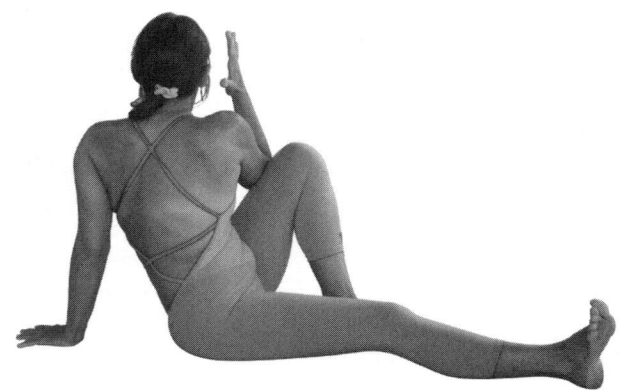

Fig. 8.12B – INCORRECT: "Seated Twist." This pose compresses discs, reverses the lumbar curve, and over stretches the ligaments connecting the hips to the sacrum.

The YogAlign "Spine Aligner Twist" (**Fig. 8.12A**) keeps the legs, hip, pelvis, and spine in an anatomically-neutral position, leaving the spine and ribs free to rotate without compression. Keep spinal twists simple, with knees bent to retain natural body design and fascia line functioning.

Be aware that putting your feet into a "braking" position pulls on lines of fascia that can compress your spine and inhibit your breathing process. When doing any pose, make sure to use foot positions that simulate how you move; natural movement involves rolling off of the ball of your foot in what we call the "stepping on the gas" foot position. Do this by spreading your toes wide while pressing through the ball of the foot rather than extending out with your heel, which restricts breathing.

In many versions of yoga "Sun Salutations", people routinely press their palms together above their heads **Fig. 8.13B.** When trying to touch the palms together, many people have to initiate from the fingertips or upper shoulders instead of moving and breathing from the center of the body.

Under these circumstances, the shoulder girdle is over-lifted and the shoulder has

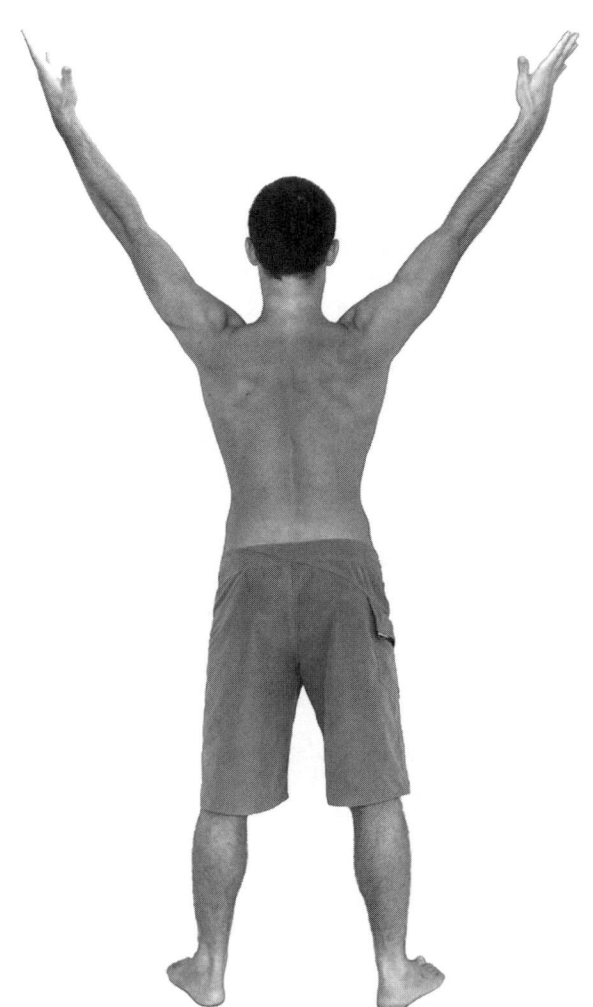

Fig. 8.13A – "Natural Shoulder Alignment"

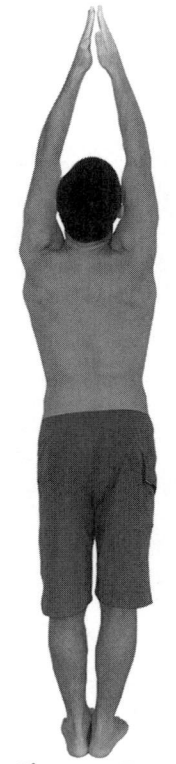

Fig. 8.13B – Unnatural Shoulder Alignment

to roll forward to allow the palms to touch together. The upper trapezius muscles have to initiate this movement and there is a disconnect from the optimal initiation of movement from the center of the body. There is also a tendency for the neck and lumbar spine to shorten and compress, accentuating forward head carriage in many people, particularly wide-shouldered strong men.

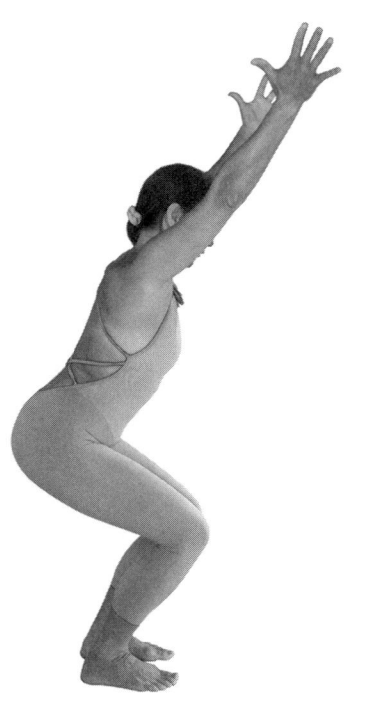

Fig. 8.14 –
YogAlign "Lightening Bolt"

ARM EXTENSION FROM YOUR INNER CORE

Try reaching up with your hands together as in the basic "Sun Salutation" shown in **Fig. 8.13B**. Begin to inhale using the Core SIP Breathing technique. Can you breathe with ease? Or do you feel restrictions in the breathing process? Now place the hands apart, as in **Fig. 8.14,** making sure you keep your arms shoulder-width apart and your fingers wide-open. Again, practice the Core SIP Breathing technique, and notice how different your breathing feels when you change the position of your hands. Your body is far better-served in functional fitness if your arms are kept apart, pulled in to the socket and engaged to the core—rather than reaching up and out—when practicing poses that require the arms to be lifted, as shown in **Fig. 8.13 A&B** and **Fig. 8.14**.

Remember, it is important to use discernment to determine if a pose allows for movement and breathing to originate from the center of the body. Always ask yourself: Is this position stable and comfortable?

EXPERIENTIAL EXERCISE #19

YogAlign Lightening Bolt

Try this pose with your feet and hands in line with your shoulders, and your fingers spread wide open (**Fig. 8.14**). Draw your arms deeply into the socket, stabilizing your shoulder blades and keeping your shoulders drawing down away from your ears. Do not lift your chin. Practice a deep Core SIP Breath when you inhale and notice the movements of breathing in your body.

Next, try the pose with the fingers tightly closed together instead of wide open. Use the Core SIP Breath again and notice how even this small effort in the periphery affects core movements of breathing, all the way back to the rib cage.

You do not use your hands functionally with your fingers tightly closed together. Keeping the fingers open wide frees up our deeper structures. It serves many of us to keep the movements of extension strong in the fingers in order to avoid the contraction process that occurs with aging and overengagement of the extremities in yoga or fitness exercises.

Another common mistake made during yoga practice is to lift the chin and lead movement with the front of the throat. This strains and tightens the muscles in the back of the neck and cuts off the flow of energy from the cranium through the spine to the lower body, as well as magnifies the postural problem of over-tensing the muscles in the back of the neck while leading from the throat. (**Fig. 8.15A**). The spine is a continuum: if you compress and flatten the *lordodic*, or convex, curve in the neck, you do the same to the lower back curve. You cannot achieve proper alignment throughout the lower back spine without paying attention to the alignment in your neck.

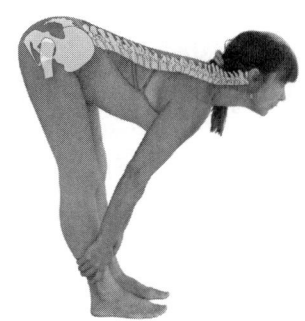

Fig. 8.15A – INCORRECT: Half–Forward Bend

When lifting the chin there is also an over-contraction of the suboccipital muscles. These muscles are connected to fascia lines which surround the fascia sheath or *dura mater* of the brain. The suboccipital muscles are also intrinsically connected to the movement of our eyeballs, and our vision center in the brain is located in the occipital region. Abnormal head positioning can cause strain and tension of the

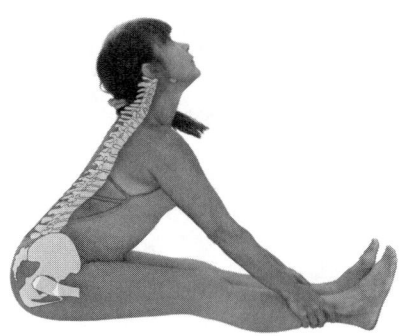

Fig. 8.15B – INCORRECT: "Half-Forward Bend", photo rotated.

suboccipital muscles and often they remain in a chronically contracted state. Tension in the suboccipital region is a major factor in headaches, eye strain, bone spurs and eventual deterioration of the facet joints in the neck. Focusing on keeping the muscles of the eyeballs relaxed as one moves the head is an important skill and one that many of us do not fully understand. *Try looking up strongly with both eyes and then begin to bend over as you retain the effort to look up. You will feel how tension in the eyes strains the suboccipital muscles in the back of the neck and lower skull area.*

Many people have a difficult time letting go of this chin-lifting habit, especially if they have done thousands of "Sun Salutations" in which they lift their chins over and over, every time they lift up their arms. Even if you keep your shoulders away from your ears (as well-trained teachers will suggest), it is nearly impossible to touch your hands overhead without over-contracting your upper trapezius and lifting the shoulders up to get your hands together. Lifting the chin and looking up repeatedly is a strain and a movement that is unnatural and forced. Keeping the head level and neutral results in better postural habits as well as strengthening of deeper core neck muscles that are vitally important to ongoing functional alignment.

The "Half-Forward Bend" shown in **Fig. 8.15A** pulls the neck and shoulder girdle forward, destabilizing the shoulder joint and compressing the posterior cervical vertebrae. Notice the strain and tension created in the back of the neck, which leads to muscle stiffness and discomfort. Any sense of pranic energy movement from the spinal column is dammed up at the base of the neck. There is not a sense of ease or comfort in the pose. If you were to assume this neck position while upright (**Fig. 8.15B**) it would clearly not be natural or comfortable, and it would certainly not facilitate the deep, unrestricted breathing you are striving for. **Fig. 8.15C** and **Fig. 8.15.D** show

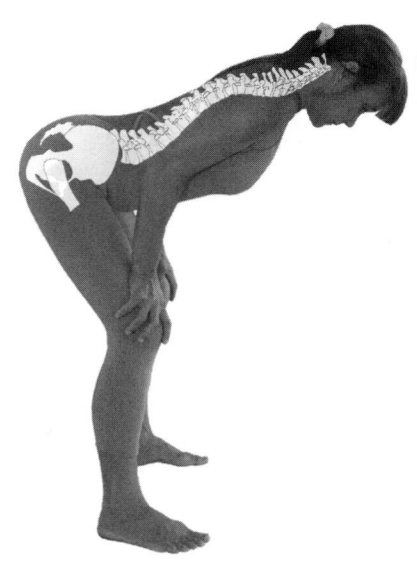

Fig 8.16C "Half Forward Bend"

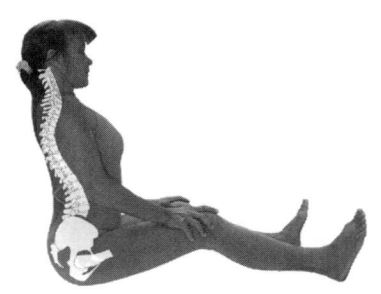

Fig. 8.15D – "Half Forward Bend", with the photo rotated, becomes the "Spine Aligner."

the "Half-Forward Bend" with natural spine alignment from sacrum to the crown of the head. In YogAlign, all poses simulate good standing postural alignment.

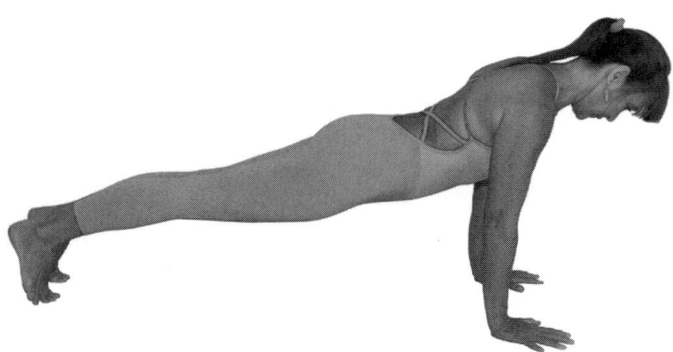

Fig. 8.16A – YogAlign Push–Up Plank

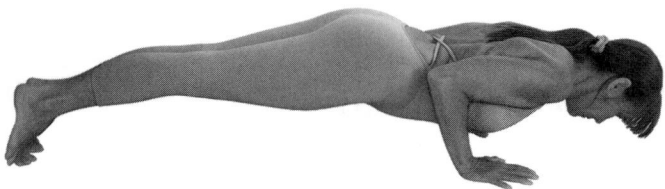

Fig. 8.16B – CORRECT: YogAlign "Push-Up Plank." Inhale down and inhale up.

When practicing intense movements like the "Push-Up" or "Plank", the internal movements of the body created when inhaling greatly support and assist spinal integrity in the body. The movements of exhalation can assist in preventing hyper-extension in the lower back. In YogAlign's version of the Push-up, the "Push-Up Plank," we engage the inhalation process as we push the body up (**Figs. 8.16A & 8.16B**). Through the Core SIP Breath, a core ring of support is generated in the center of the body that radiates out to the periphery. Once we have pushed up, we then hold the plank as we exhale, and again use the movements of inhaling to lower the body back to the floor.

This pose develops deep strength in the core of the body and establishes natural alignment executed from the deep front line. Practitioners should keep their jaw, eyes, and facial muscles relaxed, so that there is no wasted energy or unnecessary muscle contractions in the exercise — *only the right amount of effort.*

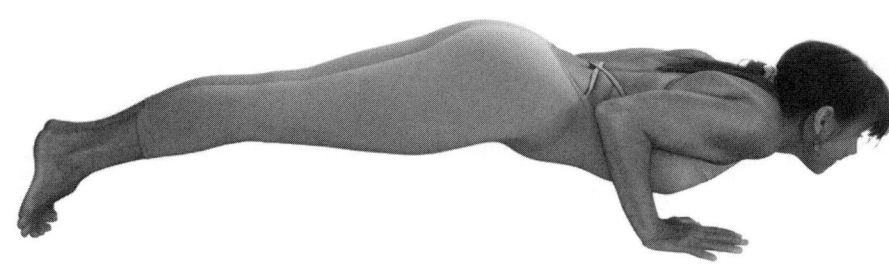

Fig. 8.16C – INCORRECT: "Push-Up Plank"

In some schools of yoga, students are instructed to keep the gaze forward when practicing this low plank pose (**Fig. 8.16C**). This inhibits proper spinal alignment, stops the flow of energy at the base of the neck, and ingrains a muscle pattern of shrugging and rounding. These incorrect positions can actually lead to more rounded shoulders, forward head carriage and ultimately compressed cervical discs. Rounded shoulders, exhaustion of the nervous system, and neck and eye tension are the cumulative effects of this style of Plank. In many cases, this is a neuromuscular reinforcement of dysfunctional patterning that the correct YogAlign Plank can re-pattern.

In the incorrect version of the "Glider" (**Fig. 8.17B**), notice the unnatural movement pattern of engaging and stabilizing the body from the front of the neck and chin, causing a shortening of the back. Would you be in proper standing alignment with your neck and head in this position? Breathing and spinal alignment are seriously compromised when practicing in this manner, which serves to strengthen bad postural habits.

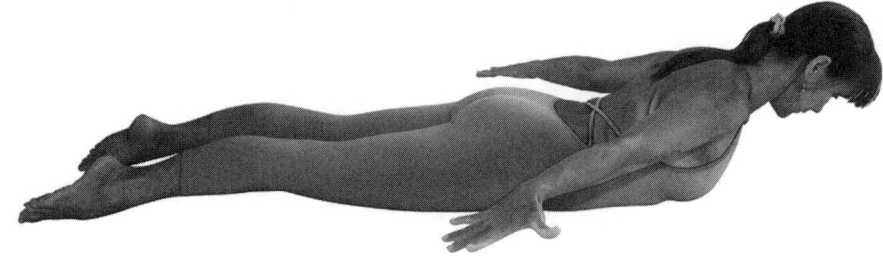

Fig. 8.17A – CORRECT: YogAlign Glider

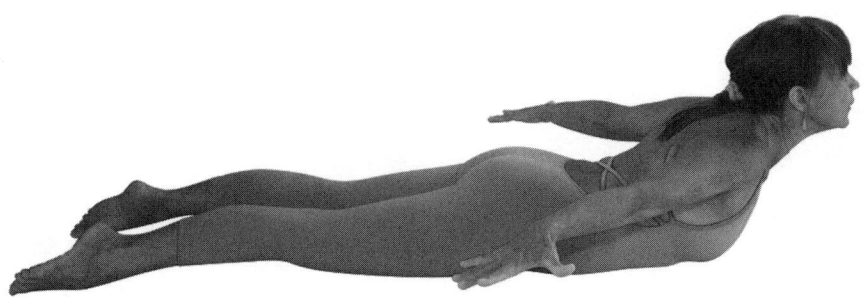

Fig. 8.17B – INCORRECT: Glider

CONCLUSION

When one practices yoga, the mindful discernment between pain and intensity can become a form of meditation. Every yoga practitioner should realize that there is a significant difference between the two. It is important to practice *ahimsa*, or non-violence, not only towards others but also toward one's self. A yoga pose that "hurts" is not serving your highest good. For instance, using a ball to support your wrists and shoulders as in **Fig. 8.18B** is the safe way to get benefits without any of the risks. Using props has been advised by many yoga teachers to reduce strain and the risk of yoga injuries. If you have been injured doing yoga, go to **www.yogainjuries.com** to take a survey on yoga injuries that will help provide all of us with a baseline of information about yoga injuries and how and why they are happening.

Listening to the messages from your body about what feels natural and aligned fosters a deep communication with your higher sense of awareness. When you are in tune with your body, yoga can become a moving meditation, allowing you to connect with your deeper awareness and allowing you to feel the essence of who you are.

The human body is ancient, and is capable of more than we can possibly imagine. Honor the intelligence of the body by giving up the need to control or force your body beyond what feels comfortable. The practice of keeping yoga safe and simple will bring you ease and comfort. You will find a sense of peace in your heart and a lightness in your step. By focusing your yoga practice on letting the movements of breath inform and align your body, you will achieve graceful movements in fluid natural alignment. In this state, you can feel the ageless energy of the human spirit and the fluid connectivity of the "kid" body, at any age.

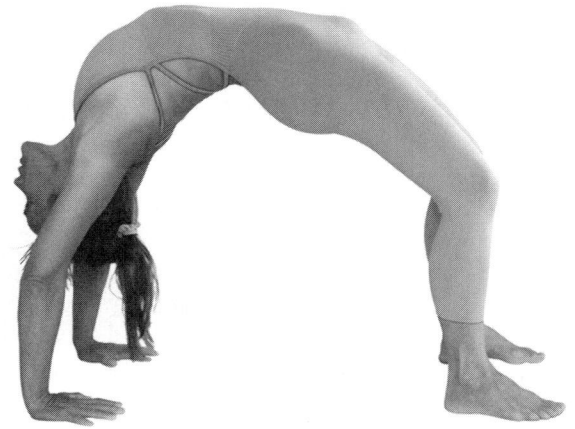

Fig. 8.18A - YogAlign "Backbend" or "Wheel"

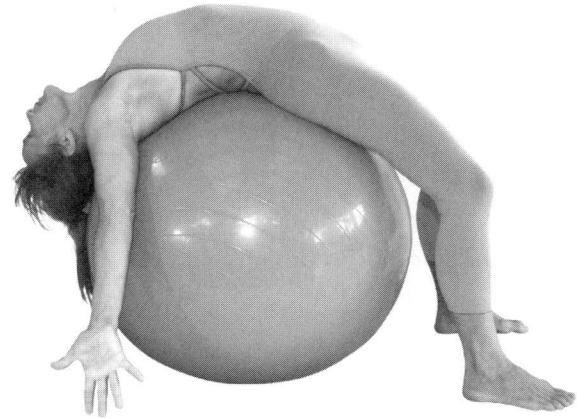

Fig. 8.18B – YogAlign "Backbend with Ball"

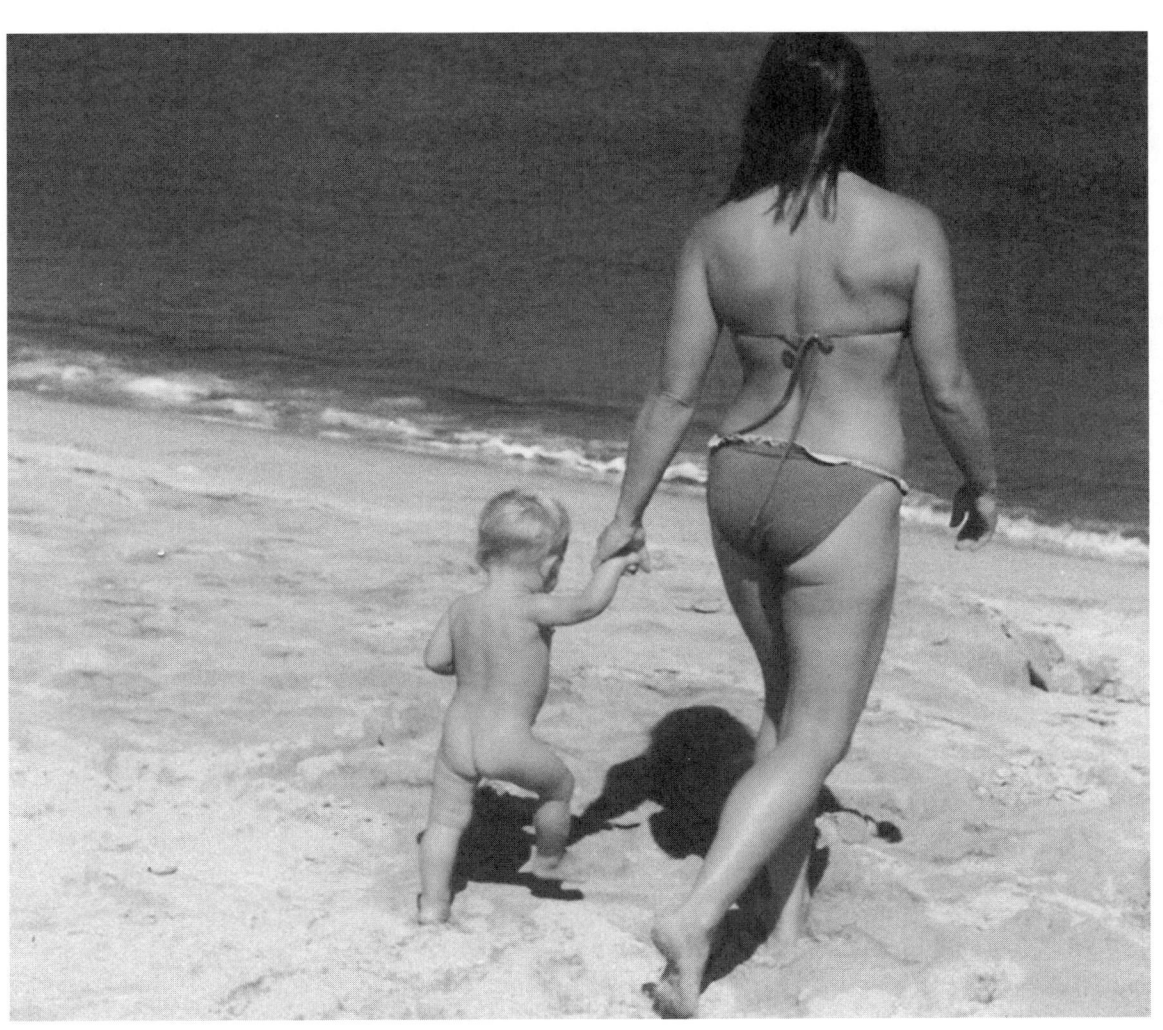

Michaelle and Baby Zack, Hanalei, Kauai, 1988.

YogAlignMent Principle #12

A pose that hurts is not serving your highest good.
Be mindful and develop the ability to
discern the difference
between pain and intensity.

YogAlignMent Principle #13

Always maintain poses that are functional
–in which your spine is aligned in good standing
posture and you feel at ease and comfortable.

*The most important yoga practice of all
is to be conscious, aligned,
and aware in your body
in every moment.*

THE YOGALIGN METHOD
70 POSES THAT PRESENT THE ESSENTIALS OF YOGALIGN—
POSES AND MOVEMENTS ORCHESTRATED BY YOGALIGN'S UNIQUE CORE BREATHING PROCESS.

The basis of the YogAlign practice is to create and maintain posture in natural alignment and therefore the emphasis is on posture, not poses. As you go through the poses in this section, focus first and foremost on your breathing process, and use these poses (as well as the *Experiential Exercises* in Part 1 of this book) to become more fit and functional in your breathing and your posture. You breathe everywhere, whether on or off the mat. This means that every moment is an opportunity for YogAlign practice!

People often ask me how much YogAlign to do, when to do it, and what poses are the most beneficial. The answer is that it depends upon you, your body, and your lifestyle. Certainly, if you can practice an hour a day, you will reap huge benefits; however, you *can* do shorter vignettes and still feel the power of YogAlign, which is to be in natural alignment all of the time. This power fosters a constant state of awareness that helps put you in the present moment, the goal of any deep yoga practice.

All YogAlign poses involve the entire body as a continuum, so you must be conscious and aware in the moment, paying attention to how you are using your body and where it is in space. Do as much as you have time for; listen to what your body tells you it needs and it will direct you.

Remember, every moment is an opportunity to do YogAlign, because YogAlign is simply the art of being aligned in your structure and breath, and you can do this every breathing moment of your life. When you do YogAlign on your mat, follow natural alignment, and use your conscious focus, the tools of PNF, and self-massage, and soon you will be aligned without "thinking." Once your body gets its new movement codes, you will no longer have to *try* in order to be aligned. You will have achieved sustainability in your own body.

WHAT DOES IT MEAN TO HAVE A SUSTAINABLE BODY?

Sustainability is the capacity to endure. It allows biological systems to remain diverse and productive over time. For humans, sustainability is the potential for the long-term maintenance of our well-being.

In YogAlign, sustainability means using our energy in movement wisely and efficiently, being our own teacher, and re-teaching ourselves functional movement patterns that heal pain and injury without surgery or drugs. Having poor alignment means muscles are working overtime and this can lead to exhaustion of the nervous and muscular systems. Having a body that is naturally aligned allows the body to use just the necessary effort in movement; the naturally aligned body has a breathing apparatus that is toned and a nervous system that is not over taxed with tension and stress from dysfunctional mental or physical patterning.

YogAlign students have demonstrated time and time again that they can become fit, toned, and energized while actually using less effort. This allows them to have more energy for what is most important in their lives. As you practice YogAlign and keep moving towards being in your body with less effort, you will begin to notice mental energy that is misdirected. Observing your thoughts without judging allows you to drop unnecessary habits such as worry, projection, judging and comparing. Freeing up your mental energy will bring forth feelings of joy, compassion, and gratitude, enabling you to better serve yourself and others.

Read through the principles below and remember to keep them in your mind as you practice. Create sustainability in your own body with YogAlign's Eight Principles of Natural Alignment.

THE PRACTICE OF YOGALIGN IS CENTERED ON EIGHT PRINCIPLES:

1. Create the Foundation with SIP Breathing. It is not what you do that is most important, but how you breathe while doing it. Optimal fitness requires learning to breathe deeply and efficiently. Breathing brings oxygen into our body, and is the most important exercise in which our body engages. Our breath creates basic structural body alignment, directs our nervous system responses, and defines our emotional well-being. Learning to breathe deeply with your inner core muscles is the most important life skill you can learn.

2. Learn to Activate the Psoas—"The Core of Your Core." The psoas group connects your upper body to your lower body, and your inner emotional body to your physical body. The psoas is involved with moving, breathing, organ support, emotions, and spine alignment. Activating your psoas in synergy with the rest of your core abdominal muscles is the key to a pain-free body and a strong, stable core. Many common abdominal exercises strengthen through flexion, or shortening, of the trunk muscles. This eventually leads to pain, misalignment, and injuries. The focus in YogAlign is to train your core muscles predominately as stabilizers of the trunk and extenders of the spine.

3. Establish Natural Spine Alignment. Establishing natural spine alignment is essential to becoming balanced and pain-free in your body. YogAlign has specific exercises that engage muscular action, which encourages natural spine alignment. When practiced in combination with core breathing, these exercises bring us into beneficial alignment patterns from the inside out. Creating natural alignment and beneficial breathing habits are the keynotes to health, happiness, and longevity. The majority of all pain in the body comes from poor posture; therefore, alignment is the primary focus of YogAlign postures. Emphasis is upon achieving natural alignment via functional yoga poses and breathing exercises that recode how we use the body at the nervous system level.

4. Learn Concentric/Eccentric PNF Neuromuscular Exercises. Beneficial spine alignment becomes intrinsic in the body as we recode neuromuscular patterning. Concentric-to-eccentric muscle engagement techniques are designed to help us quickly become strong and flexible, with no pain or strain to our joints. The way to flexibility is in the understanding that muscle tension is controlled with our brain. Proprioceptive neuromuscular facilitation, or PNF, is a powerful tool for overriding the stretch reflex, changing muscle tension, and gaining flexibility. PNF facilitations can be self-applied, or can be practiced with a partner or teacher. Learning to employ these neuromuscular techniques will give us flexibility and strength throughout our body quickly, with no pain in the process.

5. **Free Your Fascia and Know Your Anatomy.** We need to understand the anatomy of our structure and how the entire body is connected in a web. The smallest movement reverberates through our entire body. YogAlign shows us in an experiential way how our body is wired. Since the body is a continuum, the anatomy exercises in YogAlign are based on whole-body awareness. What you can sense, you can start to consciously change.

Our fascia is a web-like tissue that surrounds and guides our muscle pathways, determines the quality of our movements, and even affects our immune and hormonal systems. The unique breathing exercises in YogAlign help us to feel and engage different muscle pathways that are guided by the fascia. Fascia growth is determined by our repetitive movements and can become rigid or thickened when the body is misaligned and muscles are overworked.

Understanding anatomy of movement and learning how to optimize spinal curve mobility through breathing and muscle training are other essentials for a pain-free body. It is helpful to look at the anatomical drawings of the muscle connections and fascia pathways in our body. Once we have an outer map we can begin to practice body and sensory awareness from an inner perspective, sensing our fascia and the muscle pathways as we move about in daily life

6. **Learn Self-Massage and Sensory Body Awareness.** YogAlign asks us to make deposits in the self-love bank account. Effective self-massage is the tool for bringing blood flow, oxygen, relaxation, and sensory awareness to our soft tissue and organs.

In YogAlign we use self-massage to open the fascia that can be palpated from the outside, and we combine this with core breathing to open the fascia from the inside. The importance of practicing daily self-massage cannot be overemphasized.

YogAlign teaches *lomi-lomi*, a form of Hawaiian self-massage that is performed all over the body in each YogAlign session. Self-massage brings awareness into the voluntary cortex of the brain and out of the subcortex, or involuntary, system. Each lomi-lomi session is an opportunity to become present in our body in the here and now. Self-massage not only invites self-love and healing, but also provides an important opportunity to understand our anatomy on an experiential level.

7. **Practice Presence and Awareness in the Now.** By being present with the body, and focusing on the breath, one comes to a state of *yoga* (union) within the body, mind, and spirit. When our body is naturally aligned and the nervous system is in a relaxed state, we are more able to live in present awareness, beyond the trappings of the mind and ego. Learning to move and breathe from the center of our body and to practice full body awareness helps release us from our mind's dominance, which controls much of our experience of life. This mind dominance keeps many of us in a state of fear about the future and regret about the past. In these negative mental states, our body reflects the condition of our mind, and aging, depression, and disease begin to manifest on the physical level.

When our body feels light and comfortable, our natural state of joy emerges and we are able to reside in the present moment where life happens. Creativity and intuition can naturally flow as we connect to the inner force or source that guides all life.

By paying attention to how our body feels, we become more aware of who we are, and can access our deepest inner feelings without the normal layers of tension and fear which hold us in darkness. When we become more natural in our alignment and our feelings, our inner radiance can shine forth and we can live in the eternal present where life happens.

8. Know Your Body's Authentic Needs. Our body performs thousands of tasks everyday without us having to consciously think about them. When we walk across the room, we don't have to think about how our body will do it, because our body has a "mind" of its own. Even while we are asleep, our cells are working, our heart beats and breathing happens without any work from our conscious mind.

Our body is a gift on loan from the Earth, working 24/7 to keep all systems and organs in-sync and on-task. To connect to the present and to feel the flow of life, we need to take good care of our body, so that we can concentrate on the joy of the journey instead of on our aches, pains and problems.

Many health issues are caused by poor alignment, diet, attitude, and lack of exercise. We have the innate ability to be our own healer by taking personal responsibility to care for and love ourselves on all levels. This means avoiding drugs, alcohol, and smoking—even violent movies—and giving our body healthy food, adequate sunlight, rest, and sufficient exercise. Cultivating a deep care for ourselves, as fierce and tender as one would care for anything having the greatest value, will assure us a longer and smoother ride on this great planet Earth.

In YogAlign, Poses Are a Tool, Not a Goal

YogAlign recommends only poses which promote better posture and functional movement. The YogAlign SIP breathing process is a tool for determining whether a pose is functional or beneficial. If you cannot take a deep breath while in a pose, modify the pose until you can.

YogAlign eliminates all right-angle positions—those that put the trunk at a 90-degree angle to the legs—from the practice of yoga. These positions serve no beneficial purpose because fascial lines create a pull, compressing the spine when you straighten your legs. It is what I call a fascial fact. We are designed to move by alternately bending our knees. When both of our knees are kept straightened as we bend forward, connective tissue forces act as pulleys, creating a line of pull that destabilizes the ligament structures of the sacral and lower back region. In YogAlign, we do not sacrifice the integrity of the spine to perform a pose or a position. We do not get comfortable by being uncomfortable and it is important to pay attention to what feels right for our structure.

Practice *ahimsa* (non-violence) in your own body by focusing on positions that model functional movement and aligned, natural posture. Remember that there is a difference between pain and intensity. Sharp pains are your body's way of telling you "No!" Don't force your body to stay in an uncomfortable position; remember that you will never get comfortable by being uncomfortable. When you are aligned, your fascia and muscle trains suspend your body in a web, as if you were floating in space. With proper alignment you will not feel like one part of the body is strained or working harder than the rest.

In my years of teaching, many people have come to me with yoga injuries from practicing "Boat," "Staff," and "Forward Bend" with their legs straight. These straight-leg poses put a tremendous harmful force on your sacrum and low back area. Ligaments which provide structure and shock absorption are stretched, and the hip and sacral areas can get destabilized. The gluteus muscles cannot fire when the sacral platform is flat and your tailbone is tucked under. You lose power in the glutes, and over time tensile forces overload the hip and knee area.

PRACTICE POSTURE, NOT POSES

Those who are very flexible and find yoga poses to be easy may not feel the inherent danger of the flattening of the sacrum that occurs doing straight-leg poses. Years of sacrum stretching—whether slouching in a chair or going deeply into a straight-leg, seated forward-bend—will take a toll. Once you lose the shock-absorbing functions of the sacrum, your trunk weight will sit in the hip socket, eventually destabilizing or damaging your hip joint. If you notice your butt is getting flat from doing yoga, stop the straight leg forward bending poses and focus instead on poses that strengthen your body's ability to support your spine in its natural curves.

Your body is much like a moving vehicle. You get in your car, turn the key and drive wherever you want to go. Although you are at the wheel steering the direction of the car, you are not controlling the inner workings of the engine that make the car go down the road. In your body, all you have to do is put in the gas (food), get adequate rest, turn on your proprioception and go. You can then direct or "drive" your body anywhere you want it to go. It is the intelligence of the human body that takes the conscious idea to move into actual physical movement. Our conscious mind cannot possibly direct the millions of minute changes that must happen on a cellular level when you take even a few steps. Yet our body makes the movements happen, and we can dance with our body, sing through it, work in it, make love in it—we move it to the dance of life. How well we "drive" and care for our vehicle is going to determine the longevity and quality of our experience of living.

The YogAlign Method

POSITION #1— FULL BODY STRETCH

The "Full Body Stretch" always puts you in perfect natural alignment. Use this pose at any time during the practice to traction, align, and extend your spine. There is surprising power in this simple but profound pose.

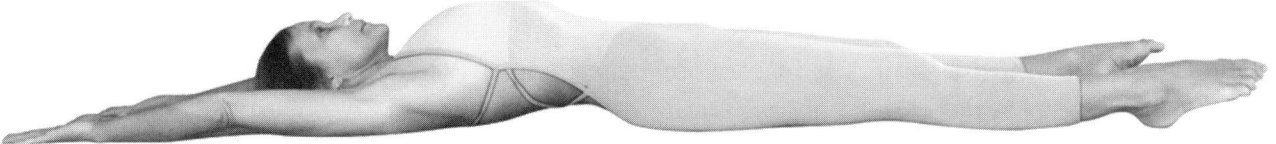

Fig. 1A – Full Body Stretch

On your mat, begin your practice lying on your back. Inhale, while reaching your arms overhead, keeping your hands at least shoulder-width apart in a Y shape. Imagine you are just awakening from a good night's sleep. While reaching, open your fingers wide and strongly point your toes. Inhale with the Core SIP Breath (discussed in Chapter 4) and feel the elongation of your body from the tips of your fingers to the tips of your toes. Keep the natural curves in your neck and lower back, rather than pressing them to the floor. Continuing to reach overhead, pull your shoulder blades down and feel your limbs originating from the center of your body.

Imagine you are pulling your arms back into the socket while keeping the elbows straight if possible. Feel the musculature of your arms engage all the way to the core of your body. Continue to keep your arms in a Y position, rather than trying to put your hands together. If you feel tension in your shoulder, do not try and press your hands or shoulder to the floor. Keep your arms lifted as you stretch or try turning your palms to face each other with your thumbs on the mat and your fingers spreading wide.

Taking a deep breath, visualize your consciousness in every cell of your body, and direct your awareness into your whole being. Point your toes like a dancer as you continue to spread your fingers wide, engaging your muscles in your arms, legs, and trunk. Use the Core SIP Breath when you inhale, drawing breath through your lips as though you are sucking on a straw or getting ready to whistle.

Retain the next inhale and tighten all of the muscles you can feel in your body from your hands down to your toes. Make fists with your hands and squeeze your butt and jaw muscles. Be sure to include your pelvic floor muscles. Hold and squeeze and sense the feeling of your muscles as they contract. When you need to exhale, let go and release all of the consciously-held muscle contractions while staying in the stretching position. Open your fingers, toes, and mouth as widely as you can, and lengthen into the stretch.

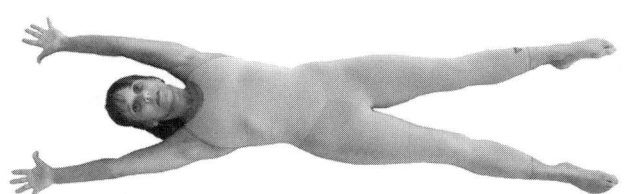

Fig. 1B – Full Body Stretch (shown from above).

Take time everyday to practice this full body stretch. As you inhale, feel oxygen nourishing every cell of your body with life force or *prana*. The "Full Body Stretch" will keep you awake, refreshed, aligned and fluid.

Position #2 — Reclining Breath Tuning

Before entering this pose, it is highly recommended that you watch the breathing segment on the DVD included with this book.

"Reclining Breath Tuning" gives you a chance to focus completely on your muscles of respiration—the core of all your movements. The core line of fascia is balanced through breathing, adding tone and lengthened support to your structure.

Breathing is an extraordinary event. Not only does breathing bring oxygen into your cells, but it also gives your organs and inner connective tissue a massage from the inside out with every breath. YogAlign's breathing exercises are designed to help you fully awaken, supercharge, and recode your breath and posture at the nervous system level.

In practicing the Experiential Exercises (in Part 1), you gain the understanding of your unique breathing process and how it defines who you are and how you move. The movements caused by Core Breathing can create deep fascial releases on the inside and outside of your entire body. By using the Core SIP Breath, you create your own internal resistance mechanism, training the breathing muscles from the inside out. This training will change deeply-rooted postural and emotional patterning.

Note: You can do this pose anywhere to make use of time spent driving, walking or waiting in lines.

Start with self-massage. Lying on your back on your mat, bend your knees and place your fingers on the lower part of your rib cage. Be careful not to over-lift your chin or flatten your lower back to the floor. The body should feel aligned and at ease with the natural curves of your spine. To awaken the muscular breathing apparatus, massage the thin muscle layer between your rib bones (the intercostals), and also massage the belly or diaphragm area just below your sternum. Tension in the scalp, ears, and neck can inhibit breathing, particularly in the upper rib cage. It is very important to massage and release these areas to facilitate deep, optimal breathing.

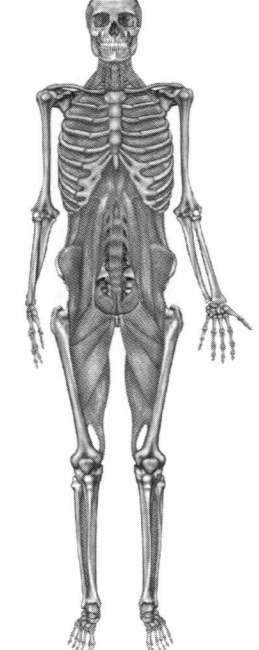

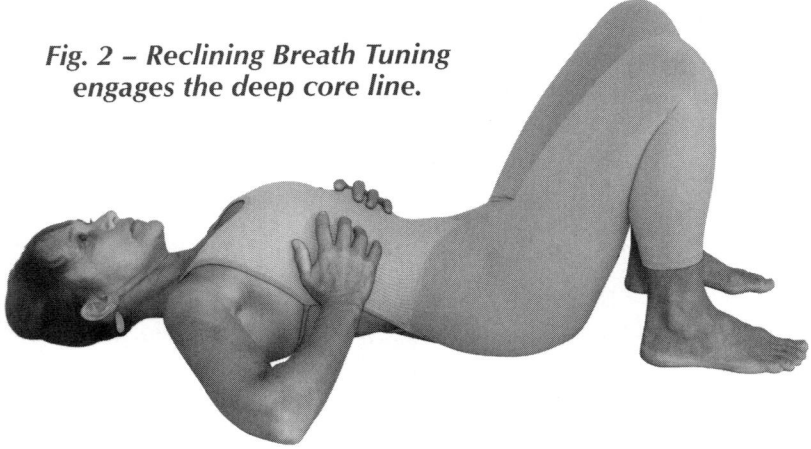

Fig. 2 – Reclining Breath Tuning engages the deep core line.

Essential YogAlign Poses

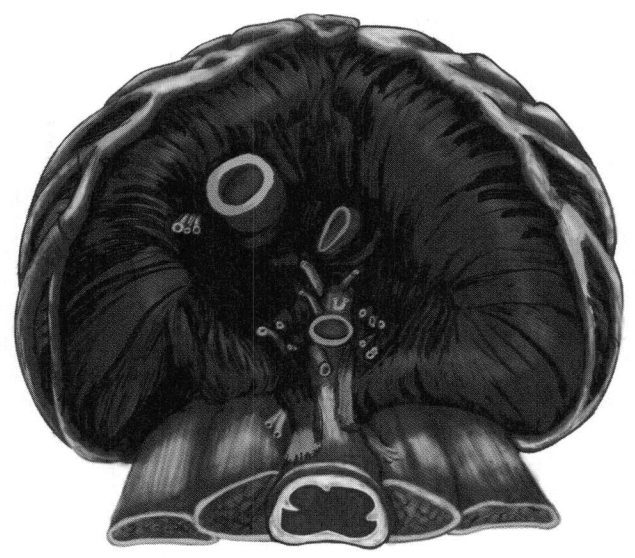

Diaphragm from the underside looking up, showing connection to the inner surface of all the ribs.

When you breathe, try moving the ribs in all directions as though you are inflating a ball. Place your index fingers between your lower ribs, feeling the muscle tissue between them. Inhale deeply using the Core SIP Breath. Notice how your outer rib muscles feel as they engage to pull your ribs apart. Keep your fingers between your ribs and exhale, noticing how the outer rib muscles have "disappeared" from your touch. See if you can feel how the internal intercostal muscles work from the inside, pulling the ribs together during exhalation to push air out of the body. Repeat the inhale with your fingers between the ribs. Hold your breath for a moment, accentuating the actions of the external rib cage muscles.

On inhalation your outer rib muscles pull the ribs apart as your diaphragm contracts downward, creating more space in the thoracic area and allowing the lungs to expand and fill with air. The center of the diaphragm has a central tendon which is fascially connected to the base of the lung tissue. The downward movement of the diaphragm during inhalation pulls on this central tendon, which helps to create an opening of the fascial sheath that connects the top of the diaphragm to the connective tissue surrounding the lungs. This creates more space in the chest area, and the air rushes in to fill the vacuum.

When you begin to exhale, go slowly by making an SSSS sound (like a snake) through your teeth. Feel the muscles of exhalation working to draw your ribs together and contract your waist and belly area. Notice how your outer belly and trunk muscles work together with the internal intercostals each time you exhale. Stop exhaling, but hold and accentuate the actions of exhalation for a moment. Let go so that the muscles relax, then repeat the entire Core SIP inhalation, accentuation, release and focused exhale series. Be aware of the feeling of your entire body as you do this.

Take a few moments to practice the inhale using the Core SIP Breath technique and feel the external rib muscles expanding to pull the ribs apart, making more space for air in your lungs. With each inhale, allow your spine to lengthen and your outer belly to stretch, while keeping the curve in your lower back. As you exhale, consciously keep the lift and space that the inhale brings to your spine and trunk.

As you exhale, notice the internal intercostals pulling the ribs back together while the outer muscles of the abdomen and waist area contract and press the air out. Feel the difference in the inner and outer rib cage muscle actions and the inner and outer trunk or belly muscles. Take some time to note that inhalation is created by the external rib muscles, and the downward contraction movement of the diaphragm; exhalation is done by the internal rib muscles and the outer trunk muscles compressing space out of the abdomen.

"Reclining Breath Tuning" is a strong exercise for the muscles of breathing, and it creates a very powerful rib cage and diaphragm that supports your structure as well as provides your cells with the respiration needed for life. People talk about getting "six-pack abs" but it may be better symbolically to go for the whole "keg" which is a fluid, powerful, and activated rib cage. Every time you exhale using the SSSS sound through your teeth or with your mouth wide open and tongue extended, you can turn the movements of exhalation into a great active exercise to tone your core from the inside out.

CRIMPING THE HOSE EXERCISE

Imagine you are in the garden and you have the hose on, but you then decide to stop the flow of water by crimping the hose together with your hand. Despite the fact that you have stopped the water, the water is still trying to flow. As you un-crimp the hose, the water that was backing up comes rushing forth.

Imagine that tightness in your abs or pelvic floor is like the crimp in the hose, stopping not water but rather the fluid movement of breath. You can use the inhalation breath, along with PNF techniques, to release the flow of breath by breaking the crimp of excess muscle tension.

Inhale with the Core SIP Breath technique. Exhale and hold the muscles of exhalation tight for a moment. Begin to inhale with the SIP but try to hold the muscles of exhalation for a second as you do it. Keep sipping in deeply as you now release the contraction of the exhaling muscles without stopping the movements of inhalation. Let your ribs just pop open as though letting go of a balloon. Focus on what you are feeling.

Now repeat the exercise, but this time, as you hold the muscles of exhalation, add the contraction of the muscles of the pelvic floor. Squeeze these muscles tightly, as if you were trying not to pee. Begin to breathe with the SIP Breath technique while tightening the pelvic floor. Keep sipping but release the muscles you are holding (the crimp of the hose), allowing the breath (the water) to expand into your body. Take a moment to sit calmly and allow your breathing to happen naturally without any force or direction.

You may notice that your breath feels more expansive after you do this exercise. Ideally, the pelvic floor muscles relax and stretch on inhalation and contract on exhalation. By holding tension in the pelvic floor (tightening what feels tight, or crimping the hose) while inhaling, we can learn how to release deep holding patterns that are affecting our breathing process. A habitually tense or tight pelvic floor can migrate all over your body and affect, in particular, your hip, knee, and leg functions.

You are your own best breath doctor, so pay attention to how you breathe. Do your ribs and diaphragm move easily or do they feel restricted? Does the movement of breathing get stuck somewhere, such as under the sternum? Do you feel your ribs evenly expanding in all directions? Do you lift your shoulders or tense your neck or jaw? Performing these exercises frees your breathing process to happen with ease, and eliminates excess effort.

POSITION #3 — PNF HIP RECALIBRATOR

*The "PNF Hip Recalibrator" (**Fig. 3**) can help release chronic tension in your hip flexors and add strength to the muscles surrounding the hip joint. To be flexible, you need to master muscle tension—via nervous system patterning—by tightening what already feels tight during stretching, thereby bypassing the stretch reflex. Tightening muscles beyond their usual contraction rate helps to reprogram the nervous system to release the muscles to a longer resting length, creating flexibility quickly and painlessly.*

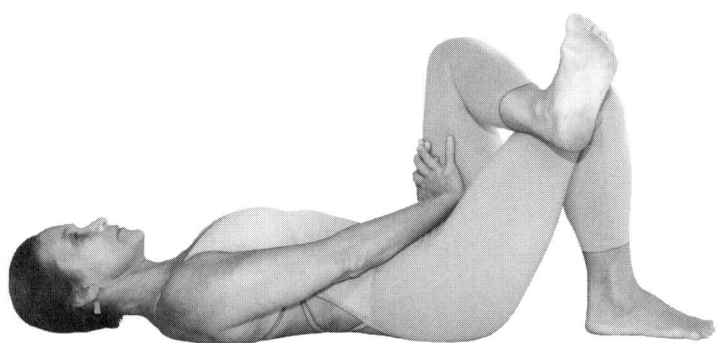

Fig. 3 – PNF Hip Recalibrator

From the reclining position with bent knees, lift your right foot and place it across the top of your left thigh. Spread the toes of your right foot and press through the ball, keeping your foot in an active position. Place both hands on your right thigh and bring your thigh up towards your belly while at the same time resisting against the leg movement using downward pressure from your hands. This PNF exercise creates a "wrestling match" between your hip and leg muscles, and your arms.

Engage via PNF: Inhale and hold the breath gently while you resist the action of your right thigh's lift by pressing it back with your hands. Feel the muscle contractions in your right leg that are activated by the movement of your thigh towards your belly. Keep your shoulders down and your shoulder blades stabilized, and practice lifting your thigh towards your belly as your hands resist the actions. Keep your arms straight and your collarbones wide. Stay in natural spinal alignment. Do not force your lower back or neck into the floor. Exhale, releasing the muscle actions in your leg, as you press back on your thigh to create openness in your hips and groin.

Repeat, adding the contraction of the pelvic floor muscles (as though you are trying not to pee). Consciously increase the muscle actions in your pelvis, leg and hip by accentuating the muscle contractions. As you exhale, open your mouth wide and extend your tongue. Relax all muscle effort in your hip, leg, and pelvis, and continue pressing your leg away from your head with your hands. Feel tension releasing in the hip, groin, and pelvic floor.

Repeat the hip press movement and feel your hip opening like warm honey pouring through your pelvis. When you exhale, feel the belly contract and pelvic floor muscles activate. Release the jaw, tongue and face on exhale. Completely relax and allow your breathing process to happen naturally without you directing it. Feel the flow of energy and sense of lightness coming into your hip area.

NOTE: For Positions 3-13, it is recommended that the series be practiced as a continuum, one leg at a time, beginning with the right leg. The entire series should then be repeated with the left leg.

Position #4 – Reclining Foot Massage

Massaging your feet and toes feels great, and positively affects your entire being, both physically and emotionally. Massage switches the nervous system to the parasympathetic mode, creating a relaxation response. Foot massage brings blood flow and awareness, helping to balance you, tone you, and strengthen your connection to the earth. Having healthy feet is essential for a pain-free, balanced body. Your feet deserve loving attention every day; you can't walk anywhere without them!

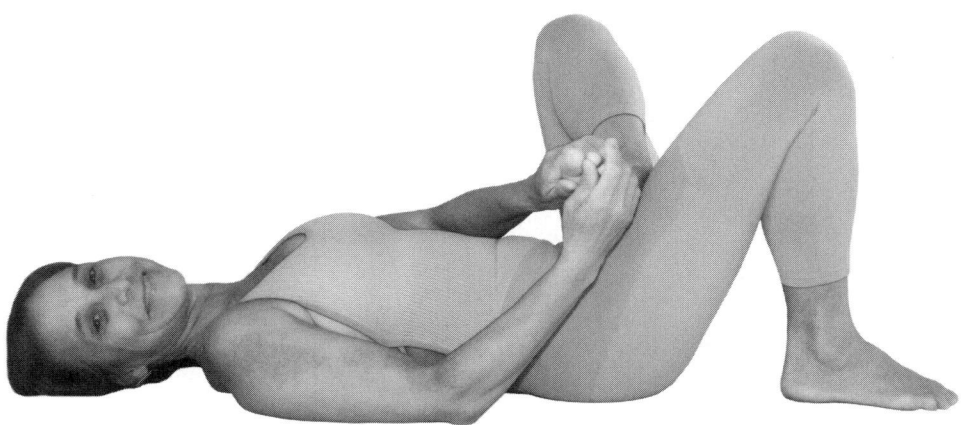

Fig. 4 – Reclining Foot Massage

Keeping the right foot on your thigh, start with both hands massaging the bottom of your foot. Stay present, be aware of your breathing, and feel your body in its entirety. **Note:** If you have trouble reaching your foot, do not lift your head or shoulders. Instead, place a block or book under your left foot to lift your right thigh higher.

Press firmly on each toenail for several seconds. Feel the blood rush into each toe when you release pressure. Roll your toes with the fresh blood and massage each digit all the way into the ball of the foot and between the toe tendons. Continue to firmly and consciously massage the ball, arch, and heel of your foot. Use your thumbs to massage your arch. Press fisted knuckles deep into the tough skin of the heel. A thoroughly-massaged foot should feel soft and warm, like kneaded bread-dough or clay. Notice if there are any problem areas in your foot, and give those more attention.

Do the foot massage with love and attention, giving yourself positive and focused energy. If there is any soreness in your feet, massage them often. Bringing in blood flow and awareness will assist your body in the healing process. Daily foot massage will bring new life and energy to your feet. Rather than taking them for granted, you will develop a keen sense of how you use them when walking, standing, or running.

POSITION #5 – TOE WEAVE AND FOOT SHAKE

Go barefoot as much as possible, and wear shoes that give your toes room to spread apart as you walk. If you notice a callous developing under the toes on the ball of the foot, this is a sign that you have contracted toes that need tendon and fascia balancing. Daily attention given to your toes is an essential part of a complete YogAlign practice, and opening your feet will add length to the the entire fascia web.

After thoroughly massaging your foot, interlace the fingers of your right hand between your toes as deeply as possible. From the underside of your foot, start with the little finger and little toe and begin weaving one finger between each toe. Bring your finger webbing as deeply in to your toe webbing as possible. Inhale and squeeze your toes together compressing your fingers. Go deeper by "tightening what is tight"—hugging your fingers with the muscles of your toes. Hold the contraction for 15–20 seconds and then exhale deeply, completely relaxing your foot and toe muscles while keeping your fingers inserted between your toes. Shake your foot rapidly and release all tension in your foot until it feels like water.

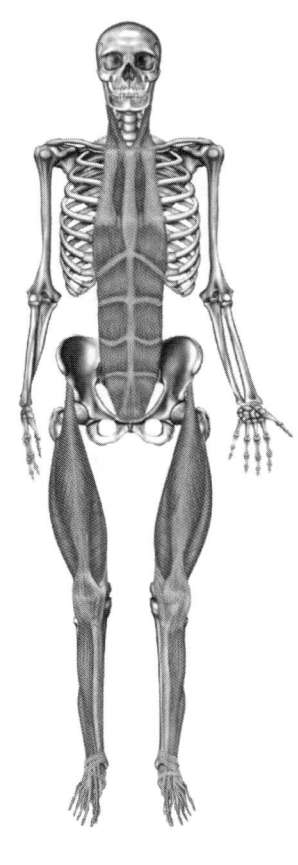

Notice the relaxation in your toes, and then repeat using the same foot.

Engage your toe webbing to hug or squeeze your fingers one more time, and on the next exhalation, open your mouth wide and stick out

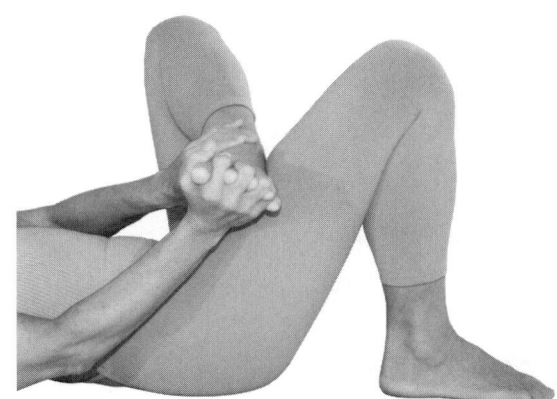

Fig. 5 – Toe Weave and Foot Shake

your tongue making an "ahh" sound as you release the foot tension. When massaging your foot, you are affecting the entire superficial front line of fascia. Visualize letting go of tension all along the front of your body. Leave your fingers interlaced as you let go of the conscious tightening of the toe webbing. Using your hand, rotate your foot in a circle pulling your toes back towards the shin.

Because the superficial front fascia line connects from the jaw to the top of the toes, tension can travel the whole length of the fascia highway. Work with your body as a whole, paying attention to fascia connections, and you will be pleasantly surprised to notice your toe webbing soften and open, creating balanced action through your feet.

POSITION #6 — LEG MASSAGE

Self-massage is an act of self-love, and when you take the time to do it, you make significant deposits into your health equity account, while establishing loving communication with your body. Daily leg and foot massage will keep your muscles and joints healthy, and provide much-needed blood flow to areas that are often sore and over-contracted. Massage increases your awareness of pain and misalignments you may otherwise not have noticed. Self-massage can also be a type of meditation when you practice conscious breathing and body awareness at the same time. Having time to connect with yourself in the moment creates a habit of paying attention to the subtle language and feeling of your body.

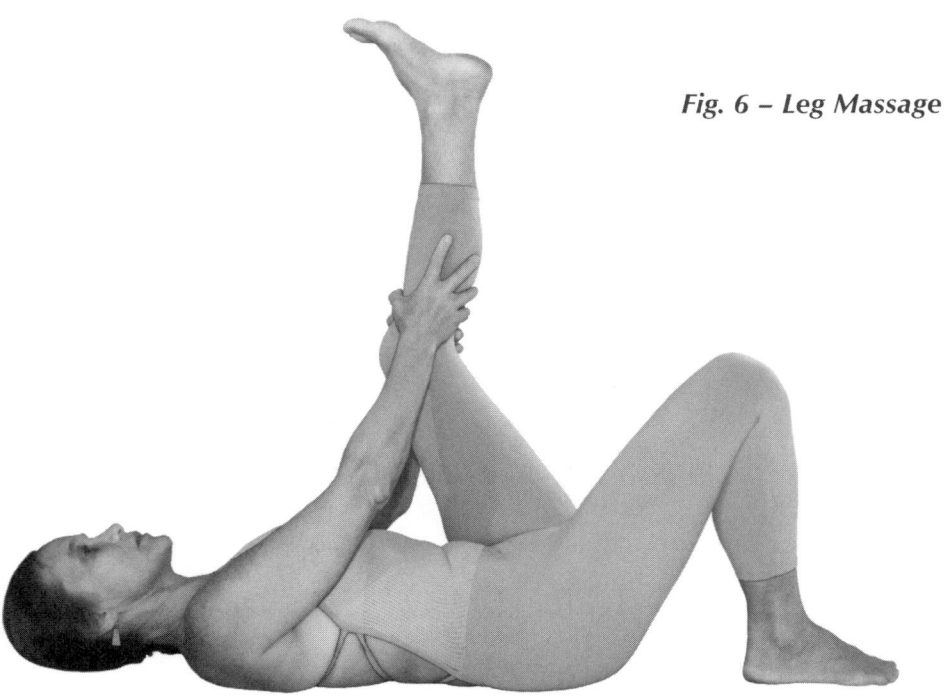

Fig. 6 – Leg Massage

Extend your leg toward the ceiling and massage it firmly and vigorously, bringing blood flow and attention from your calf all the way to your sit bones, which is where the hamstrings attach to your pelvis. Massage around all sides of your knee, paying attention to any pain you may notice. Keep your knee bent if you feel your lower back pressing into the floor. Spend time massaging around your knee, and separating the layers of leg muscles from one another.

With your toes wide open and flexed, twirl your foot around in a circle for several rotations and then reverse. Notice the range of movement in your foot and ankle. Stay in natural alignment as you practice breathing and being present while you massage your entire leg. Pay attention to your breath, your energy level, the feeling of your body, and the sounds that are occurring around you.

POSITION #7 — THIGH SQUEEZE

This pose helps to release tight muscles in the hips, thighs, and butt area. Consciously practicing "tightening what is tight" helps retrain the brain to let go of extra tension, freeing your hips and toning your butt.

Slide your right thigh over your left thigh, and lift your feet from the floor. Hold your knee caps in your hands. Straight elbows will keep you from pulling your knees in too closely towards your chest, which would compress your spine. Rolling your knees too far towards your head flattens and compresses the lumbar curve. Keep your knee caps right above your hips in order to keep the curve in your lower back. Squeeze your thighs together tightly. Keep your toes spread and your feet in the "pressing on the gas" position, while keeping your head and neck relaxed and at ease.

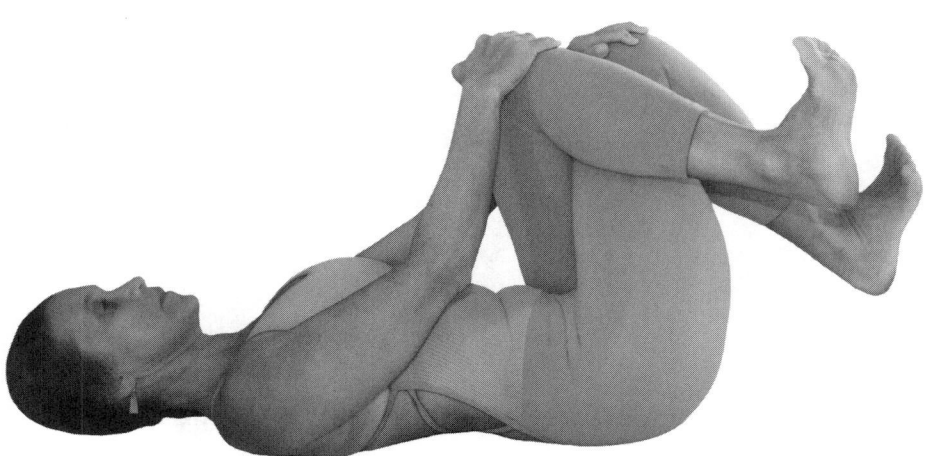

Fig. 7 – Thigh Squeeze

Inhale, and focus on keeping your lumbar spine lifted from the floor, making every attempt to maintain the natural curve of your back. Squeeze your buttocks and pelvic floor muscles. Release them and repeat the squeezing action while holding your breath. Feel your hip rotators, in particular the deep muscles of your butt that rotate your hip, pulling from the outside leg to your sacrum. On the exhale, release your thighs and buttocks while keeping your toes extended. From this position, proceed to the next pose, adding a twist.

POSITION #8 — TWIST MASSAGE

This pose is a wonderful way to stretch the lateral, spiral, and functional lines of fascia. Self-massaging the body in a side-lying position enables you to get to the lower back, sacrum, hip, and butt muscles with no compression to your spinal column. While massaging, the focus is on using the breath and the breathing process to open the fascia from the inside out, freeing the rib cage and enabling fluid movement all over the body.

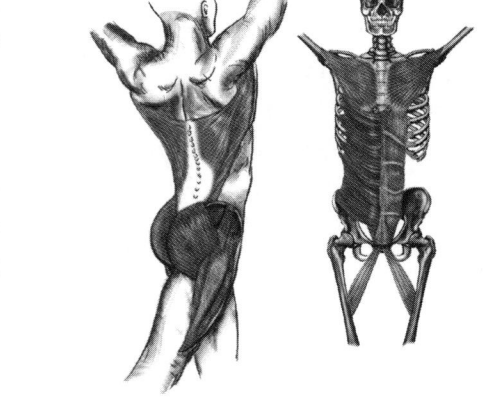

Keep your thighs crossed as you roll onto your left hip. Ground both shoulders to the floor to accentuate the twist. Feel your spine lengthen. Use the Core SIP Breath to lift the sacrum and accentuate the lower back curve. Massage your hip, buttocks, and lower back to bring blood flow and awareness into your body. You can also

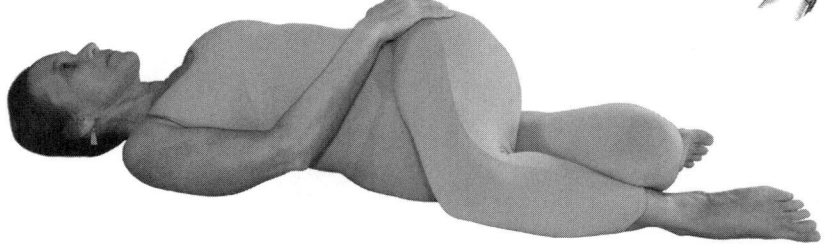

Fig. 8 – Twist Massage

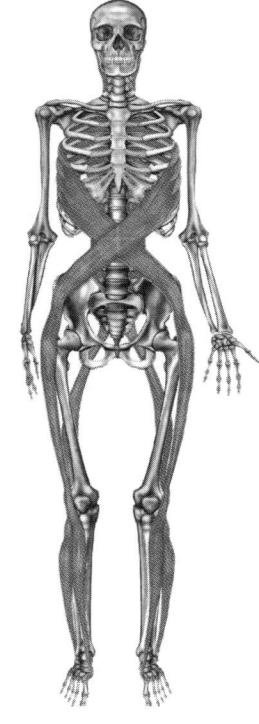

massage your rib cage in this position, paying attention to the intercostal muscles between the ribs.

Work with the lateral fascia line by reaching your right arm overhead, feeling how your wrist connects to your hip. With your arm extended overhead, twist your right hand around. Keeping your arm extended alongside your ear with your elbow straight (but not locked), pull your shoulder back into the socket by engaging your lateral trunk muscles and shoulder blades. Always keep your shoulders down and away from your ears. Focus on connecting the inner part of the arm to the socket while the outer fascia elongates. Feel your arm connect back to your hip, spine, and sacrum. Take a Core SIP Breath and feel your rib cage—and the entire side of your body—open. Take another breath and hold it, as you consciously contract your breathing muscles for about ten seconds. As you let go, open your fingers and jaw wide upon the exhale, releasing tension.

POSITION #9 — LEG AND FOOT RECALIBRATOR

The "Leg and Foot Recalibrator" balances the action of the leg and restores functional alignment from the pelvis, through the knees, to the feet. This pose installs new muscle and fascia patterns that enable the knee joint to hinge in natural alignment. It also helps alleviate chronic knee and foot pain while protecting the joints from injuries related to postural imbalances. The "Leg and Foot Recalibrator" tones and lengthens the entire superficial back line of fascia.

Stay on your back and extend your right leg towards the ceiling, perpendicular to the floor. Be sure that you are in natural spine alignment, and that the curve of your lower back is not pressing into the floor. Inhale deeply and extend from the tip of your spine through the crown of your head. Adjust your chin so that it is level with your forehead without flattening the natural curve in your neck. If your chin points upward and the front of your throat feels tense, you can put a small pillow or towel under your head.

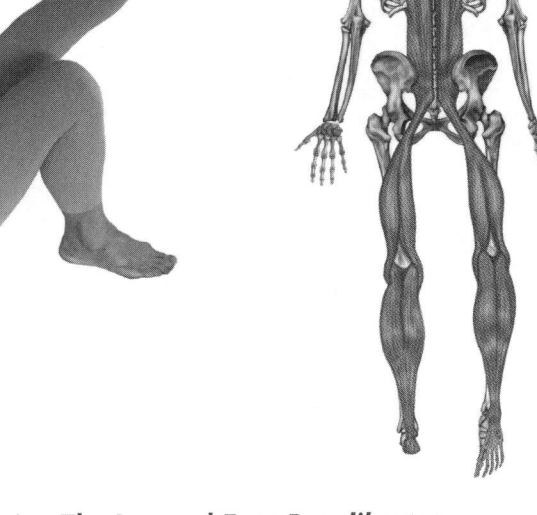

Interweave your fingers behind the back of your raised leg, below your knee. Keep your elbows straight and gently pull your shoulder blades down while you extend the heel towards the ceiling. Do not pull your leg back towards your head, but simply extend your heel up while keeping the hips on the floor.

Fig. 9A – The Leg and Foot Recalibrator

Do not straighten your knee if you feel your lower back pressing into the floor; instead, keep your knee slightly bent in a position that maintains the curve in your lower back. Remember that the superficial back line of fascia connects from your spine to your leg, so be aware that straightening your leg can cause the fascia lines to pull, compressing the sacrum and lower back curve.

In all of these movements, it is vital to maintain the integrity of your spinal curves. If your legs and hips are very flexible and you can straighten your leg without losing your spinal curves, pull your leg in closer to your trunk, moving your hands up and grabbing your calf muscles.

Foot position is a huge determinant of posture, breathing, and alignment. The position of your foot changes the tension in the fascia lines affecting how well you move, balance, and breathe in the whole body. Because of their connection from head to toe, foot tension can inhibit inhalation, and releasing the jaw can help relax the foot. The parking brake foot position (shown in **Fig. 9B** below) contracts not just your toes but the entire front of your body in a way that inhibits the breathing process from the top of the foot all the way to your belly and up to your jaw.

If you have tight toes, sore arches, or flat feet, practice only the dancer foot or gas pedal foot positions.

In this pose, you will be using several different foot positions. Remember, if you have pain in the heel or bottom of the foot, avoid lifting with the heel and practice pointing or flointing instead. It may be difficult to do either at first, but in a short time your feet will become more like your hands: nimble and strong. If you do experience cramping when you try to point or floint, extend through your heel for a moment and tighten the area that is cramping. Relax, do more foot massage, and then repeat using the same foot.

Inhale as you spread your toes wide, extending up through the heel and pulling the toes towards the shin. Do the Core SIP Breath while lengthening through the heel, noticing how breathing activates the deep core fascia line and engages the leg and back muscles deeper into the movement. Inhale, hold your

Pointing or dancer foot   *Flointing or gas pedal*   *Heel pressing
or parking brake*

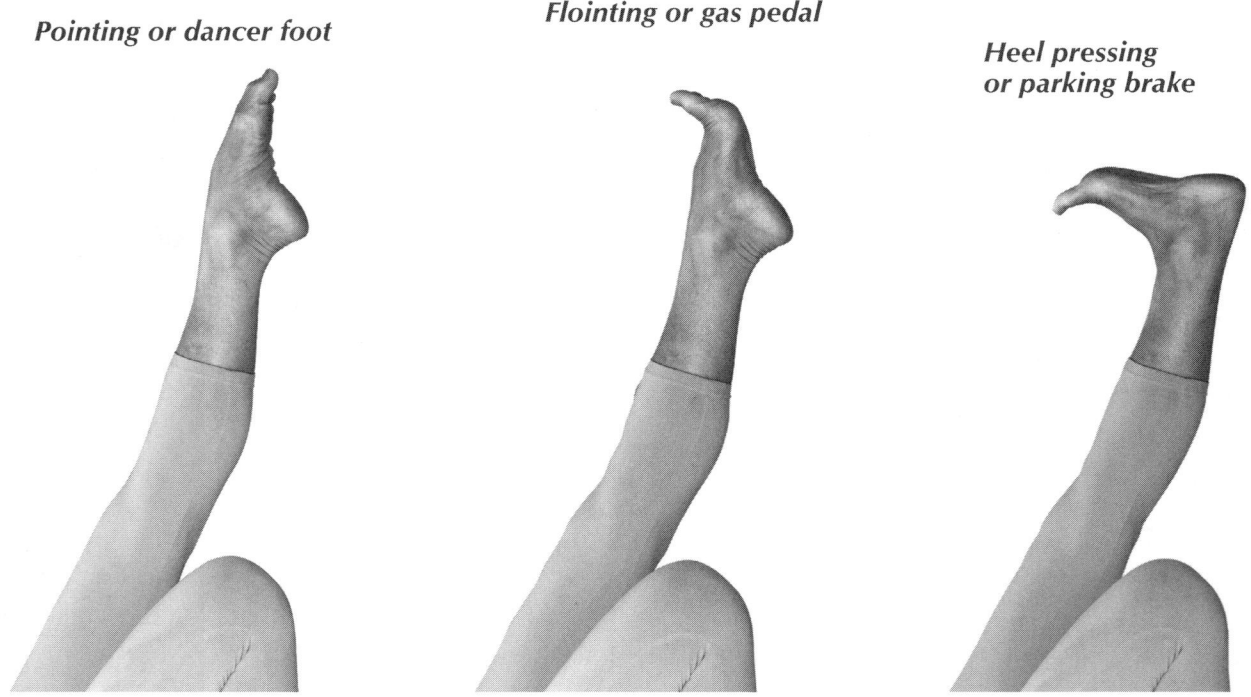

Fig. 9B – Focus on Foot Positions

breath, and accentuate this muscle action. Exhale and continue to lift through the heel, but release the excess muscle tension. Move your hands further up the leg towards your foot, and feel the new flexibility and looseness in your muscles. Practice this for a few breath repetitions, extending up through the heel, tightening what is tight in the back and core of the body and then releasing into the stretch, without adding tension.

Continue the exercise, but change your foot position to pointed toes. Notice the new muscle engagements in the front of your leg and the arch of your foot. Contract your leg muscles so that they tighten and engage deeply. Inhale with the SIP Breath technique and, while pointing the toes like a dancer, accentuate the muscle tightness in the front of the leg. Hold your breath for a few seconds and tighten your leg muscles further. Exhale, releasing the extra tension in the legs, hip, and back, but continuing to point your toes. If you are able, move your hands farther towards your foot. Repeat this action of pointing, noticing the action, accentuating the action, then holding the point while releasing the accentuation.

By actively engaging the foot with pointing and the gas pedal foot, your feet become strong and flexible in the way that you use them in real life. When combined with the internal movements of YogAlign breathing, you wake up your deep inner core line of muscles and free the fascial restrictions coming from your center. At first your feet may feel awkward, stiff, and unresponsive, but after a short period of time your feet will come alive, giving you a keen sense of balance and movement awareness. Your feet will change shape, your arches will be activated, your toes will spread open, and your feet will feel strong and relaxed. As your body shifts back to the supple responsiveness of youth, you will see improvements in your ability to point, extend, and engage your feet.

Inhale using the Core SIP Breath, and now try the exercise using the "floint" or "gas pedal" position. Hold and accentuate tightening in the muscles that engage, then release the tension, but keep your foot engaged in the floint position even through the movements of exhalation. Notice how your foot feels now. Remember you are mostly water and space and your feet can be easily shaped to a new form. Your foot can acquire a toned arch, relaxed strong toes, and stable ankles if you focus on doing these poses daily.

Toe flexion or Toe extension?

Many people use the word "flex" as a verb to describe muscle actions. You've certainly heard someone say "flex your muscle" or "flex your bicep." However, this is an incorrect usage of an anatomical term that is actually intended to describe the actions of joints. Muscles do not flex! Joints flex; muscles contract or release.

When the toes are pulled back toward the shin (as in the parking brake position), the toes are extended, but the ankle is flexed. In the dancer foot (or pointing foot), the toes are in flexion, and the ankle is extended. In the flointing (or gas pedal foot), the toe and ankle joints are both extended, which simulates most closely how we use our feet in daily life.

Although we are not all ballet dancers, using the point or dancer foot while reclining can help us build strength in the arches and the muscles that extend the ankle, without running the risk of compressing the bones of the ankle.

In contrast, the parking brake foot is part of the right-angle template that is unnatural for human movement, and therefore should be avoided entirely, or only used in combination with widely-spaced toes. Remember: the tension-balance in your feet both affects, and is affected by, your entire body.

POSITION #10 — CORE CONNECTOR & LEG CIRCLES

Optimal alignment of your whole body can be achieved quickly, with just a few days' practice of the "Core Connector." In this exercise, we explore how core breathing—combined with specific foot positioning and leg movements—stabilizes and strengthens the muscles of the inner core, while naturally aligning the body's posture from head to toe. This pose works like magic, connecting the movements of your breath from your diaphragm to your psoas group, out through your legs to the arches of your feet; at the same time it balances the muscular and fascial forces of your arms and brings your head to neutral. The psoas is the only connecting muscle between the diaphragm and the legs, joining the upper and lower body. Vitality in breath and movement happens quickly when the psoas and diaphragm connection is awakened and activated by doing this pose. The psoas is our main hip flexor but also an accessory muscle of breathing, a spine stabilizer and the initiator of leg movement in an optimally tuned body. This pose activates the psoas in an eccentric contraction, in which a muscle paradoxically lengthens as it contracts, releasing tension in the lower back and stabilizing the spine and sacrum.

This full-body exercise aligns the neck and shoulders, balances the fascia lines, and helps to correct forward head carriage and poor posture. In addition to strengthening the core by toning the psoas as well as the breathing muscles, this exercise also increases foot awareness. The slightest change in foot position can constrict breathing and shift the fascia lines that dictate structural positioning of your spine and sacrum. Most people are surprised that foot position affects breathing, and that it is also a determinant of sacral and spine alignment.

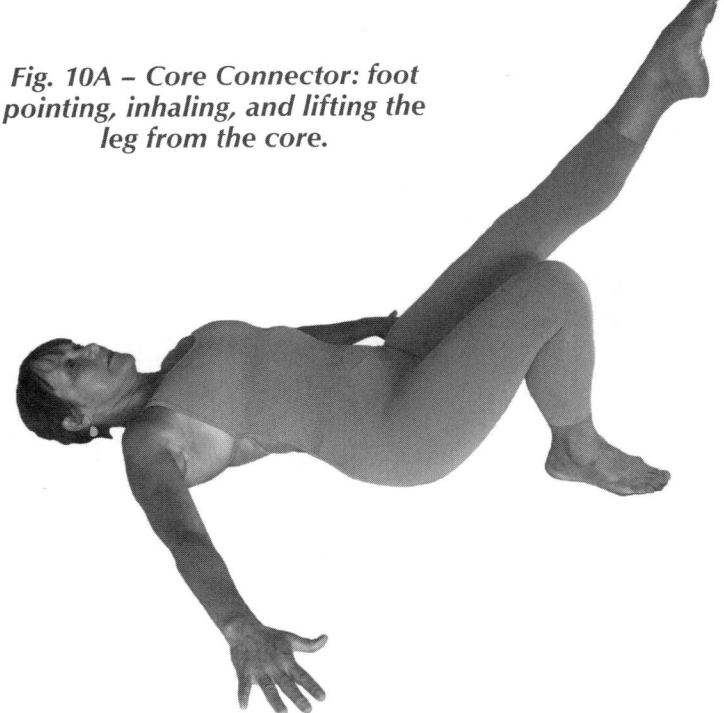

Fig. 10A – Core Connector: foot pointing, inhaling, and lifting the leg from the core.

Caution: Make sure that you point your foot as you inhale and lift your leg. Exhaling while leg-lifting with extended toes pulls on fascia/muscle lines that contract the muscles of the abdomen and rib cage. When your navel is drawn in from exhaling, this also flattens or flexes the spine taking the curve out of the lower back. Exhaling while lifting your leg puts you at risk for overstretching and aggravating the ligaments of the sacrum and lower back.

The movements of exhalation create a shortening of the spine, so in YogAlign we *always* inhale while doing single leg-lifts, in order to maintain an inner-extension of our core.

Using the Core SIP Breath while lifting the leg (with pointed toes) keeps the spinal curves in a neutral position, and programs the core trunk muscles to work in synergy, engaging in a stabilizing fashion through eccentric contraction. A toned, but flexible psoas keeps the spine stable and the hips flexible, freeing your body to move from the inner core with less effort from other peripheral forces. Using inhalation when contracting the psoas and hip flexors to lift your leg will activate your psoas/diaphragm connection. Doing the "Core Connector" wires the movement of your leg to initiate from the very center of your body. The eccentric programming of the core muscles accentuated in this pose frees up the muscular forces in your entire structure, releasing unnecessary tension throughout the body. This tension was a legacy of muscles performing functions that they were never designed to do. The fascial restrictions that grew to support that tension begin to reorganize, creating a balance of dynamic tensile forces throughout all of the fascia lines that support optimal posture and movement. When the "Core Connector" is practiced for even just a few days, people begin to see and feel their waist and neck lengthening, and experience a huge release of tension that frees the dynamic kid body. With the awakening of the psoas/diaphragm connection through breathing, one begins to move naturally from the center without extra effort in the periphery. Many say they feel as if they are "floating."

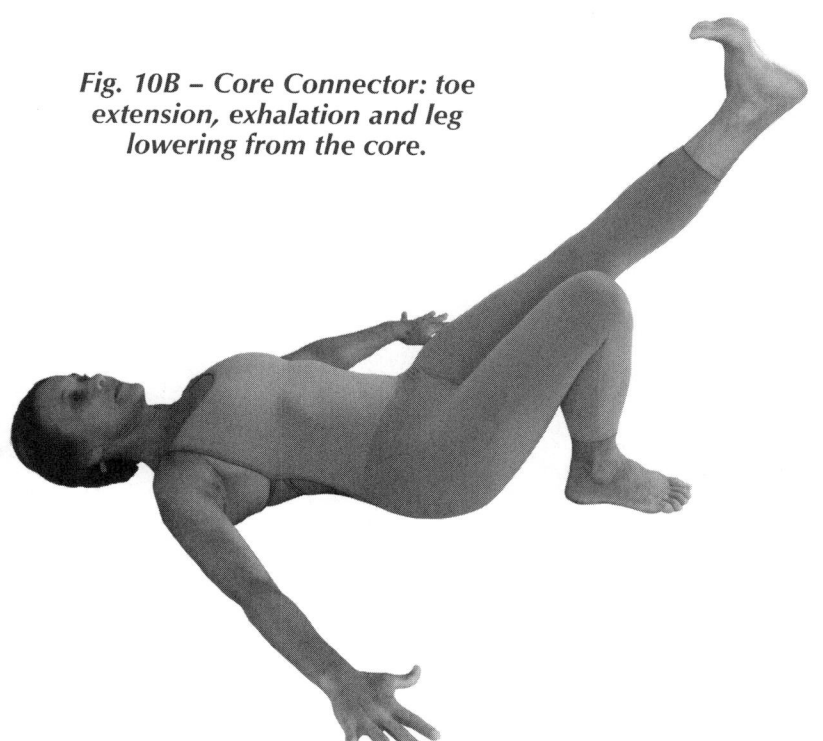

Fig. 10B – Core Connector: toe extension, exhalation and leg lowering from the core.

DOING THE CORE CONNECTOR

Beginning with your fingers spread, press your palms to the floor with your arms in a downward "V" shape (or 45-degree angle) from your trunk. Stay aware of your whole body as you anchor your shoulder blades and palms to the floor. Keep your shoulders down, relax your neck, and lower your collarbones away from your ears, being sure to keep the natural curves in your neck and lower back. Draw the tips of your shoulder blades down towards your hips.

Point your foot and begin to use the SIP inhalation technique. Start the inhalation a few seconds before you initiate the movement of lifting your leg. Go slowly and consciously, making sure to keep your toes pointed like a dancer. Stay aware of how you feel as you engage your breathing muscles. Keep your foot actively engaged through every toe, sensing the contraction of your muscles as they hug-in towards your leg bones. On your next exhale, slowly lower your leg toward the floor, while extending through your heel with your toes spreading wide. When your foot is about 12-18 inches above the floor, point or floint your toes, and begin your next Core SIP Breath, before drawing your leg back up towards the ceiling. Remember to always initiate your movements with the breathing process. Practice feeling the link between the psoas and the diaphragm by connecting your leg movement to your breath.

Now exhale. Reach again through your heel with toes spread wide. and lower your leg down toward the floor. Inhale, point, and then breathe as you lift the leg upward. Lift your leg towards a 90-degree angle, but keep your leg lower if your hip begins to lift, or if your lower back presses into the floor.

Do eight to ten of these leg lifts, stopping with your leg in a 45-degree angle to the floor. Proceed on to the "Leg Circles / Hip Lubricator" exercise.

POSITION #11 — LEG CIRCLES / HIP LUBRICATOR

This pose not only feels good, it also keeps your legs looking great. Leg circles strengthen the diaphragm, psoas, and the inner-thigh-to-foot line of movement. Through this exercise, the adductor (or inner thigh) muscles are strengthened and lengthened, bringing balance to the actions of the knee and hip rotators. "Leg Circles" increase synovial fluid (or joint lubrication) and nourishment to your hip joint; at the same time, the sacrum and hips are massaged and energized by the circular movements. See the DVD included with this book for a visual demonstration of leg circles.

Inhale, point or floint your toes, and circle your extended leg out to the side and then up towards your head. Lower it back towards the floor on the exhale. Continue to breathe, circling your leg on each inhale. Make sure to start the circling leg movement with a deep core inhale, keeping your leg muscles firm and your foot active by pointing your toes or using the gas pedal position. Keep your shoulder girdle stable against the floor, but let your hips swivel as your leg circles. Move slowly at first, developing more speed when you can move deeply and fluidly without any jerking.

Fig. 11 – Leg Circles / Hip Lubricator

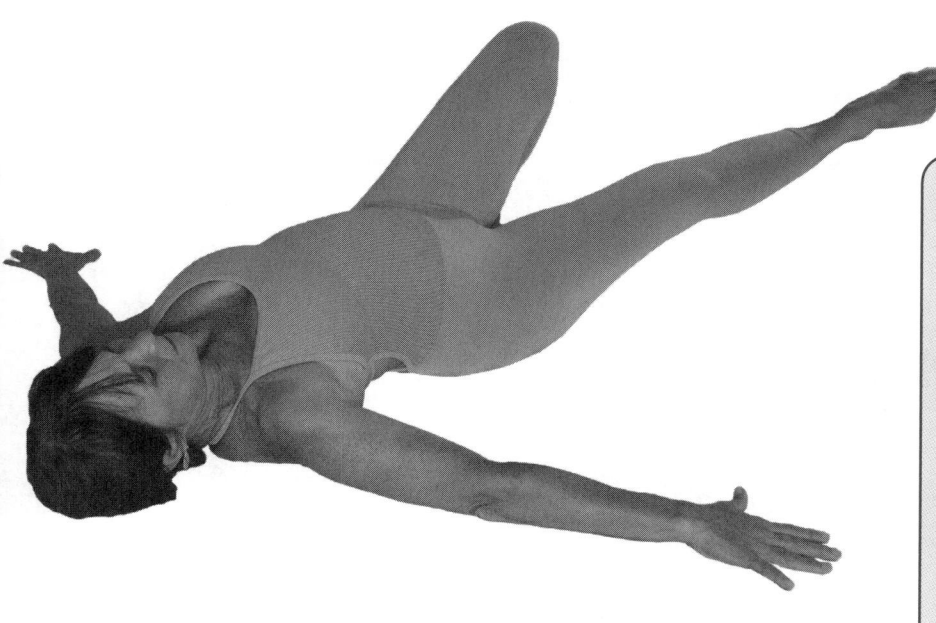

Caution: If your hip makes a popping sound you might be circling your leg in the wrong direction. The right leg should be circled in a counter clockwise position and the left leg in a clockwise manner. Make sure to engage the leg circles with a strong point or gas pedal position in your foot, while keeping your opposite knee bent and your foot on the floor. Make smaller circles at first, and be careful to avoid tension or strain in your groin.

POSITION #12 — LEG WRESTLE: ENGAGE, RESIST, RECALIBRATE

The "Leg Wrestle" uses PNF techniques to reset the resting length of muscles, particularly in the superficial back line. Through this exercise, the tension of the erector spinae muscles is reset, the spine lengthens, and the nervous system switches to relaxation mode. Tension in the lower back muscles—which can be present even in those who are very fit—can create a muscular vice-grip keeping us in a state of pain and compression. Your kidney and adrenal organs are suspended in your lower back muscles. When back muscles are strained, there is a lack of blood flow in the muscles which also affects kidney and adrenal functions in the long and short term. To eliminate this tension, you can use the "tighten what is tight" principle, consciously releasing and resetting the resting muscle length of the entire back line.

Part A: Engage and accentuate muscle actions

Interlace your fingers behind the back of your left leg, and put your foot in the gas pedal or floint position. While holding the back of your leg, pull in with your arms as you move your leg away from your head. Let your arms pull your leg back towards your head while you resist and engage the muscles of your leg. With this move you are "wrestling" your leg muscles against your arm muscles. Hold your breath gently for a moment while resisting. Close your eyes and notice the action of your leg and back muscles, and how they engage to keep up the "match." As you exhale, release the extra contraction you added and go deeper into the stretch, drawing your thigh back towards your belly. Bend your knee and go deeper.

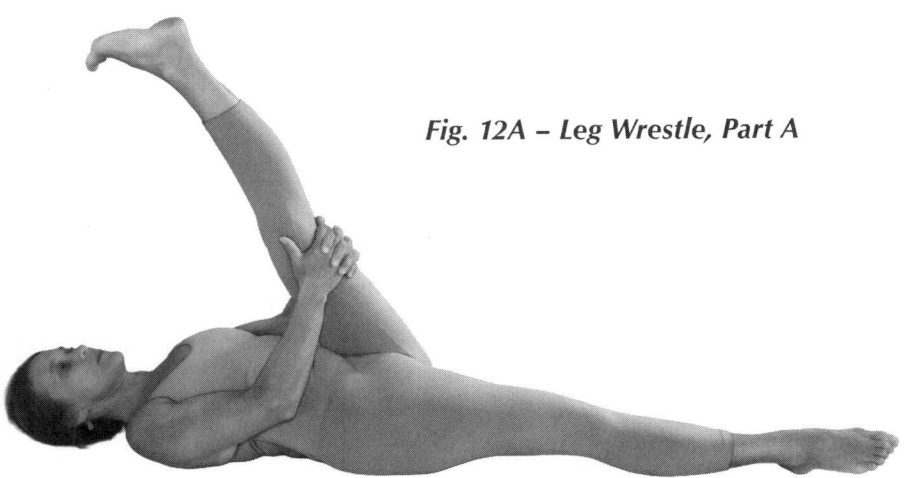

Fig. 12A – Leg Wrestle, Part A

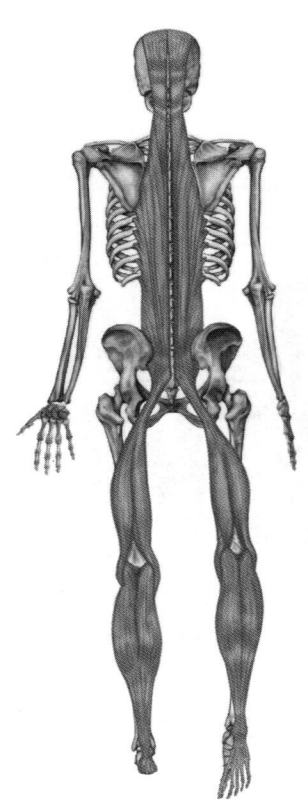

Part B: Release the action of the leg—bending the knee if necessary—while letting go of tension in your back.

Repeat the "match" again. While holding the pose, consciously increase the actions of the leg muscles, and hold for several seconds. Inhale and hold your breath gently for a moment as you continue to pull back on the leg with your hands, keeping your feet in a pointed or gas pedal position. Hold and accentuate for a moment, then relax the actions of your leg as you draw your

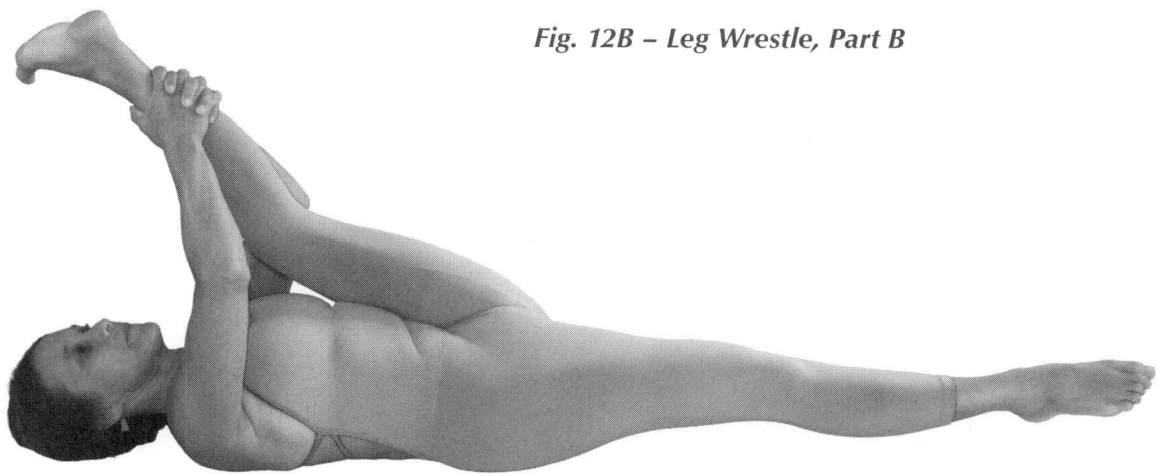

Fig. 12B – Leg Wrestle, Part B

leg in towards the armpit, sliding your hands up towards your calf muscles and allowing the muscles of your back to relax and lengthen.

Let the knee bend softly, and feel the muscles in the back side of your body lengthen and soften. Straighten your other leg, (the right one) while keeping your toe pointed and your foot raised above the floor. Draw your shoulders down and roll your body from side to side. This will traction your spine and, at the same time, the rolling movements will provide a wonderful self-massage that uses the weight of your own body.

This is a great pose to do with a partner. Lean into your partner's lifted leg as they resist against you. Do not push into the back of the knee. Place your hands above and/or below the knee. Be gentle on the exhale/release and encourage your partner to lengthen in the back and release tension in the jaw. The back of the neck should be lengthened and the cervical curve maintained.

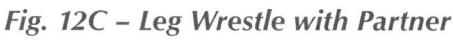

Fig. 12C – Leg Wrestle with Partner

POSITION #13 — * STAR *

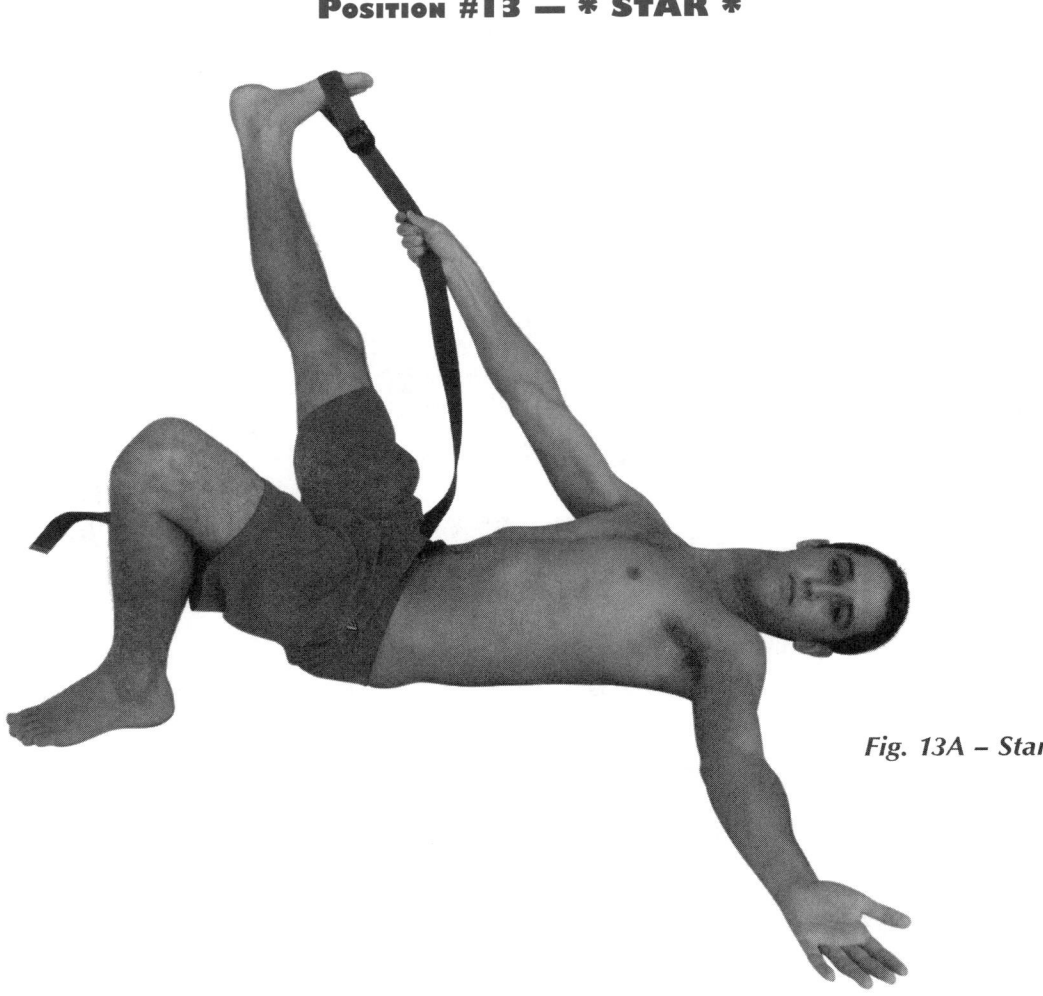

Fig. 13A – Star

Still reclining, place a strap around the ball of your right foot or hold the ball of your right foot with your toes pointed or flointed. Keep your knee extended if possible with your toes actively spread or pointed. Do not pull hard on the strap, and avoid putting any pressure or strain on your knee area. Inhale deeply, tighten your left hand into a fist, and squeeze your arm and leg muscles tightly. Hold 10–15 seconds. Engage and accentuate the actions of your muscles. Tighten what is already tight, including your gluteus (buttock) and pelvic floor muscles.

Exhale, and bring your right leg out to the right side, drawing your right foot towards your right ear. It is important to keep your left hip on the floor as you complete this motion. Your inner right thigh should be gently rotated internally to maintain a balance of actions in the hip rotators. Maintain muscle actions rather than falling out of the socket and hanging from your ligaments. Turn your head to

Caution: If you feel a pulling pain or sensation in your groin, do not take your leg as far out to the side; instead, work within a smaller range of motion.

the left as you exhale, spreading your fingers and opening your mouth wide with your tongue extended. As you exhale and release the right leg out to the side, imagine that you are drawing your arms and legs deeper into their sockets on both sides, connecting into the core. To stretch effectively, your body must feel safe, with the joints stabilized. In YogAlign we accomplish this by creating the effort to draw the limbs back in toward center, rather than by reaching the limbs out and away from the socket.

As you hold your leg out to the side, inhale and feel your limbs and the muscles of your entire body engaged back toward the center of your body. Sense that your body feels like a star, as you extend your arms and legs out from the center of your body. When you need to exhale, open your mouth as wide as possible, and extend out with your tongue.

Do a "Full Body Stretch" after completing this pose. Notice the difference in both sides of your body, and notice how energized, lengthened, and relaxed your right side and right leg feel compared to your left side. Repeat the exercises and self massage techniques from positions 3-13 now on your left side and then end with another "Full Body Stretch" taking a few moments to notice how your body feels in its entirety.

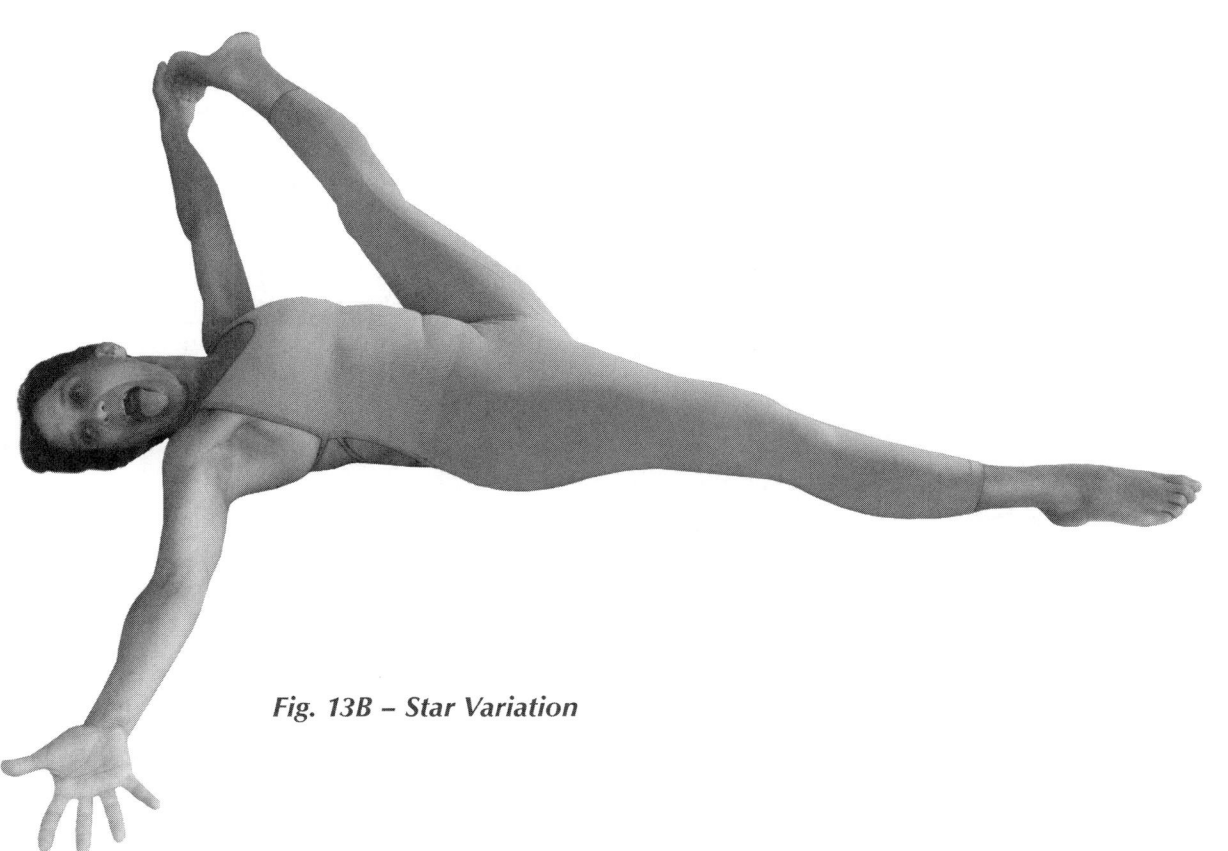

Fig. 13B – Star Variation

POSITION #14 — SIP-Ups: Ab-Work without the "Crunch"

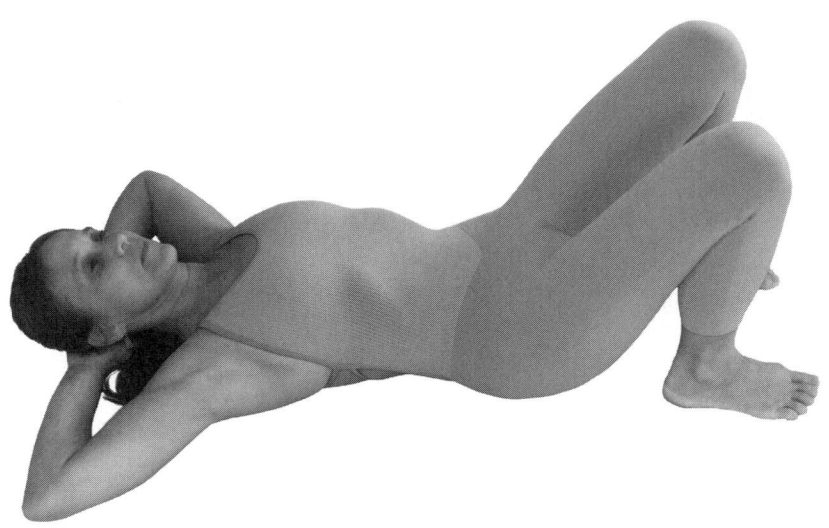

Fig. 14A – SIP-Ups

Why do the SIP-up instead of the Sit-up?

SIP-up exercises synergistically train your core trunk muscles—abs, psoas, QL, and other core and spinal muscles—to lengthen rather than shorten as they contract. Using the movements of inhalation while contracting your abdominals reprograms the muscles to extend and stabilize your spine in all movements. You get strong, toned, and elongated in the core rather than short, tight and in the vice-grip. The deep core fascia/muscle line is also toned and lengthened, giving you the tools to move and breathe from the center of your body. Toning these muscles in synergy gives you a muscular ring of support that stabilizes your spine, lengthens your waist and provides more space and support for your abdominal organs.

SIP-ups teach you how to use less externalized effort in your body and attain comfortable, relaxed, natural alignment. SIP-ups also build core strength while preventing the tightness and over-shortening caused by most ab crunches and sit-up exercises, all of which typically instruct you to exhale as you lift, or exhale as you fold. Remember that exhalation is a body movement that shortens the trunk; when combined with sit-ups this exhalation contributes to an excessive shortening of the front of the body as well as a lot of compression on your spine.

The focus in these exercises is on breathing-in with a Core SIP Breath, as you contract the abdominals. This combination brings tremendous tone and length into your trunk, releasing tension from the abdomen, and mitigating any compression of the spine. The movement to lift your trunk should always be initiated by first doing a few seconds of the SIP inhalation technique. This will create a lengthening of the trunk, even as you contract your abdominals at the same time.

Exhaling as you do sit-ups creates shortness in the front body, leading to more pressure on your spine and internal organs. As the spine compresses and shortens, the space between your ribs and your hips decreases until you lose your waist. Your organs are then "homeless," so they protrude out in the front, giving you a pot belly despite all of the sit-ups and ab-work you might do. The secret to toning the core is focusing on exercises that increase stabilization. Let go of the desire for hard six-pack abs, and embrace your kid body. Remember, the tighter you make your front, the tighter you make your back. A tight belly will only restrict movement, breathing, and feeling all over your body. What you want is fluidity and tone, not chronic tight and tense belly muscles.

Tuning in. . .

Lie on the floor with your fingers on your rib cage area. Practice Core SIP Breathing with your eyes closed for several breaths. Feel your ribs move and separate during inhalation, expanding outward in all directions. When you exhale, use the sssss sound and notice how the ribs are pulled together from muscular actions that work from the inside. Inhale and feel the external rib muscles and inner core (diaphragm, psoas and QL) turn on. Exhale and feel the inner rib cage, outer belly and waist squeezing in. Breathe in using the SIP Breath and breathe out using the ssss sound, a wide open mouth or through your nose (for clogged noses, see below). Expand the ribs like an accordion, as open as possible, through breathing. Tuning into the breath will help you remember that how you breathe is the most important part of the "SIP-up."

Stabilize your scapula. . .

Stabilizing the scapula (shoulder blade) is key to core stabilization, natural alignment, and proper breathing during this exercise.

Preparing to do the SIP-Up

Lying on your back, bring your elbows down along your sides and your forearms and hands up as though you are pushing on low ceiling. This is the "stick 'em up" position from a reclining position designed to help you train your mid back muscles to stabilize your scapula. Pretend that you are pressing up with your hands, but do not move your arms. Feel your scapulas activate and draw together in your back. Keep your shoulders down and away from your ears. Take a deep breath and notice how your chest and ribs are more open when the scapulas are "fixed."

> **Note:** If your nose is clogged for the exhale, first try sinus massage to open your nasal passages. If breathing out through the nose is still difficult, exhale through your mouth using the ssss sound or wide open with an extended tongue. Focused movements of exhalation tone your abdomen, bring blood flow to your organs, and increase your sense of awareness in your solar plexus.

SIP-Up. . .

Now, interlace your fingers behind the back of your head. Breathe in, keeping the natural curves in your lower back and neck while drawing the tips of your shoulder blades down. Exhale making the ssss sound through your teeth. Relax your eyes, face and jaw. Keep your elbows wide and your arm muscles firm. Inhale using a Core SIP Breath, and lift your head and shoulders slowly off of the floor. Exhale through a wide open mouth with your tongue extended. As the exhale is ending, slowly lower to the floor, feeling your ribs drawing together and your belly pulling in towards your spine. If you want to add more intensity to the "SIP-Up," make a soft "ssss" sound as you exhale, while accentuating the contraction of your exhalation muscles.

Do five lifts with your eyes gazing straight up towards the ceiling. Remember to use the movement of the inhale each time you come up, and to slowly exhale yourself down to the floor, while keeping your elbows wide. Don't let your elbows move towards each other; also keep your shoulders away from your ears, and your shoulder blades drawing towards your hips.

On your next inhale, continue to use the breath for lifting, but add a twist to one side as you complete the inhalation. Exhale down to center, and then inhale up to the other side. Do five lifts to each side. If you want to work harder, stay up in the twisting position as you exhale, retaining a lifted position rather than letting the movements of exhalation compress your body. Start a SIP inhalation and twist to the other side, keeping your neck long and the entire body extended. Each time you exhale, go to the floor or stay twisted to one side. Do not move or twist while in the exhalation process. Go back to the floor on your next exhale and rest.

Massage your diaphragm and rib cage area and then move back into the basic position, with hands behind your head, ready for the next exercise.

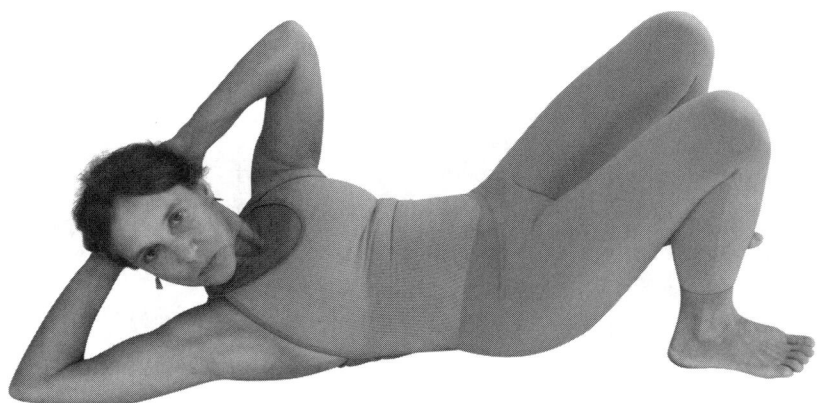

Fig. 14B – SIP-Up Twist

Caution: If you feel tension in your neck, bring your head and shoulders back to the floor each time you exhale. Remember to always stretch your elbows wide as you bring your head and shoulder girdle to the floor. Keep your throat and arm pits open. Do not pull on your neck as you come up, and use the movements of breath to guide and lift you.

POSITION #15 — BICYCLE SIP-UPS

The "Bicycle SIP-Up" brings the psoas into action, creating full-body movement from your core. It balances the spiral line of muscle and fascia which directs lateral and twisting rotations of the body. Through this exercise, the deep front line is balanced from head to toe. If you have low back pain, be sure to keep the bent-knee leg on the floor while extending through the other leg.

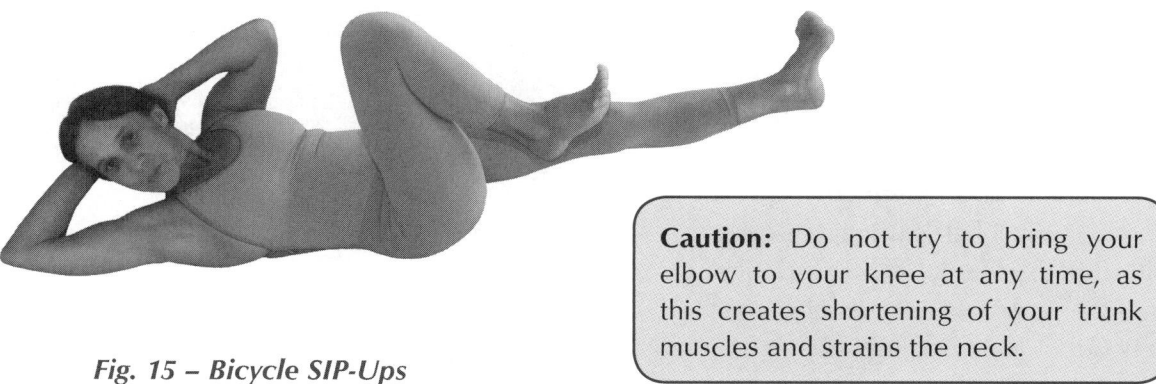

Fig. 15 – Bicycle SIP-Ups

Caution: Do not try to bring your elbow to your knee at any time, as this creates shortening of your trunk muscles and strains the neck.

To begin, lift both feet off of the floor, keeping the knees above the hips. Inhale using the Core SIP Breath, and extend your left leg straight-out, about two feet above the floor. Keep your foot flointed or pointed. Still inhaling, lift and twist to the right. Remember, you are not trying to touch your elbow to your knee. You are simply lifting and twisting with your inhalation, maintaining length in the spine. Exhale, lowering the upper body to the floor and bringing both knees back above the hips.

Repeat on the other side, this time straightening-out the right leg, inhaling, lifting and twisting to the left, then exhaling back to center. Make sure that you do a complete exhale and come all the way to the floor between repetitions. If you feel strain, lift the straightened leg higher and/or keep your left foot on the floor to stabilize your hips.

Keep your elbows wide, shoulder blades down and neck spine long, but not flattened. Imagine that you are breathing into the arch of your foot as you stretch into your leg, spreading your toes wide open. Keep your foot level and balanced.

To increase intensity and core balancing, hold the elevated twist, and press your head back into your hands without allowing it to move. Release the action in the neck and inhale, twisting to the other side. Notice how you are now using less effort. Feel the neck release as you breathe in.

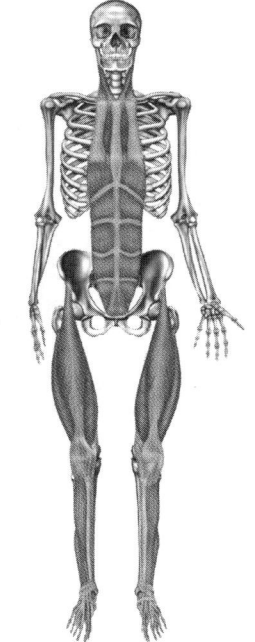

Exhale the knees back to center, reclining the shoulders back to the floor. Try linking several twists together, breathing in for as long as you can. See how long and slowly you can inhale while bicycling the legs and twisting the trunk. Do not hold your breath. Return to the floor when you need to exhale. Massage your breathing muscles and be aware of the increased energy flow in your center and the expansion in your ribs and diaphragm.

POSITION #16 — CORE SYNERGIZER (ADVANCED)

This pose strengthens the deep core line of breathing, while toning and strengthening your inner core.

Lie on your back with fingers interlaced behind the back of your head and shoulder blades pulled down. Put your heels together with toes spread and extended towards your shin. Inhale using a deep SIP Breath, lifting your head and shoulders up while extending your

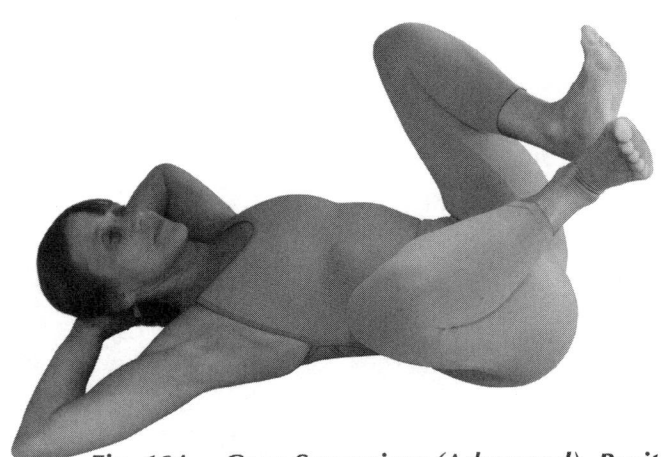

Fig. 16A – Core Synergizer (Advanced), Position 1: Exhaling, bring the heels together.

legs out at least two feet above the floor. Keep inhaling and squeeze your inner thighs and butt as you now point your toes. Keep your heels pressed together. Begin to exhale out your nose or with an "ssss" sound from your mouth, and slowly return to Position 1. Complete the exhalation, and feel your belly muscles draw tightly together.

Always inhale as you lift up. Do five sets lifting your trunk straight up, a few inches off of the floor. You can then add several more sets, lifting and twisting to each side with straight legs. Focus on breathing into your pointed toes, engaging the inner thighs and squeezing and contracting your gluteal muscles.

Fig. 16B – Core Synergizer (Advanced), Position 2: Inhale with core breathing, squeezing the inner thighs and buttocks.

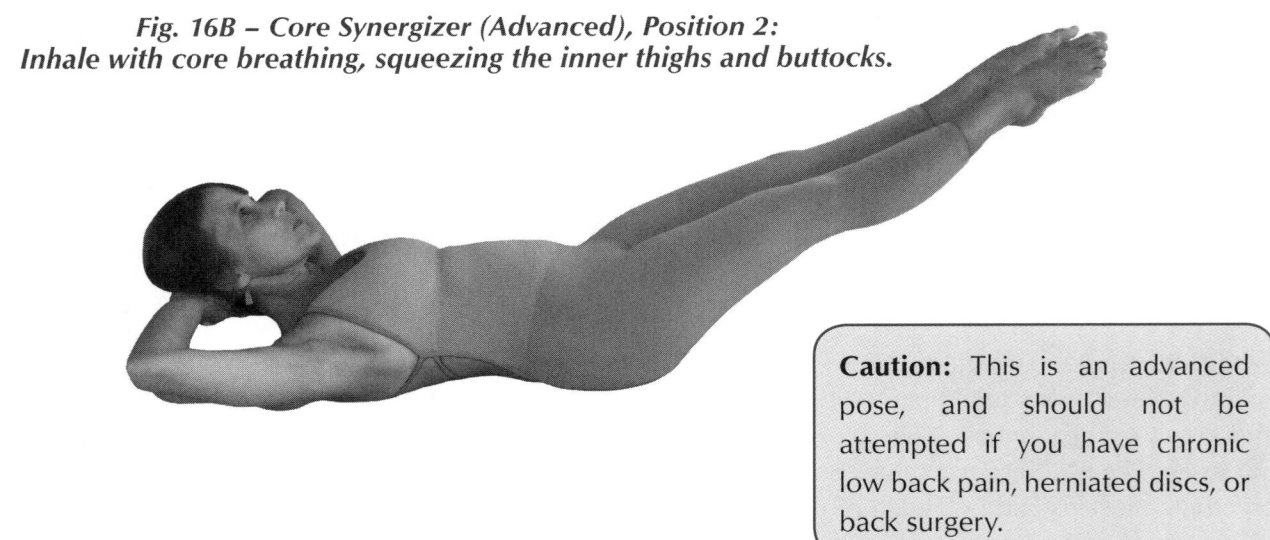

Caution: This is an advanced pose, and should not be attempted if you have chronic low back pain, herniated discs, or back surgery.

POSITION #17 — SPINAL ROLLS

Spinal rolling gets you in touch with your kid body. Spinal rolls are fun, they give you a great back massage and they teach you to trust your body and move without fear. Rolling also tones your core, massages your organs, and helps relieve built-up pressure in the colon (acting as a gas expeller).

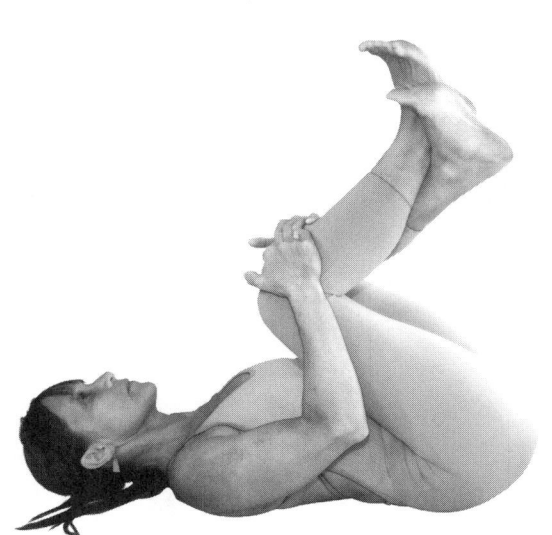

Fig. 17A – Exhale and relax with knees above hips.

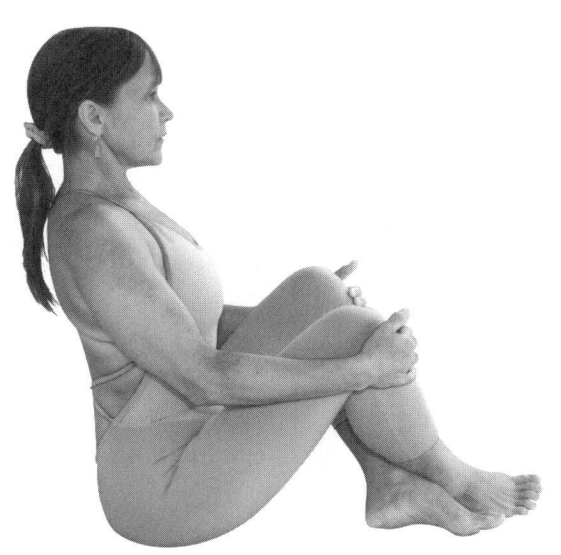

Fig. 17B – Inhale and rock up, keeping the lower back curve and sacral lift.

From a lying down position, take a deep Core SIP Breath. Roll up with a lift in your waist, and hold your knees or shins with your elbows straight. Keep a feeling of leaning back as you balance on your sit bones. Feel the lift in your waist and the lengthening in your spine that is created from deep core breathing. Exhale, relax, and roll back onto your mat. Focus on letting the weight of your body pressing against the mat create a massage of the back muscles that run along your spine. Inhale and roll back up into a sitting position, balancing on your sit bones and staying in natural alignment. You can use a mirror to ensure that your position is supporting the curve in your lower back, which protects the natural tilt in your sacrum.

When you are in the sitting-up position, your head should feel as though it is resting atop your spine with no effort. Lean back and draw your shoulder blades down your back, using your lower trapezius and rhomboid and serratus anterior muscles. Think about pulling down with the tips of your shoulder blades and keeping your upper shoulder blade wider at the top. Drop your collarbones to bring your shoulders away from your ears.

Repeat the exercise: exhale and roll back, inhale and roll forward. Each time you roll up, lean back slightly and feel your spine and waist lengthen. Use the SIP inhalation to create an inner lift that provides the curve in your lower back, taking pressure off of the sacrum. Be sure not to round your upper back, as this will cause you to lose this lower-back curvature. Inhale and feel your breathing muscles lengthen, supporting the front of the spine and engaging your breathing tube as an inner support system for your body.

Exhale and relax as you roll back. Feel your spinal muscles being massaged by the weight of your body as you roll. Be sure to have a mat surface padded enough to prevent feeling any pain in your spine. Pretend that you are a child, rolling up and down, just for the sheer fun of it. Breathe yourself up each time you roll to the sitting position. Focus on how it feels to breathe, and how your breath lifts and supports your entire body.

Each time you breathe, feel the inner ring of muscular support getting stronger, as you tone from the inside out. Notice that as your inner primary breathing muscles strengthen, your upper neck, jaw, and shoulder muscles are freed from holding up the weight of your head. You can also inhale as you roll both ways. Make sure that you use inhalation to come to sitting up and then exhale while keeping the gift of the lift. Focus on keeping the lift of your waist as you exhale and do not let the movements of exhalation take the curve out of your lower back or shorten the length of your neck or waist.

POSITION #18 — ARCH TUNER AND ANKLE ROLLER

The "Arch Tuner" is a one-stop-shopping pose, as it balances, massages and tones your feet and ankles, as well as aligns your spine, tones your core, and opens up your chest and arms. This is the best sitting position to use whether meditating, eating, chanting, or watching TV. Staying out of your chair and doing this pose often will keep your spine healthy and aligned. Use a mirror to check your alignment from the side: you should be able to envision one line running from the center of the ear, through the shoulder, and down to the hip.

Arch Tuner

Kneel on your mat, sitting upon one or more yoga blocks in order to keep pressure off of the tops of your feet and knees. Make sure your position is comfortable. If you feel any pressure at all in the top of the feet or your knees, add another block or small pillow. Do not do this pose if it causes any sort of pain in your knees or feet; if this is the case, you can massage and tone your feet while reclining on the floor.

Check that your feet are parallel to each other, and that your toes are pointed straight back. Press into the mat with the tops of your feet and toes. Take in a breath and hold it. Close your eyes, and increase the pressure you are exerting onto the mat with your toes and feet. Feel the muscles involved in this action, and then further intensify the pressure. After 10–15 seconds, exhale and relax the muscles in your toes and feet, feeling the blood flow and energy that has been created by engaging the foot muscles and then relaxing the effort.

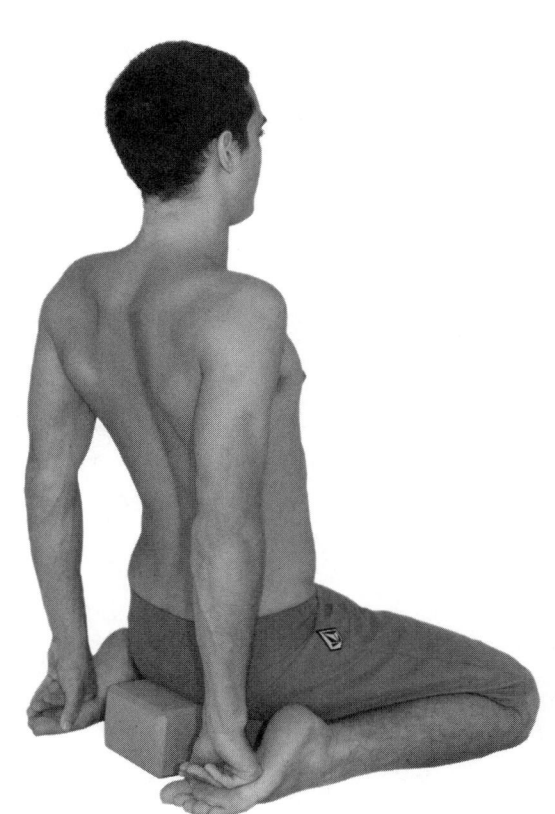

Fig. 18A – Arch Tuner

Make fists with your hands, and press them into the arches of your feet. Roll your fists with your arms straightened, while pressing your body weight back into your feet. Follow the principles of natural alignment, keeping your scapula pulled down and your spinal curves neutral. Lean back, draw your shoulder blades down, and feel the opening in your chest. Use a mirror to view your posture, and be sure you are keeping the natural curves in your spine, and that your head is balanced correctly at the top of your spine. Breathe open your rib cage, hold this inhalation for a moment, accentuating the inhalation muscles, then release as you lengthen your trunk.

Ankle Roller

To do the "Ankle Roller," start from a kneeling position as shown in **Fig. 18B**. Begin to slowly lean back, pressing your fists deeply into your feet in order to put more of your body weight into the massage of your arches. Take your hands behind you with your fingertips pointing back towards your hips and try lifting your knees off the floor **(Fig. 18C)**. From this position, roll forward onto your shins, then rock back and forth, massaging the tops of your feet from the ankles to the toes. Keep your chest lifted, shoulder blades drawn down, and your head in neutral standing alignment. If there is any pain or discomfort, try rocking just one foot at a time. Don't do this exercise if you experience any pain or discomfort; the shape of some peoples' ankles or feet simply may not allow the bones to articulate comfortably in this movement, so don't force it if you are one of these people. Remember: there is nothing to gain with pain, and you do not get comfortable by being uncomfortable.

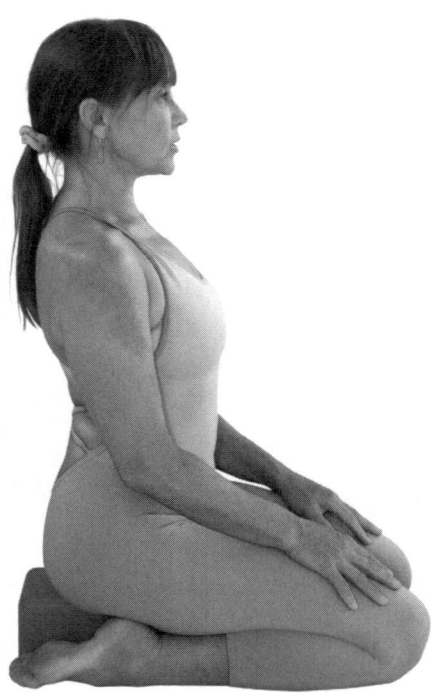

Fig. 18B – Ankle Roller

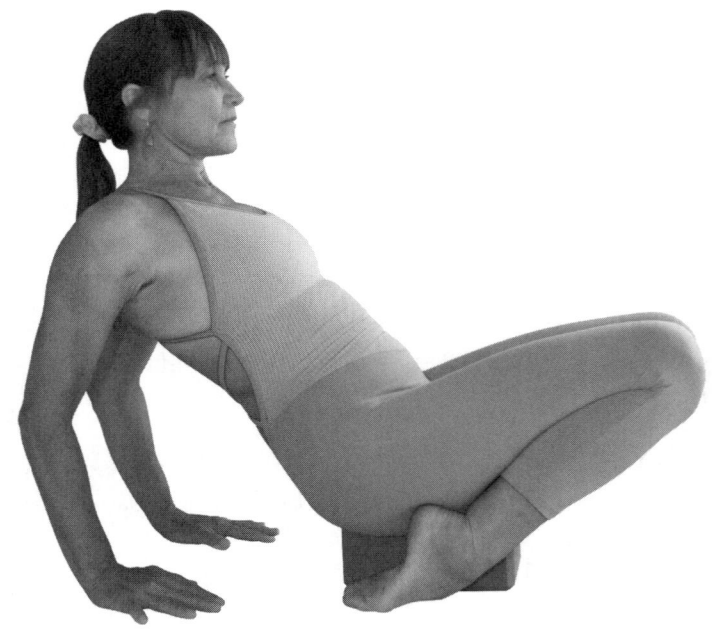

Fig. 18C – Ankle Roller

POSITION #19 — WRIST OPENER AND ARM MASSAGE

The "Wrist Opener" gently tones and stretches the wrists and fascial arm lines, while creating a deep connection from the fingertips to the core of your body. This pose helps to relieve pain and stiffness associated with computer use and repetitive strain. Go slowly and pay attention in order to protect the integrity of your joints.

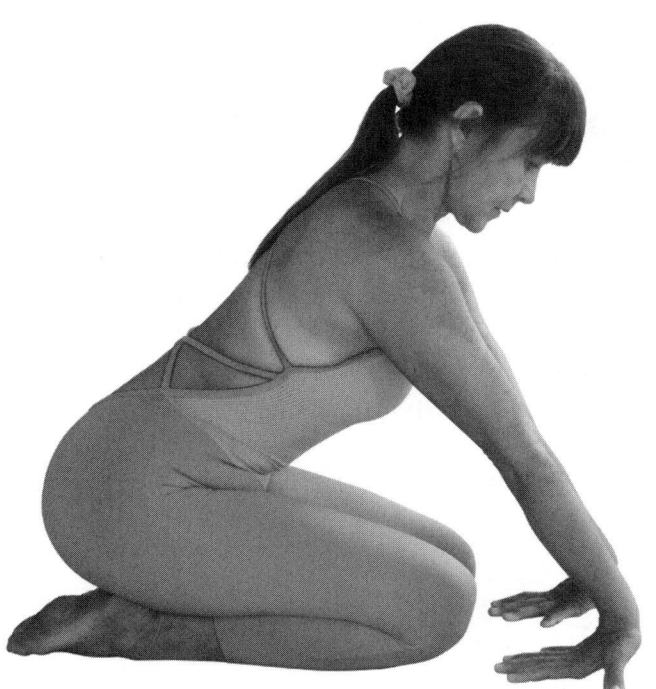

Fig. 19 – Wrist Opener and Arm Massage

Continue to sit on the block(s), or remove it if you are comfortable without it. Begin by massaging your right hand, starting with the palm and then kneading and rolling each finger. Press firmly on each fingernail stimulating blood flow into your fingertips. Work into your wrists, forearm, elbows, and all the way up to your shoulder. Let both arms hang down and notice how much lighter your right shoulder feels. Repeat the massage on the left side. Never underestimate the power and benefits of daily self-massage.

Place your hands on the mat with your palms down and your fingertips facing your knees. Keep your spine in natural alignment, with your shoulder blades and lats engaged down and towards your hips. Use inhalation to extend the trunk and feel the spine growing long from the sacrum to the neck. Do not lift your chin or let your shoulders ride up towards your ears.

Inhale and press the heels of your hands gently towards the floor. Notice where there is resistance; stop and then increase the tightness of that resistance for a moment. As you exhale, release the added contraction. As your muscles release, gently press the heel of your hand closer to the floor. Ensure that you are not pulling on ligaments by keeping your side body strong, with your arm bones drawn back into your shoulders.

Contract your arm muscles and feel the arm line fascia connections all the way into the shoulder and beyond to the rib cage, spine, and the crest of your hips. Inhale, keeping the neck neutral, and practice keeping length in your trunk as you exhale, gently extending the heel of the hand further towards the floor.

Now sit back (onto the block, if you are using one) and bring the backs of your hands together with your fingers pointing down. Rotate the fingers in towards the body, down and around, bringing the palms together, and repeat. Squeeze your wrists one at a time and then release. Drop your arms to the side, and notice the flow of energy in your arms.

Finish the exercise by raising your arms up towards the ceiling, make fists with both hands and squeezing tightly. Inhale, then hold your breath while sensing your body in its entirety, as you tighten and activate your muscles. Exhale with mouth and jaw wide open, tongue extending out, and your fingers wide. Pull down with your shoulder blades and feel the energy extending from the core out to your fingertips. Let your arms hang back down at your sides and notice the flow of energy in your body. Turn your head side-to-side, and briskly rub your scalp and ears with your fingertips.

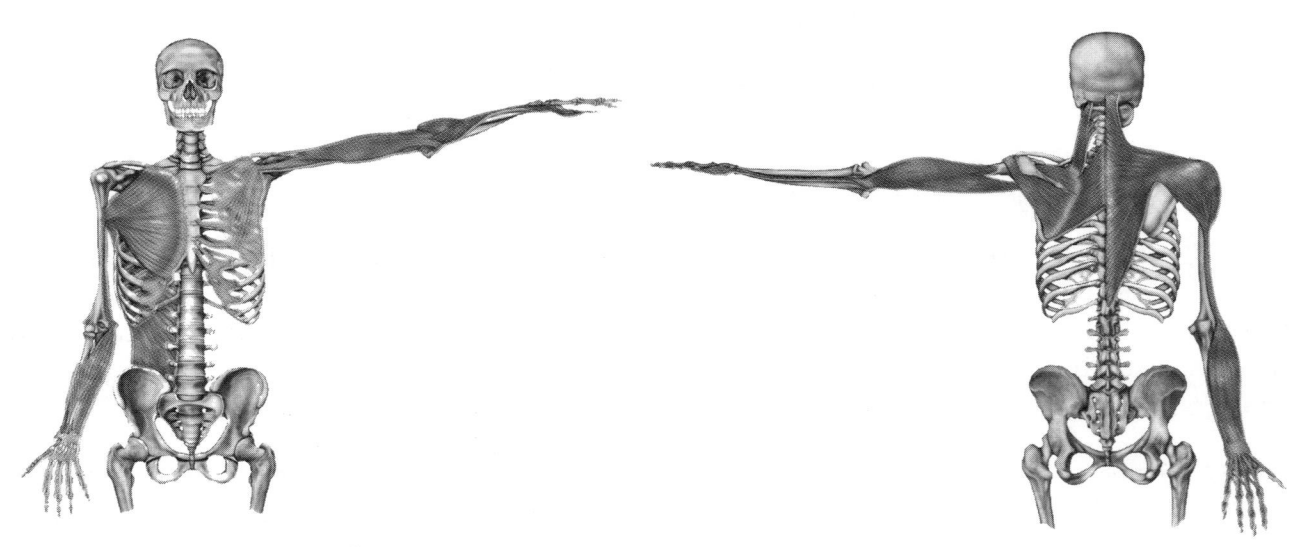

POSITION #20 — ROTATOR ROLLS TO SPINE ROLLS

This self-massage technique is very effective for relaxing, toning, and bringing blood flow into your gluteus and hip rotator muscles, such as the piriformis group. If you suffer from sciatica or piriformis syndrome, "Rotator Rolls" are a great self-healing tool that helps to balance tensile forces in the functional fascia lines. The rolls release tension, and at the same time build toned and balanced rotating power in the gluteus and other hip-rotating muscles. You will be toned, relaxed, and at-ease when you practice these "bum" rolls.

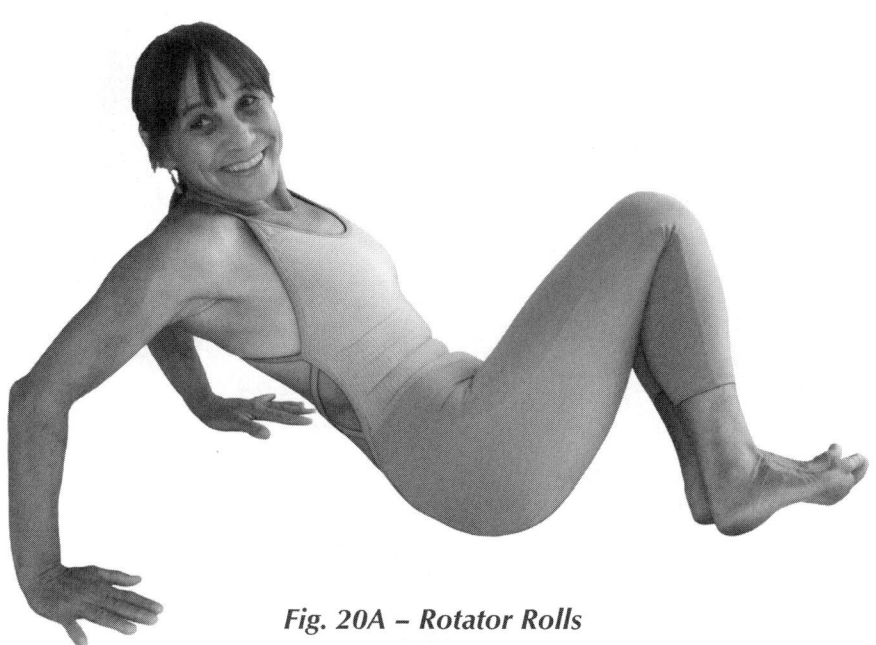

Fig. 20A – Rotator Rolls

Begin at the back of your mat. Lean onto one side of your buttocks with your hands behind you, palms down and fingers pointing back towards your hips. Keep your knees bent and your feet lifted off of the ground with your ankles crossed. Roll from one side of your buttocks to the other, and then back again. Continue rolling side-to-side, inching yourself all the way up to the front of your mat. Keep your butt muscles loose and relaxed as you swing from side-to-side. Stop on one side of your buttocks muscle making small outward circles in order to massage your muscles using the weight of your upper body. Make micro-movements, using your body weight to move into different areas of your glute muscles, staying longer in areas that ask for more attention. Keep lifted in the chest and draw down with your shoulder blades to assist this action. Roll onto the other side and repeat.

Reposition your body, moving onto your hands and knees. In this position, move your hips around like a hula dancer. Notice the openness and energy flow in your gluteals and hips. Then place yourself in the "Spinal Roll" (Position #17) and roll-up to standing. You are now ready to balance the arm and neck lines.

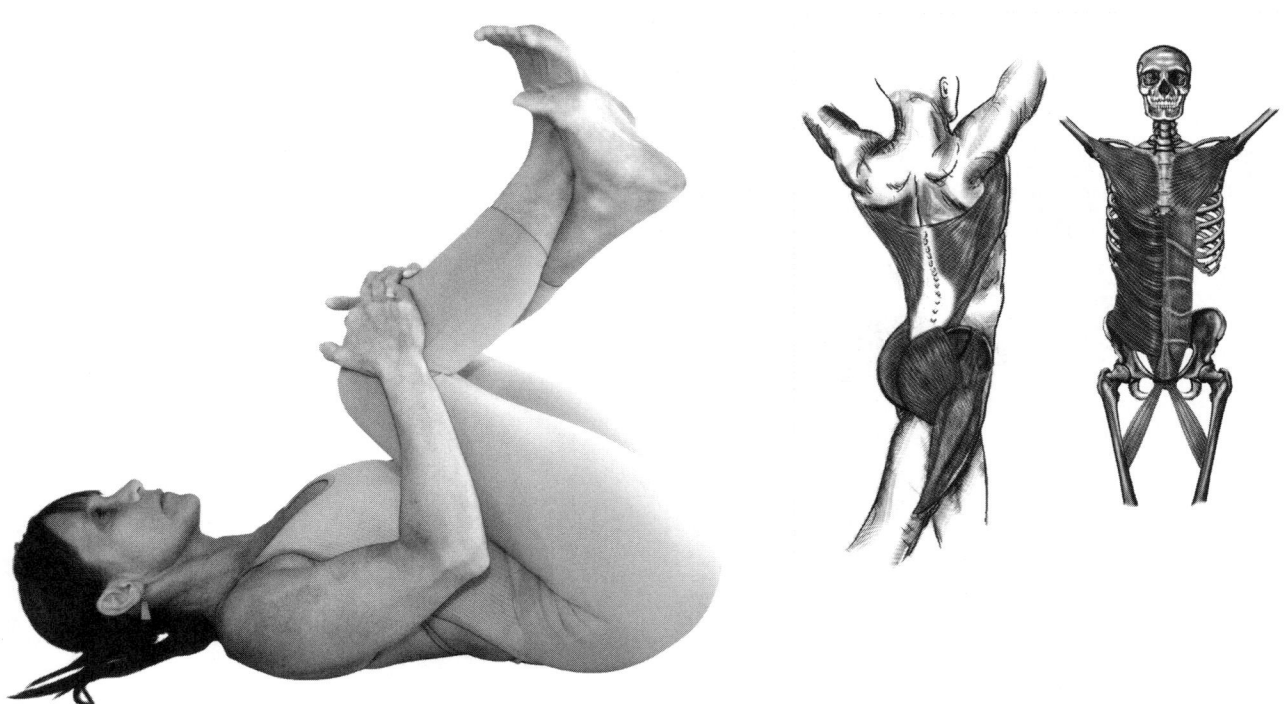

Fig. 20B – Spinal Roll (Position #17)
Exhale and roll the knees overhead.

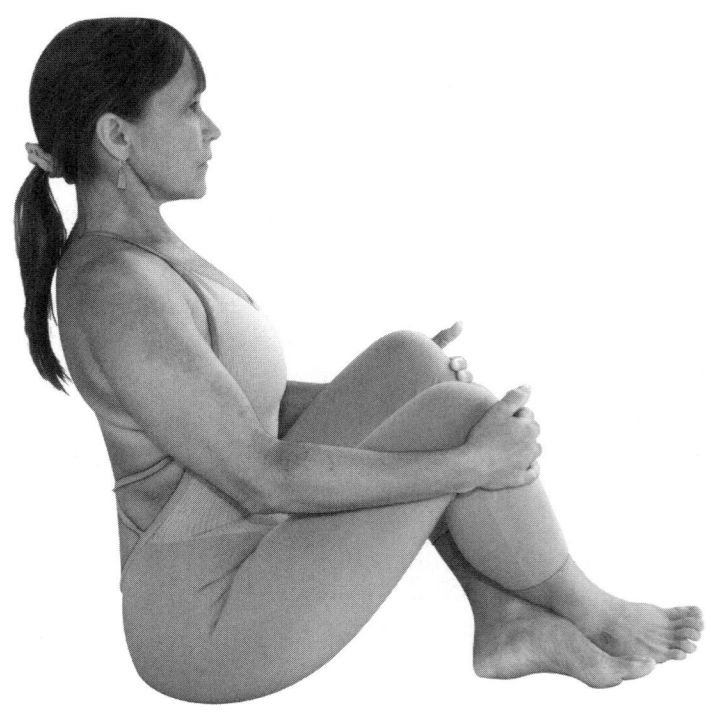

Fig. 20C – Spinal Roll (Position #17)
Inhale while rocking up.

POSITION #21 — SELF-MASSAGE TUNE-UP AND POI POUNDER

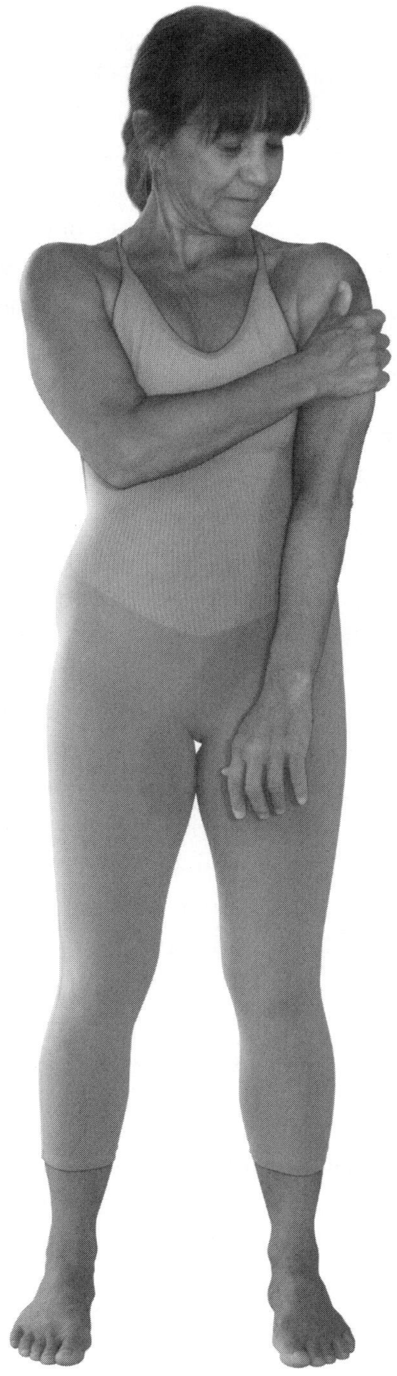

Self-Massage Tune-Up

Stand with your feet hip-distance apart, while evenly pressing into the four corners of each foot **(Fig. 21A)**. With your knees slightly bent, quickly shake your knees sideways for about 30 seconds. Shake your legs front to back like you are walking quickly for another 30 seconds. Stop and close your eyes, sensing your body in its entirety. Sense the movement of energy, and connect with the feeling of truly residing in your body. Feel the tension in your legs and hips disappear, leaving you relaxed and grounded in ease.

Inhale, and roll your shoulders up and back in circles. Begin massaging your right arm by starting with your hand and fingers. Bring attention and blood flow to each finger. Be thorough, and pay attention to any aches or pains you feel as you continue to massage your entire arm, all the way up to your shoulder and neck. Stay present in the moment, listening as your body tells you where it needs more massage attention. Massage the top of your shoulder, into your upper trapezius, and along the side of your neck. Rub around your collarbone, as well as along the front and upper intercostal muscles, which are between the rib bones in your chest.

After thoroughly massaging your right arm, let it hang loosely by your side. Notice the difference between the right and left shoulder areas. Now shift your attention to your left arm, and massage its entirety, with the same amount of awareness. Massage all the way up into the left side of your neck. Bring your attention into the collarbone and upper intercostal areas on this side as well.

Fig. 21A – Self-massage Tune-up

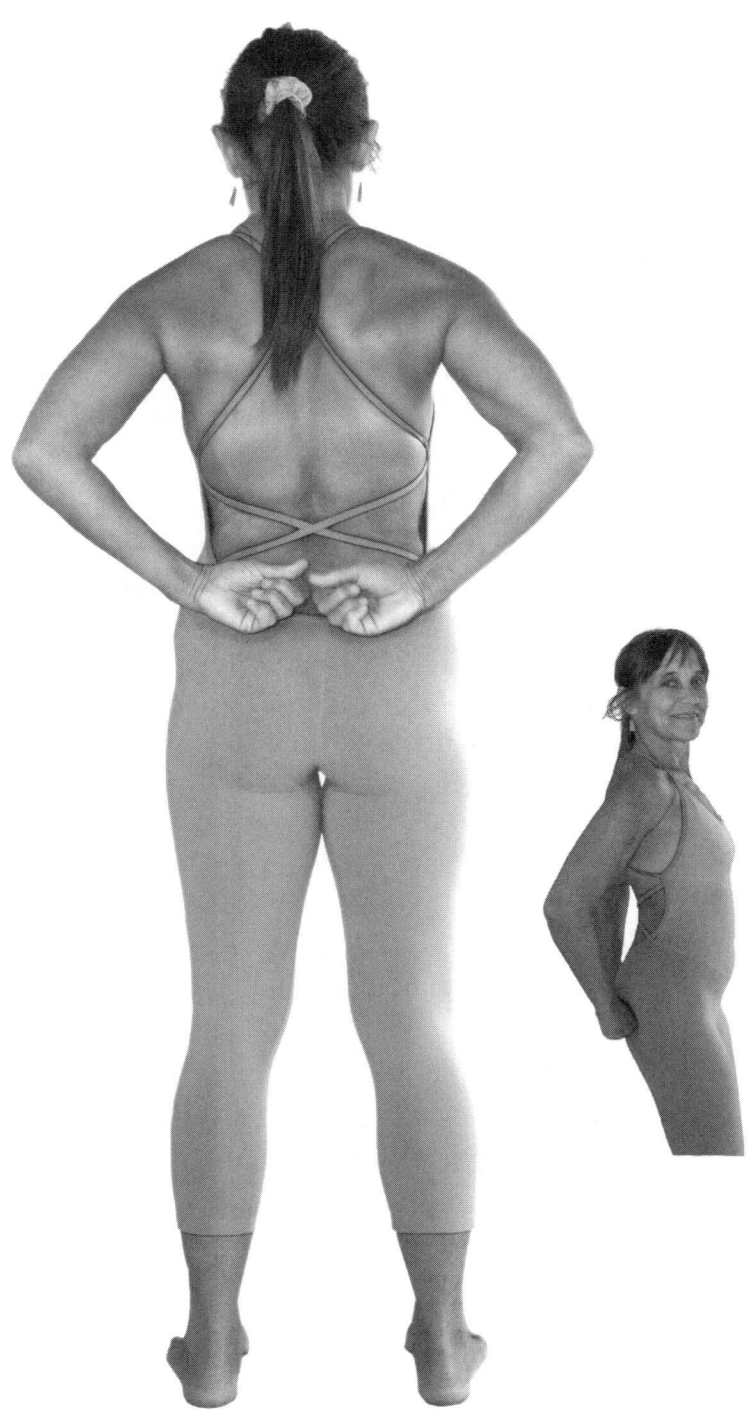

Fig. 21B – The Poi Pounder

The Poi Pounder

Now make fists with both hands, reach around behind yourself and begin to rub your middle and lower back, up and down, from your lower ribs to your hips. Feel the massage waking up your kidneys, adrenal glands, and sore back muscles. Tighten your gluteals and pound them like a drum **(Fig. 21B)**. Loosen your gluteals and continue to pound softly. Continue this drumming for a minute or so, while you continually contract and release your glutes.

Now, release your fists and use your fingers to massage your belly, starting from the bottom, out to the right side, across the diaphragm area to the left, and then down the left side. Imagine that you are massaging warm oil into your belly. Continue in a smooth circle up the right (ascending colon), across the top (transverse colon), and down the left side (descending colon). Do any emotions arise as you massage your belly? Unconscious pain and fear are sometimes held in the belly. This added tension can contribute to indigestion, the holding-back of emotions, and breathing restriction. Acknowledge and release emotions that are not serving you.

Send a blessing of gratitude and wellness to your internal organs. Thank them for the miraculous work that they do, which keeps the body running 24 hours a day, seven days a week.

POSITION #22 — SWAYING TREE

The "Swaying Tree" recalibrates and lengthens the lateral myofascia line and tones the latissimus dorsi muscles. Through this pose, rib cage muscles and fascia are stretched and toned from the inside out, creating a powerful and expressive kid-like body. Poor breathing habits developed from sitting in chairs are overcome, and the waist and neck areas are toned and lengthened.

Stand with your arms hanging down by your sides and your feet pressed into the earth. Avoid either hyper-extending or pushing in on the back of your knees. Use a deep Core SIP Breath to align your rib cage above your hips and bring extension into your trunk. Notice your head floating atop your spine, and focus on breathing while maintaining natural alignment.

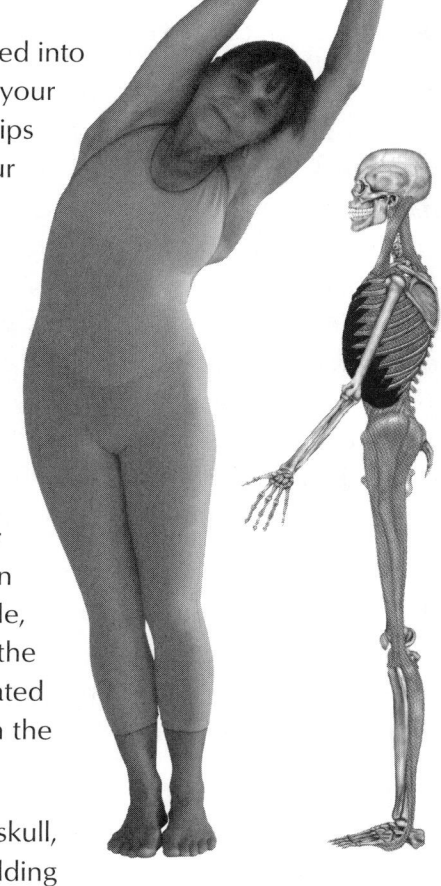

Reach your arms overhead, and inhale with your fingers spread wide-open. If you have tight or injured shoulders, you may bend your elbow and hold area of your arm above your elbow. Make a fist with your right hand and grab the right wrist or elbow with your left hand as you lean and lift to the left side **(Fig. 22)**. Hold your breath gently, tighten your muscles and keep your arms pulled back towards the socket. Maintain length and extension on both sides of the waist and neck and resist back to the center with your trunk muscles while your arm pulls your body in the other direction at the same time. Focus on this "wrestling match" and accentuate or intensify the actions. Exhale, and release the additional muscle contraction, but stay extended in the stretch, allowing yourself to lengthen even further without the accentuated muscle action. Be aware of your spinal alignment, taking care to retain the natural curve of your spine and natural tilt of your sacrum.

Focus: Sense your lateral fascia line that runs from the side of your skull, criss-crossing down your side to the bottom of your foot. While holding this lateral stretch, take another Core SIP Breath through pursed lips, expanding your rib cage muscles as you inhale. Hold the inhale for a few

Fig. 22 – Swaying Tree

seconds, and as you exhale, open your fingers wide, exhaling forcefully out your mouth, sticking out your tongue. Lift and extend through the spine even more through this exhale, remembering that the exhaling process can cause a shortening of the trunk. Focus on staying long and extended. Inhale back to center, then exhale, bringing down your arms. Notice the difference in feeling between the two sides of your body.

Now, repeat this exercise on the other side. When the other side has been exercised, roll both shoulders up, around, and back. Notice the sense of added space in your torso, and added length in your waist and neck.

POSITION #23 — NECK ELONGATOR

The "Neck Elongator" teaches bodily sustainability, by showing you how to "turn off" the excess muscle effort that we all hold in the neck and jaw area. Because of this extra tension, many people suffer from headaches, TMJ, and vertigo. The root of these problems is the lack of proper inner core support, which leads to the over-engagement of the muscles of the upper shoulders and neck. Being forced to perform functions they were not designed to do, these muscles soon become chronically tense and sore.

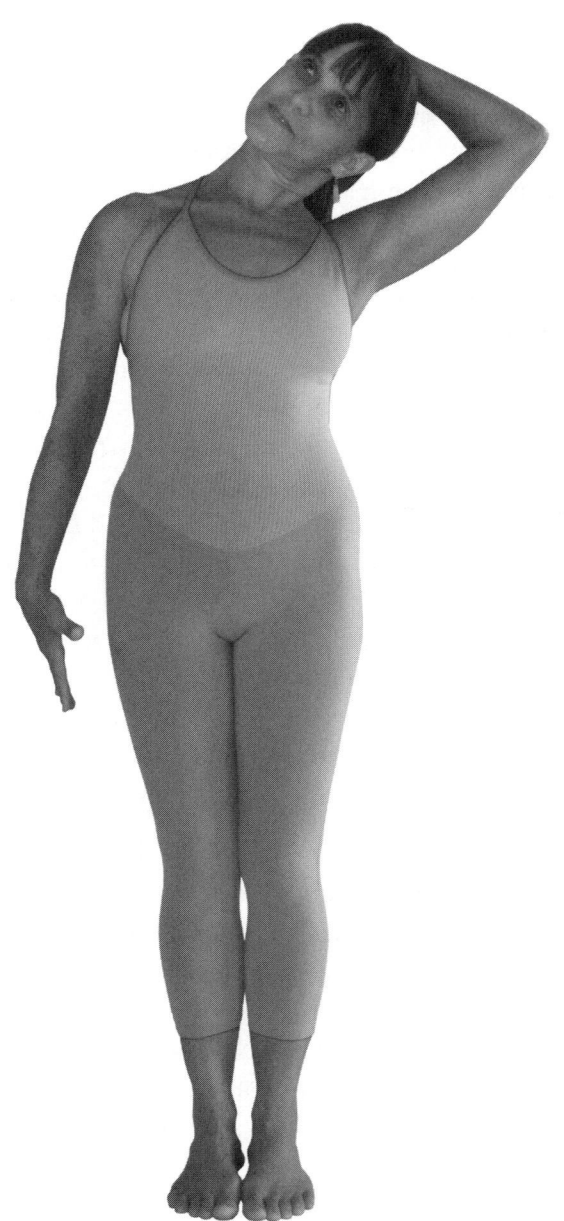

The "Neck Elongator" pose targets the scalene muscles that run under the collarbones and connect your neck spine to your rib cage. Tight scalene muscles create tension in the deep core line of fascia, causing strain and pain that can migrate all over your body. In order to stop the pain, one must get aligned and find support in the core, as well as teach the overworked muscles to let go of their stored tension. This pose trains your nervous system to turn off all of that extra effort, and find balanced support from the core. Your head will start to feel like it is floating atop your spine, and your chronic pains will start to lessen or disappear.

Before beginning this pose, take a few moments to gently and thoroughly massage your neck, face, and upper shoulders. Focus on bringing blood flow and awareness into these areas.

Stand with your feet either hip-width apart or slightly closer together. Ground your legs, pressing evenly through your feet, without locking your knees. Maintain extension in your body, focusing on the "gift of the lift" that happens naturally by way of inhalation. You can use a mirror to review your alignment, and ensure that you are maintaining naturally-aligned posture.

Inhale with a Core SIP Breath, and focus on keeping body-wide extension as you tilt your head gently towards the left; keep both sides of your neck and waist long. Reach across with your left arm, and put your left hand near your right ear, applying gentle

Fig. 23 – Neck Elongator

resistance to the actions of your neck while keeping the intention of bringing your right ear towards the ceiling. Extend your right hand towards the floor with your fingers spread wide-open, keep your wrist in line with your shoulder, and engage your hand forward as if you were pressing forward but being stopped by an imaginary wall. If you want more traction, you can loop a strap under your right foot and pull up with your right hand creating a stronger force of traction in your neck. Exhale, drop your shoulders and pull your head to the left, lifting the right side of your head and ear towards the ceiling. Inhale and feel the deep strap muscles in your neck contracting; then tighten them further for a few seconds. Exhale, and release the extra contraction, but keep the stretch alive, engaging the forces of extension in your inner core as you deeply root your legs and right shoulder down toward the earth.

Take another breath and hold it, resisting your head against your hand by pulling your ear up toward the ceiling and your head towards center. Feel your muscles contracting again and now tighten them even more–even your jaw muscles. Even though you feel the intense stretch of the right side of your neck, focus your awareness on your entire body while keeping the length in both the right and the left sides of your neck and waist. Throughout the entire process, keep your shoulders pulled down and away from your ears. Now, exhale with your mouth wide open and your tongue extended. During the exhale, keep the extension in your spine while opening the fingers of your right hand towards the floor. Stay in the stretch and feel the head-to-toe connection of the lateral fascia line, which runs from the jaw all the way down the side of your body, to the outside of your heel.

Feel how breathing and resistance engage your scalene muscles. Slowly release the hand on your head, and inhale while you bring your head back to center. Does the left side now feel shorter, as though your muscles are pulling your head towards your shoulders? If so, you may be carrying extra tension that depletes your energy and inhibits your freedom of movement. This tension is almost like the constant hum of an appliance that you don't notice until the appliance is turned off and the noise stops. This exercise is a perfect example of how you sometimes have to engage what you don't want, in order to let it all go.

Now repeat this exercise on the other side, inhaling as you bring the right hand to your left ear. When you finish exercising both sides, gently massage your neck and walk around, noticing how free your neck feels and how your head is almost floating.

POSITION #24 — BENT-KNEE FORWARD BEND

❝*Toe touching puts undue stress on one of the main supporting ligaments in the spine, the posterior longitudinal ligament. It is also possible to injure a disc by putting your spine in this dangerous position.*❞

Dominguez, and Gajda, *Total Body Training*

Preparation for the YogAlign "Forward Bend"

Keeping the knees straight is not a natural position for the human body, whether one is flexible or not. In yoga asana and other fitness exercises, people are generally instructed to exhale as they fold over, and this movement is done repeatedly when practicing poses such as "Sun Salutations" and "Forward Bends." The dangerous position of the spine created by leaning over with straight knees is further compounded by the front-shortening actions of the exhale. Therefore, it is essential to inhale as you bend over, and practice keeping the "gift of the lift" when you do exhale.

By practicing forward bending with a conscious effort to stay long in the front, while keeping the knees bent to release fascia pulling, forward bends can be safe and effective. However, they can pose a great threat if the spine is compressed. Many people are fairly flexible and feel okay in the forward-bent pose, but are unaware that the pull in the low back is actually creating a dangerous stretching of ligaments in the sacrum and lumbar area. When practiced over a period of time, this ligament stretching yields unattractive, flat, and weak buttocks, as well as a sacrum that is flattened and no longer able to fulfill its role as one of the main shock absorbers in the body.

Your legs connect to your sacrum and lower back through the back line of fascia. Overstretching of the spinal column (and especially the sacrum and lower back) destabilizes your structure. Without the natural ligament tension that creates a 30-degree angle and tilt of the sacrum, the weight of the upper body compresses into the hip socket and knees, leading to a gradual degeneration of the hip and knee joints. Many yoga and stretching practitioners are finding out too late that doing forward bends with straight legs has dire consequences that are not obvious when one is flexible. Hip and knee replacements can result from the cumulative effect of years spent doing poses and positions that over-stretch important ligaments that should be providing support to our structure.

Practicing forwards bends with bent knees simulates how you move in real life, and allows awareness of the pull of fascia lines and how they affect the quality of your movements. Why bent knees? The only time we can effectively move in the body with both of our knees straight at the same time is when we swim, or jump up in the air. When we do jump or swim, we are floating in space. Our toes are naturally pointed or flointed in the gas pedal position. When we jump up to do something like hit a volley ball, we could never get off the ground if we had our toes extending back towards our shins. As we jump, we press off the ball of our foot. Swimming would be at a standstill if we didn't point our toes and extend through the balls of our feet. Try swimming with your toes pulled up towards your shins and you will be "dead in the water." You may also notice how the extended toe position in swimming causes tension in your lower back and sacrum area.

Pulling up (extending the toe muscles) is a body movement that happens automatically as a startle reflex when we become fearful. This could feasibly be why some people drown; they become frightened, which invokes a startle reflex that causes muscle shortening from belly tightening that pulls up on the toes. When this shortening happens, the frightened individuals panic as they are unable to propel themselves through the water. This leads to more panic and a possible drowning when one is frozen in a fear response that puts the brakes on the propelling movements of the body.

Bend your knees to stay safe when bending forward.

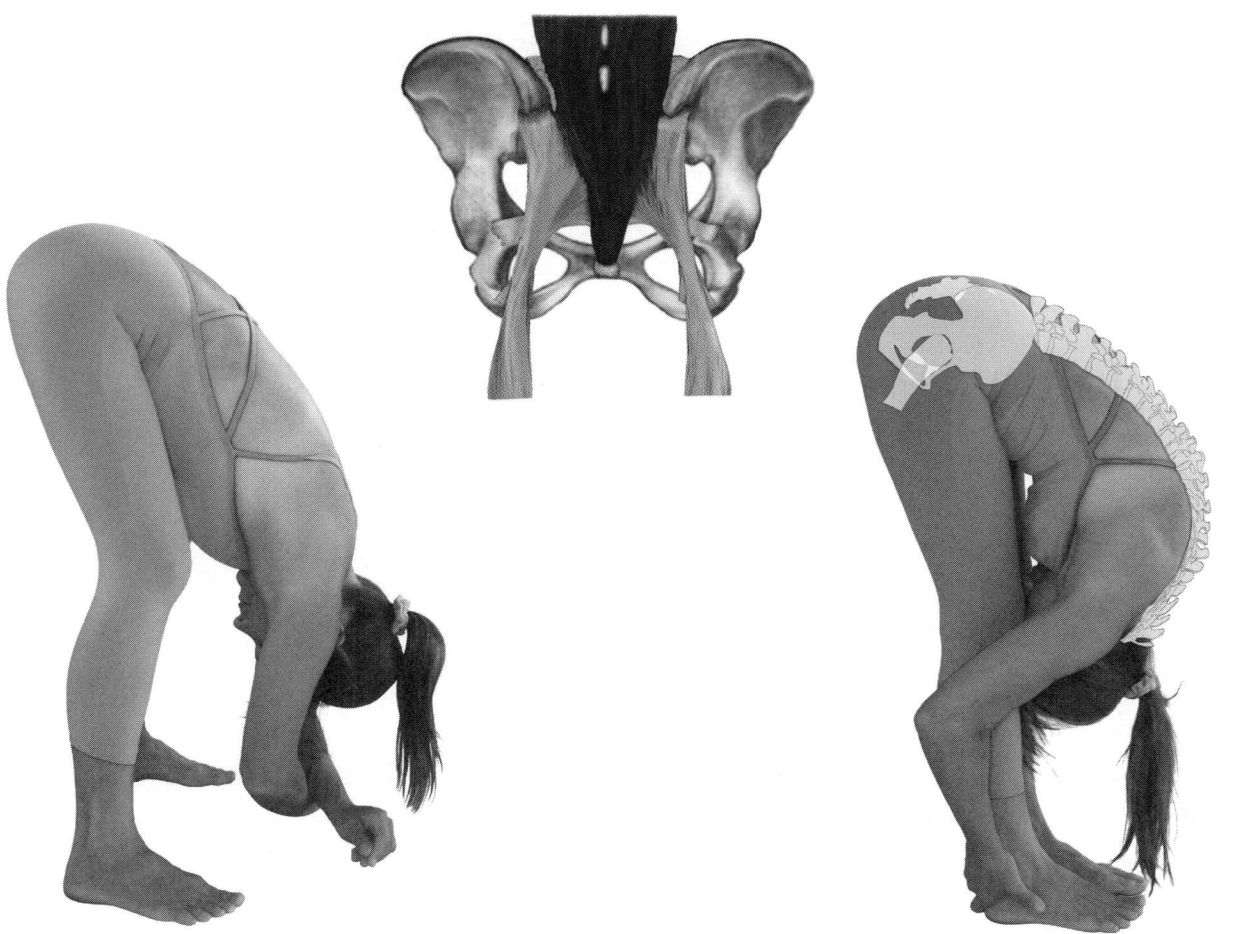

Fig. 24A – CORRECT: Bent-Knee Forward Bend

Fig. 24B – INCORRECT: Forward Bend with straight knees and the head pulling forward puts serious stress on the spine.

This "Bent-Knee Forward Bend" (**Fig. 24A**) is an inversion that tractions your spine, tones your organs, and stretches the entire backside of your body without inducing pain or spinal compression. In this pose, the focus is on keeping length in the front of your spine in order to protect the discs in your lower back from compression. Keeping length in the front body also prevents your sacral and posterior longitudinal ligaments from overstretching. To be safe, keep your knees bent, and the front and the back of your spine elongated. The YogAlign way of bent knees and elongated spine protects you from injuries that often occur by forcing your head and chest towards your legs, or by locking your knees, as seen in **Fig. 24B.**

Now you can practice doing a safe forward bend:

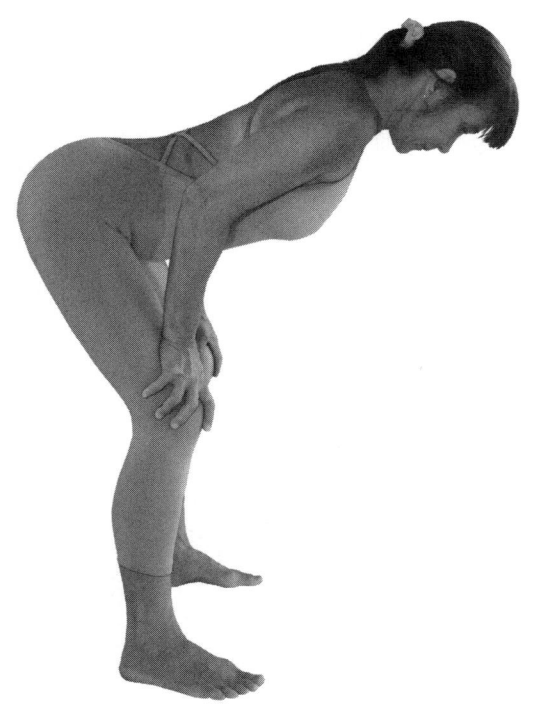
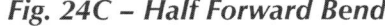

Fig. 24C – Half Forward Bend

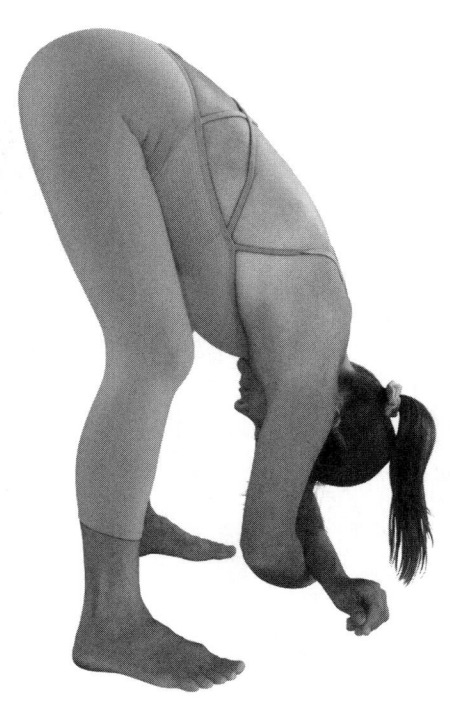

Fig. 24D – Full Forward Bend

To practice the "Forward Bend," stand with your feet at least hip distance apart, and keep your knees bent. Take a slow Core SIP Breath, extending and lengthening naturally with the inhalation process. Do only one or two of the Core SIP Breaths, and then begin to breathe through your nose, exhaling out of your mouth if needed. Start to lean halfway forward (**Fig. 24C**), supporting yourself with your hands on or above your knees. Stay long and extended in your spine even as you exhale, keeping the "gift of the lift." Fold halfway forward, inhale and feel your breathing tube muscles elongating and supporting the front of your spine. To retain length in the front and back of your spine, continue to feel your abdomen lengthening as you exhale. If, at this point, you can retain the natural curve in your lower back without the vertebrae strongly protruding, continue breathing yourself all the way over, allowing your head to hang relaxed as in **Fig. 24D**. Many folks need to stay in the position shown in **Fig. 24C**, supporting the weight of the trunk by putting their elbows on their thighs or their hands on their knees, rather than going all the way over.

With knees bent and your head hanging, keep your neck muscles relaxed. Begin to turn your head side to side, releasing jaw tension by opening your mouth wide on the exhale. Imagine that your head is heavy like a bowling ball, and your neck is a small string that the ball hangs from. Do not push your face towards your shins or your chest towards your knees but just stay focused on being long in the front of your spine.

If the ends of your toes are turning white, you are over-contracting not only your feet but also your entire superficial front line, all the way to your jaw. Relax your feet, jaw, face, and neck, and let gravity traction your entire spine

Caution: Be sure to bend your knees and put some weight on the inner edges of your feet. This action will contract the medial hip rotators and the adductors along the inner thighs, taking pressure off of your sacrum.

Stay in the forward fold as long as you are comfortable, but notice when you feel ready to come up. Move consciously, with your knees bent while you slide your hands back onto your thighs or knees as in **Fig. 24C**. Keep your legs, feet and buttocks strong, and your knees bent. When your belly is parallel to the floor (and your head is even with your hips), move your hands back to your knees for support. Keep the curves in your spine, and lift from your core using the breath. Don't lead or lift with your chin or throat. Focus on moving and breathing from the center of your body. Do not round your upper back as you come up, as this puts unnecessary pressure on your lower back.

Stay in the halfway-up position for a moment, sensing your body and connecting to the core through your breathing. Breathe through your nose as you come up to a standing position. Take a moment to feel the shift in your energy and root your feet as you grow upwards with your trunk.

Position #25 — Forward Bend and Head Massage

This pose is a wonderful mini-yoga session that takes just a few minutes. Here you get a huge stretch to the entire superficial back line of fascia at the same time that you open your chest and arm lines. In one exercise you get an inversion, chest opening, a leg and back stretch, neck traction, self-massage, a breathing tune-up, and a new hairdo, too! Massage is potent medicine that can increase blood flow, both arterial and venous; improve lymph drainage; decrease swelling; and break up scar tissue and decrease adhesions. Practicing self-massage daily makes large deposits into your health account, and soon you will be filthy rich with vitality!

Follow the instructions for the "Bent-Knee Forward Bend" (Position #24), but this time add self-massage of the head and neck region. Press on the inner edges of your feet to keep your sacrum and lower back safe. Exhale with your mouth wide open and your tongue extending out as far as possible. Feel tension leaving your jaw and face. Massage your entire head, your neck, your ears, and scalp while letting your head hang down with no tension in your neck. Work over the points in your skull where there is tension, paying particular attention to the rectus capitis muscles, which are located at the point where your skull attaches to the base of your neck. Keep your eyes relaxed and the back of your neck lengthened. This is a powerful pose to practice when you first awaken in the morning. Brushing your hair in this position distributes your natural oil into your hair and increases blood flow to your hair follicles. It can be a meditation if you stay present with your breath, the feeling of your entire body, and the awareness of sounds occurring as you massage. Stay in the position as long as you feel comfortable, then follow the instructions from the "Bent-Knee Forward Bend" (Position #24) to safely come up to a standing position. As you stand upright, feel the glow in your head and neck.

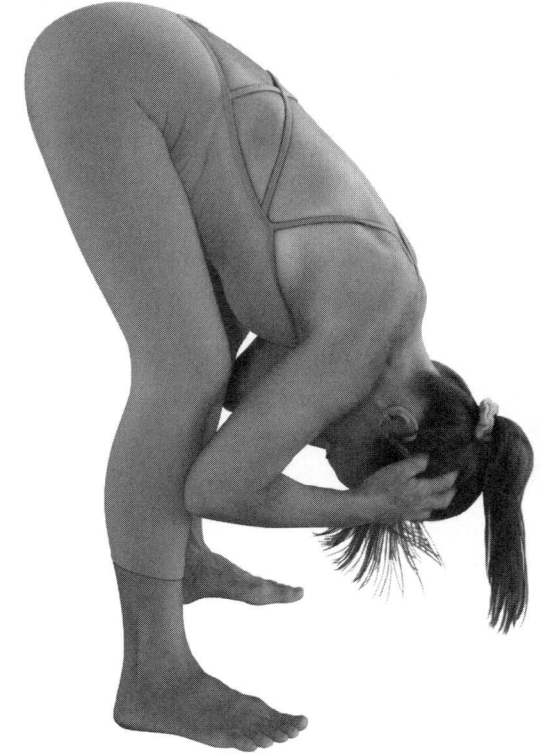

Fig. 25 – Massage your scalp while you traction your neck.

POSITION #26 — INVERTED SHOULDER BALANCER

If you want to have great posture quickly, this pose works like magic. Do this shoulder-balancing exercise to stabilize, strengthen, and tone your shoulder girdle, balancing the fascial actions between your front and back fascial arm lines and streamlining your nerve pathways and movements. This pose exemplifies how concentrating on the movements created by the act of breathing can stretch and balance your fascia lines from the inside out.

This pose will tune your whole body in just a few minutes. I call it "one stop toning" because it addresses all of your toning needs: leg muscles become toned and lengthened, the back-body is lengthened, the neck receives traction, inversion is created for your spine and organs, muscles are re-balancing in your neck, back, and shoulders, and a huge amount of tension is released in the upper trapezius, neck, and jaw. All this without any special gear or gadgets.

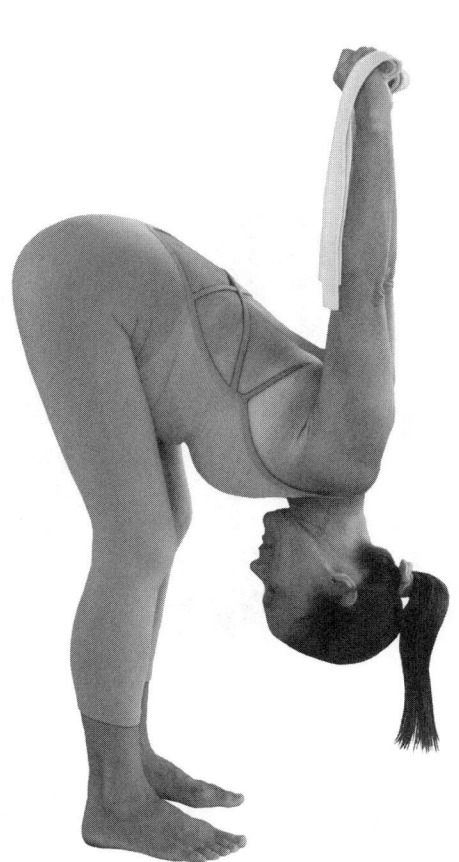

Fig. 26C – Inverted Shoulder Balancer

Before you begin, take a moment to assess your current posture. Stand and look in the mirror, noticing the symmetry of your collarbones. Are they even and level? Or, does one side look higher than the other? Stand sideways and observe the top of your shoulder. Is it aligned with your head or pulled forward? If your collarbones are lifted and your shoulders are rotated forward, it is essential to practice this pose every day to balance out your neuromuscular patterns and fascia pathways. This imbalance is holding you in postural positions that can cause chronic pain and eventual acute injury to your shoulder joint. The "Inverted Shoulder Balancer" pose will give you the tools to balance the muscular and fascial actions of your rotator cuff, balancing your shoulder, and allowing you to use your entire arm with less effort, avoiding pain and arthritis in the elbow, wrist and fingers.

The scapula is held in place by a delicate balance of tension in the many muscles that pull it in different directions. Some of these muscles connect to your neck, spine, and skull. If your neck muscles are over-engaged, your scapula will be elevated and destabilized, causing painful arm and shoulder movements as well as neck tension. You have already rid yourself of unnecessary muscular effort in your neck and head region by doing Positions #22–24. Remind yourself of this new sense of lightness by turning your head side-to-side. Pay attention to what you are feeling and remember to eliminate any extra effort that you don't need to be making. Establish that feeling of "sustainability," by using only necessary effort in your body.

Massage deeply under one side of your collarbone near the intersection of your arm, and feel for the coracoid process (located at the head of the collarbone). This bone is a finger-like protuberance that is actually part of your scapula, or shoulder blade. Protruding out from under your collarbone near your shoulder, it provides an attachment site for muscles in your arm and rib cage. Three major muscles attach here: the pec minor, coracobrachialis, and the shorter head of the biceps brachii. If any of these muscles are tight and shortened, they will pull the coracoid process forward, changing the delicate angle of the scapula and shoulder girdle. The angle of the coracoid process can also be elevated from overengaged muscles in the neck and upper back. Most people with this muscle/scapular imbalance have chronic neck, shoulder, back and arm pain. As a result of the constant tension, conditions develop such as forward head carriage; shallow, weak breathing muscles; severe neck tension; migraines; TMJ; and vertigo.

To begin, stand with your knees bent and your feet at least shoulder-width apart. Your feet can be slightly

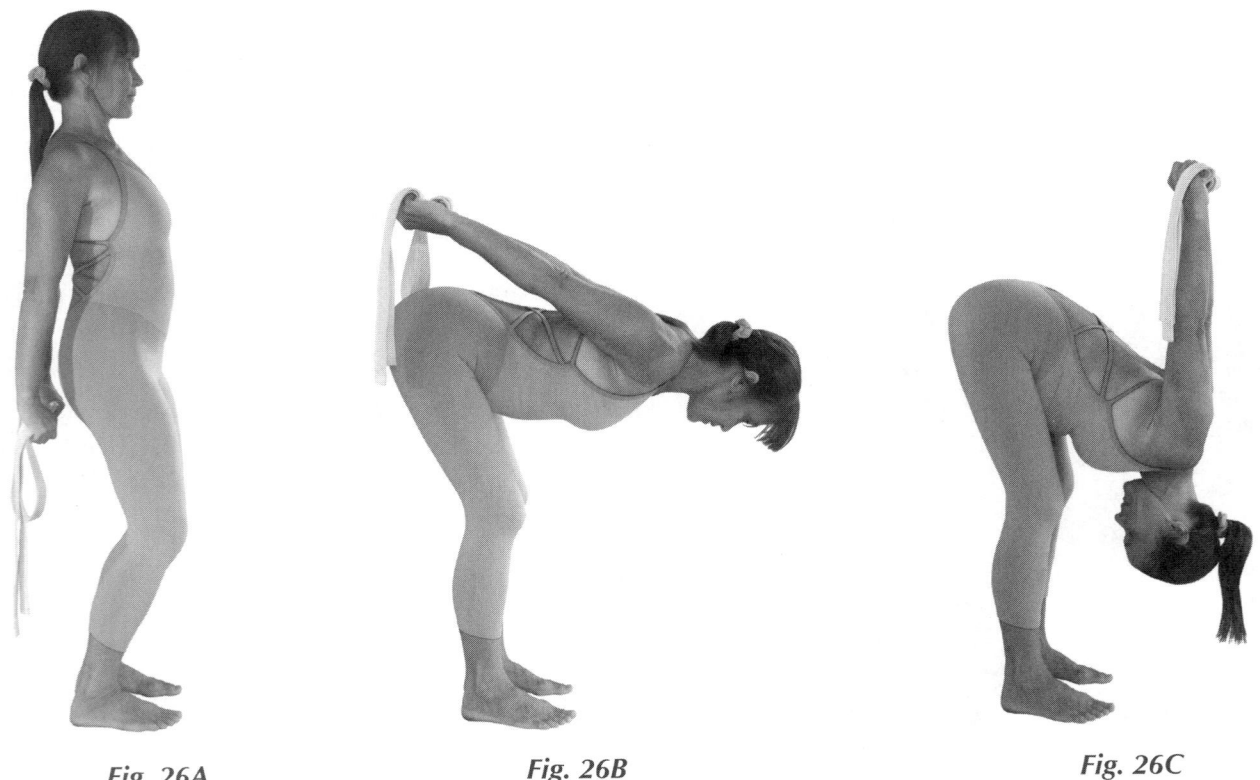

Fig. 26A   *Fig. 26B*   *Fig. 26C*

Sequence of movements for the Inverted Shoulder Balancer

turned out, or parallel to each other. Spread your toes and root firmly into your feet. If there is pressure in your lower back, put slightly more weight on the inner edges of your feet to engage the inner thighs and hip rotators, balancing the tension on your sacrum. Hold a strap behind you, palms facing out from your trunk, and arms shoulder-width apart. Keep your wrists in line with your shoulders or wider, to protect your rotator cuff. Draw the bottom tips of your shoulder blades downward toward your hips and pull your hands apart on the strap **(Fig. 26B)**.

Take a Core SIP Breath, feeling your how your breathing muscles engage and how the expansion of

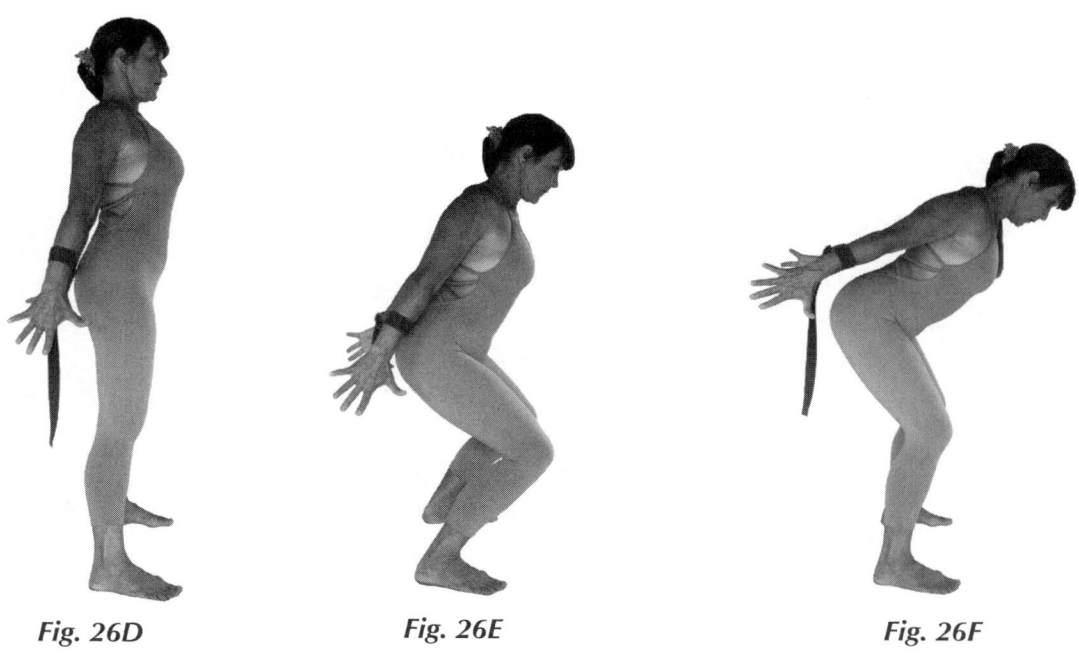

Fig. 26D   Fig. 26E   Fig. 26F

Sequence of movements for the Inverted Shoulder Balancer

your ribs stretches open your pectoral muscles. Without lifting your shoulders, draw your arms into the shoulder socket. This action strengthens and balances the deep rotator cuff muscles, and prevents you from overstretching the ligaments that keep your shoulder joint strong, stable, and safe.

Take another Core SIP Breath, and notice how the pectoralis minor assists with inhalation by opening the upper chest. Feel the engagement of your upper costal muscles between your ribs assisting with the movement of your rib cage. To feel these actions, you must keep the rhomboid muscles between your lower shoulder blades contracted. These actions stabilize your shoulder blades, which keeps the chest lifted. This allows the pectoralis minor to assist with the movements of breathing.

Note: Try holding the strap with just the action of your thumb, leaving your other fingers free to expand open. If you have a buckle on the strap, you can make a shoulder-width loop and put your wrists inside the circle made by the strap. The loop will allow you to have your hands free and your fingers extended as shown in **Fig. 26D–F.**

Note: The computer imagery in the breathing section of the accompanying DVD will help you gain a better experiential and anatomical understanding of how the pec minor begins to work as a breathing muscle when the back muscles that stabilize the shoulder blades are engaged.

With your next inhalation, still pulling the hands away from each other on the strap in back, lean slowly over with bent knees. To prevent compression or overstretching in the lower back and sacrum, maintain length in the front spine as you lean over. At first, go only a quarter or halfway over, retaining an open chest and the "drawing in"

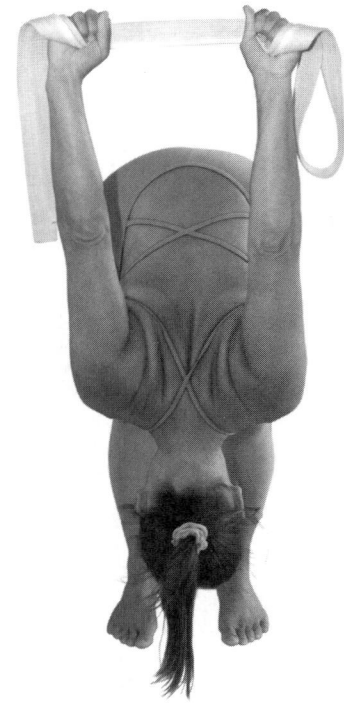

Fig. 26G – CORRECT

of the lower shoulder blade while keeping the curve in your lower back. Keep the front of your spine extended **(Fig. 26B)**. If you can maintain spinal integrity and comfort in your body, lean all the way over, keeping your knees bent, and your neck relaxed **(Fig. 26G)**. Allow your head to hang straight down, with the back of your neck long and your arms extending straight up overhead. Imagine that there are two straps suspended from the ceiling, and you are pulling on them as you resist downward, pulling your shoulders away from your ears.

Keep your shoulders pulled away from your ears to avoid shrugging in the pose and to avoid letting your chest drop.

Are you maintaining openness in your chest? Imagine that you are trying to squeeze a pencil between the lower parts of your shoulder blades, "pinching" inwards. Check that your shoulders are pulled away from your ears, avoiding the incorrect posture as shown in **Fig. 26H**. Inhale and see if your chest is still open, and if your upper rib cage muscles are engaging when you breathe. Exhale, open your mouth wide and release your jaw with your tongue extended out. Inhale and exhale again in this position. Bend your knees, lengthen the front of your torso, and ground with the actions of the muscle in your feet, making sure your toes are not turning white.

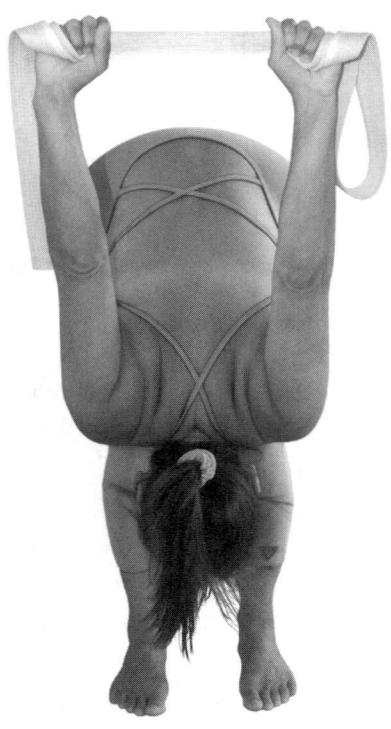

Fig. 26H – INCORRECT

Still inverted, inhale and turn your head all the way to the right, letting your arms reach over to the left. Hold for a moment and increase the contractions of your arm muscles. When you need to exhale, maintain the stretch, but release the extra tightness in your muscles.

Come back to center. Inhale as you turn your head all the way to the left, swinging your arms to the right and repeating the tightening as you hold for a moment. Exhale, maintaining the stretch but relaxing the extra tension you were holding. Inhale back to center, letting your head hang down for a moment. Inhale through your nose as you come up. Keeping your knees bent, act as though you are starting to sit in a chair dropping your hips towards the floor. Engage your buttocks and leg muscles as you lift with your breastbone to stand upright. Do NOT lead with your chin or keep your knees straight as you come to standing.

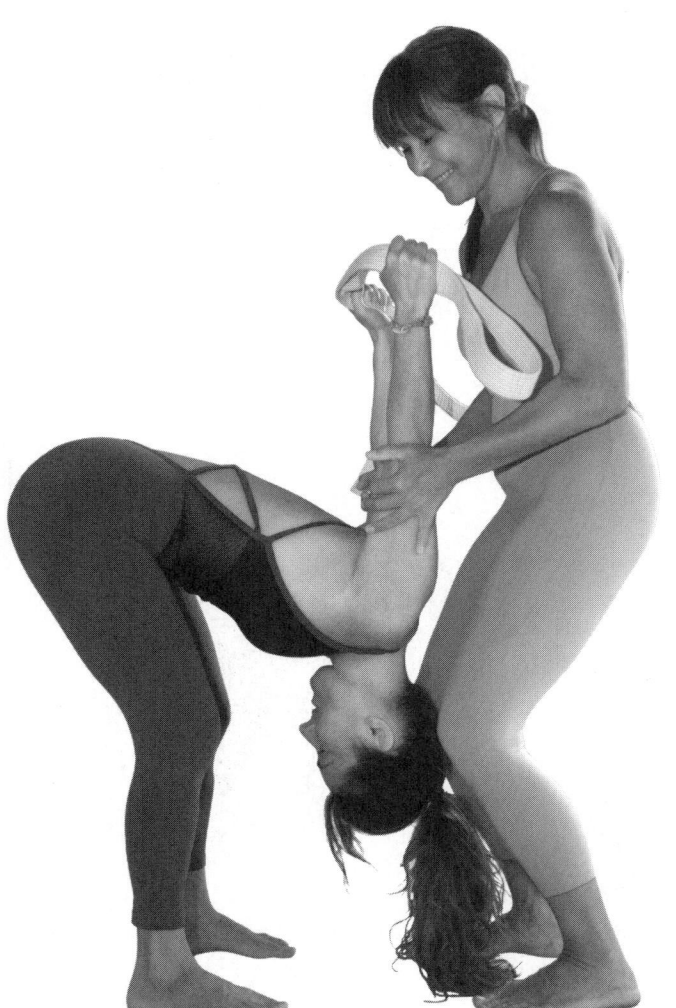

Fig. 26I – Inverted Shoulder Balancer with a Partner

Note: You may feel slightly dizzy the first few times you do this, so come up slowly and carefully. If you continue to feel dizzy breathe only through your nose as you invert.

Stretching the myofascia of your arm lines and re-balancing the muscular forces of your shoulder girdle restores strong joint functions and effortless movement in your arms and shoulders. After studying the illustrations of your arm's fascial connections on the next page, visualize the feeling of the arm lines when you do the "Inverted Shoulder Balancer" pose.

When working with a partner, I sometimes use my knees to gently move their head from side to side, so that they will actually "let go" of excess tension in their neck. As seen in **Fig. 26I**, I am helping Amy "turn off" the upper traps and neck by helping her let her head hang like a ball suspended by a string. While inverted, she focuses on keeping her chest open and strengthening the back extensors and arm lines. Working upside down takes more effort against gravity and leads to more strength in the lower trapezius and rhomboid muscles, which balances the position of the shoulder blades.

Learning to relax your neck is the key to releasing tension in your shoulders. Sometimes the best way to program beneficial neuromuscular patterning is to go upside down and make new patterns. While inverted, you will be more conscious of engaging only the muscles that you need. Relaxing your neck muscles while your arms are contracted will help you learn to move with less effort in your daily life. Using an open–mouth exhale helps people feel neck and jaw tension and then release it. Do this pose everyday and you will be Peter Pan.

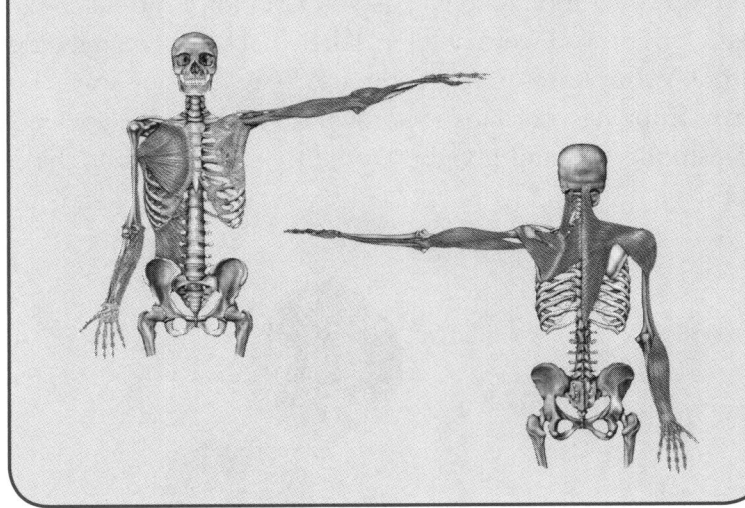

Your arm lines cover the front and back of your arm, and affect movement pathways all the way to the center of your body.

Trapezius Muscles

Keeping the lower part of your trapezius muscles contracted balances the actions of the muscles as a whole.

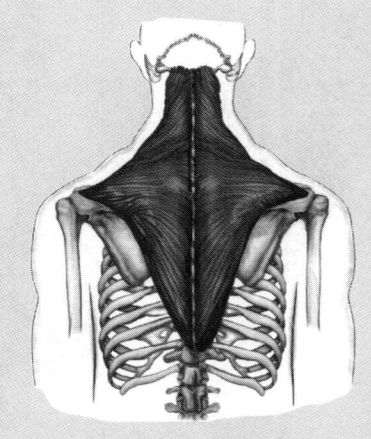

While inverted, draw your shoulders away from your ears using the mid-back muscles that stabilize your shoulder blades or scapula. This action activates a downward flow of the trapezius muscles that balances the muscular actions between the upper and lower sections. This can alleviate the postural problem of being "top heavy" in your shoulders and tense in your upper back muscles. In this postural issue, your head is pushed forward from the overengagement of the upper trapezius and you literally feel "trapped" by your upper trapezius.

Essential YogAlign Poses

POSITION #27 — THE RAINBOW

"The Rainbow" pose tones and balances your chest and arm fascia lines. The movements of breath expand the heart and connect out through the arm lines into the fingertips. With this exercise you can balance the front and back fascial lines, and correct misalignments resulting from repetitive motion, poor sitting habits, or other exercises that pull the head and arms forward of natural alignment. Breath is linked to movement, and functional breathing patterns are regained when fascia lines are stretched and movement arises from your core. Emotional-holding in the heart and rib cage are released, and a rainbow of energy and lightness permeates from the breastbone and lower back all the way out to the tip of your fingers.

Do all previous arm warm-ups (Positions #20–25), before beginning this pose. Keep yourself safe by warming up with massage and the movements of deep breathing. Any residual neck tension will hamper range of motion for the shoulder, so relax your neck in order to free your shoulders whenever you feel "stuck" in this pose. If possible, stand sideways to a mirror in order to monitor your alignment. Check for the curve in your lower back, and keep your rib cage aligned above your hips. Check that your head is not pushing forward when you lift your arms up and begin to move them back. To protect your rotator cuff muscles, always pull your arms in towards the shoulder socket when you engage the shoulder blades down towards the hips.

Also be sure to keep your arm muscles firmly engaged and active, in order to stabilize your shoulder joint and protect ligaments from overstretching. Avoid locking your knees and over-arching your lower back. Your head should rest atop your spine with very little neck effort. Your breath will determine

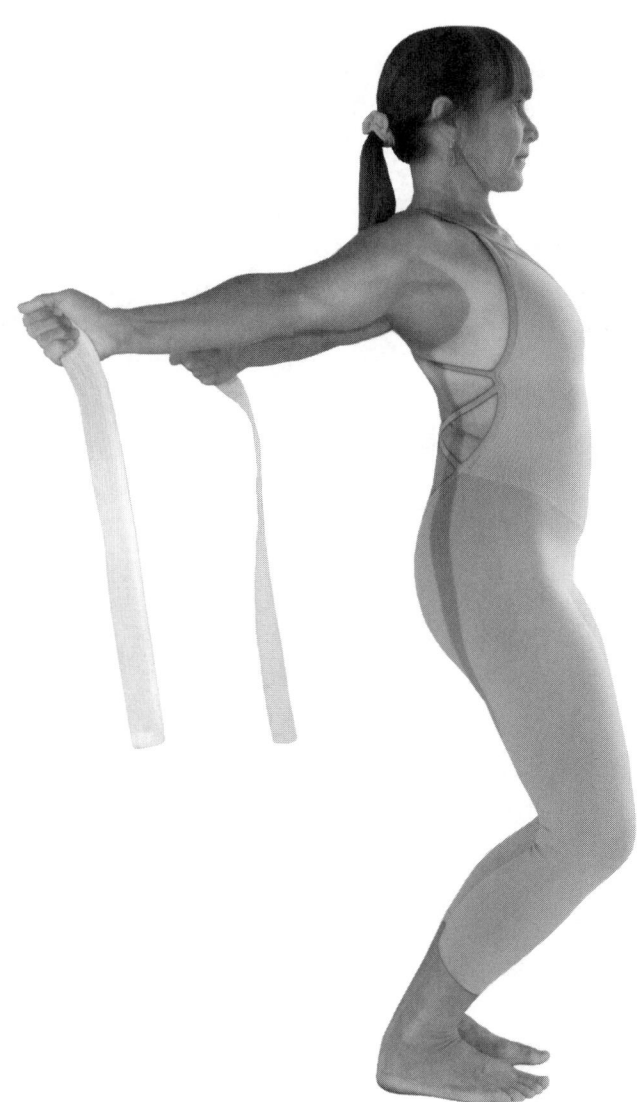

Fig. 27A – The Rainbow

your success in this pose; if you initiate your breath with your upper shoulders, you will not be able to move your arms behind you. Remember, it is not what you do but how you breathe when you do it that determines movement quality and range of motion in your joints.

Lastly, if you have a severe shoulder injury, you should use the alternative version of this exercise, as outlined on the next page.

Stand with your feet hip-distance apart. Exhale as you hold a strap overhead, palms facing forward, with your hands greater than shoulder-width apart. Draw your shoulder blades down, bend your knees, and inhale while you bring the strap behind your back. Keep your elbows straight, and move fluidly until your arms are behind your back and lowered toward your hips.

Let your hands slide to a wider position on the strap if you are straining or bending your elbows. Stay still for your exhale, pulling on the strap to tone your arm muscles while keeping your shoulder blades down. Inhale using the Core SIP Breath as you bring your arms back up alongside your ears, keeping your shoulders down and your neck long. Exhale bringing the arms down in front of you (or keep them overhead), and then repeat the entire sequence several times. Always inhale when moving the arms in

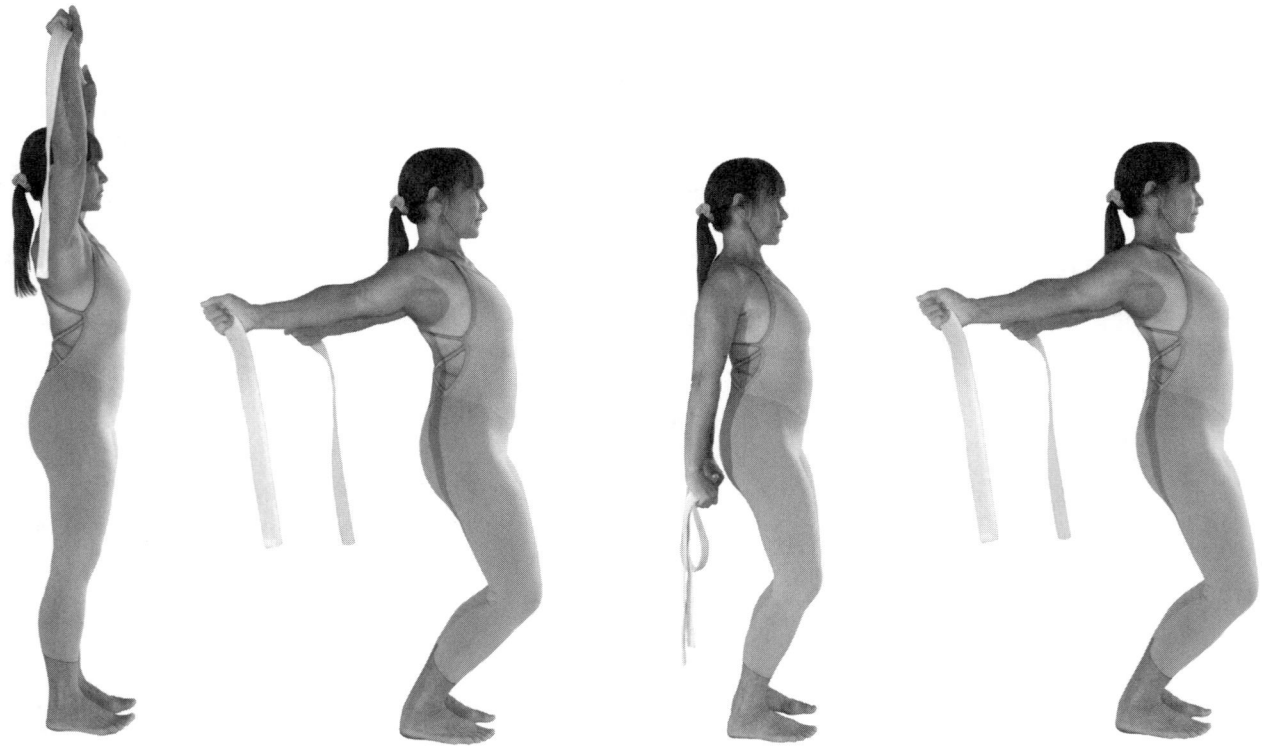

Fig. 27B – The Rainbow

Exhale, overhead.   *Inhale, arms back.*   *Exhale, arms stationary.*   *Inhale, arms up.*

either direction, and exhale when the arms are in place behind your back, or after you have lifted them back overhead. If you are circling your arms, make sure you are simultaneously using the SIP inhalation to create deeper movement and extension in the inner body.

THE SHOULDER/ARM LINE TUNE-UP

Caution: Anyone with a severe shoulder injury or pain should should try this alternative pose to tune the arms rather than doing the "Rainbow" pose. With one arm extended out to the side, open your fingers wide and hold your hand (palm facing up) against a doorway or post as shown in **Fig. 27C** while keeping your shoulder blade down and your posture elongated. If this is too much pressure on the front of your shoulder, press your hand flat to the post, palm down. Use the SIP Breath to create ideal alignment, and avoid locking your knees out or letting your head be in a forward position. Keep your fingers wide open as you press your hand into the wall as you simultaneously draw your arm bone back towards the socket. Inhale and feel the extensor muscles of the back engaging, while the front body is stretched and opened. Hold and accentuate the muscle contractions in your arms and back using the PNF techniques. Exhale and release the extra tension, but retain the pressing and stretching. If you do not feel much intensity, turn your body and step sideways to create more stretch in your chest muscles. Do each arm separately in this fashion and focus on keeping the arm pulled back towards the shoulder joint and the shoulder blades moving down the back. Start with your arm in a postion with the wrist lower than the shoulder. Do the pose with the arm in line with your shoulder. On the third round, step in close to the post and bring your arm extended up towards the ceiling as shown in **Fig. 27D**. Stand up high on the balls of your feet and practice tightening the muscle actions and keeping your arm bone pulling back in the socket with your back muscles stabilizing your

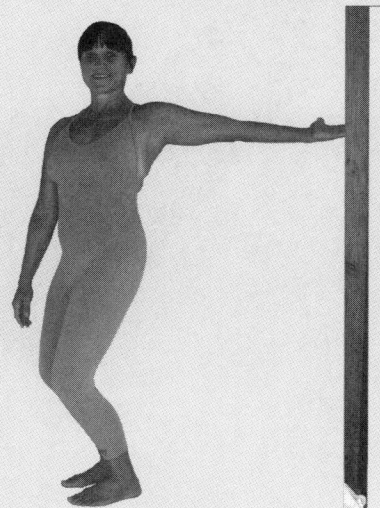

shoulder blade. Hold the body position and an inhalation for a few moments and then exhale out of the mouth, open the fingers wide and draw the shoulders deeply away from your ears. Stay in the position with your scapula stable as you release the extra muscle actions added. Engage with the lift and connection that you feel in your body. Come out of the pose and walk around the room seeing if you can keep the gift of the lift found in this pose.

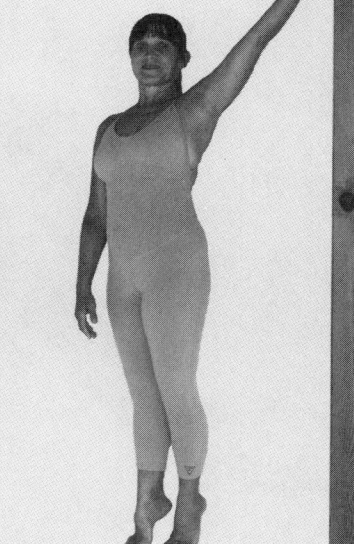

Fig. 27C

Fig. 27D – "Arm Line Tune-Up" on the balls of the feet.

THE DOWNWARD DOG SERIES

POSITION # 28 — HIGH DOG

The YogAlign "High Dog" is a wonderful inversion that tractions and aligns your spine while stabilizing the actions of your core and the integrity of your joints. Here you will gain balanced core strength, tune your fascial pulleys, strengthen the arches of your feet and gain stability of your shoulder joint at the same time that you release tension in your neck. The "High Dog" is a variation of the downward dog pose, one of the keystones of modern Yoga Asana. The problem with the traditional "Downward Dog," as we discussed at length in Part 1 of this book, lies in the traditional form of keeping the heels pressed and the back "straight." This makes the "Downward Dog" a right angle body position done upside down, with all of the postural problems that entails. There is a tendency for many flexible practitioners to compress the spine and overstretch the sacral and shoulder ligaments when they are instructed to push their chest or head towards the floor and get their knees straightened with their heels pressing down. In the YogAlign "High Dog," your heels are kept lifted, simulating how you actually use your feet when moving while avoiding the overstretching of ligaments in your feet needed for structural support.

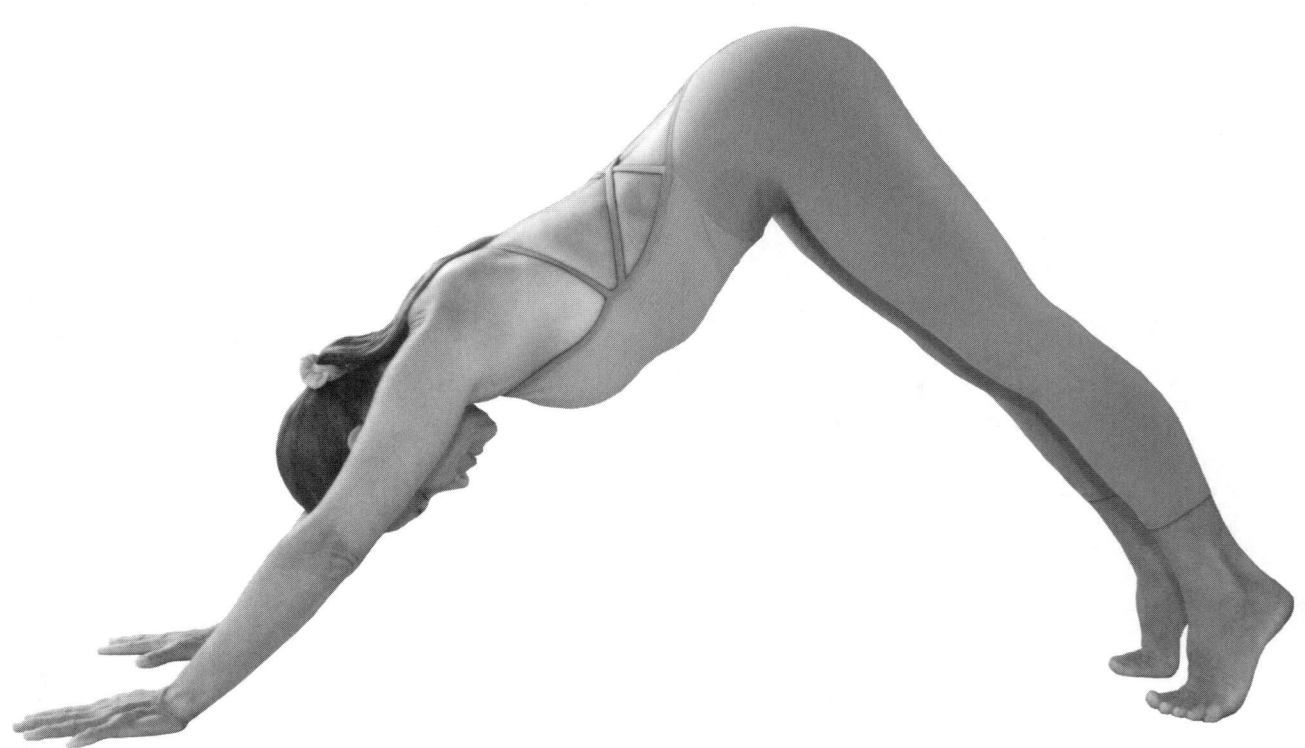

Fig. 28 – YogAlign High Dog

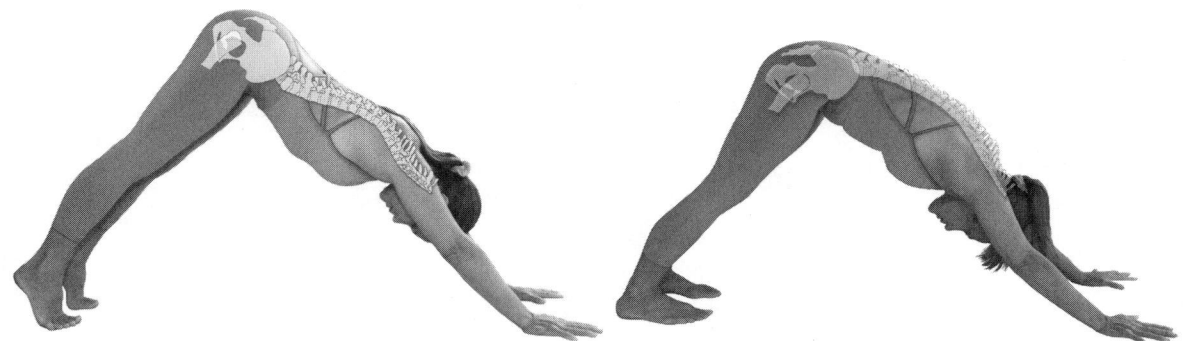

Fig. 28B – CORRECT and elongated | *Fig. 28C – INCORRECT and compressed*

In **Fig. 28B**, you can see how in this pose the natural curves of the spine are present and the postural relationships between the head, shoulders and hips are maintained, even when the body is inverted. In **Fig. 28C**, the heels are pushed down and the front of the body is short, creating a rounding in the upper back. Continued practice in this poorly-aligned position creates muscle actions that strengthen muscle imbalances and poor posture in general.

When practicing the "High Dog," use a mirror, and make sure your trunk is aligned as though you were standing with good posture.

Begin the exercise on your hands and knees, with your feet hip-distance apart, and your hands shoulder-width apart. Inhale as you lengthen your neck and draw your shoulders down and away from your ears. Spread your fingers wide, stretching the webbing between your fingers as you press your palm into the floor. Roll the crease of your elbow forward so that your upper and lower arm bones line up and your elbows are straight. Engage your forearms towards each other as you keep your upper arm bone lifted and your armpit hollow. If you have hyper-mobile elbows, do not twist into extreme extension. Keep your arm muscles firm and active.

Without pushing your shoulders or chest towards the floor, keep your ears in line with your arms. Tuck your toes under, press into the ball of your feet and inhale as you lift your hips up towards the ceiling into a V shape. Keep your heels lifted as high off of the floor as possible.

Continue pulling your arms into the shoulder socket, connecting deeply with your breathing process. Inhale with a Core SIP Breath as you extend your neck, engaging your core trunk muscles. Keep your waist long while creating more space between your shoulders and your ears.

Again, it is beneficial to practice this pose sideways in front of a mirror, so that you can make sure you are maintaining the four curves of natural spine alignment. If your lower back is flat and your upper back is rounded, you need to bend your knees until you feel your sacral tilt and lumbar curve return. Practice sensing your entire body as you press your wide-spread fingers and the balls of your feet into the mat.

POSITION #29 — TRACTION DOG

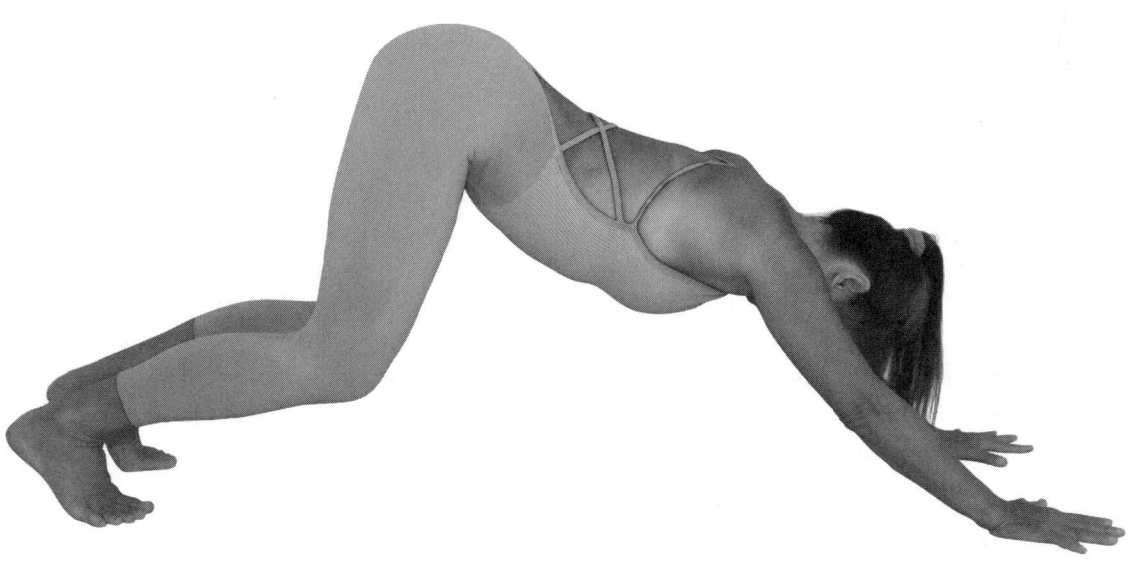

Fig. 29 – Traction Dog

Now bend both knees to move into "Traction Dog." Pull up your hips and back, extending through the crown of your head. Inhale into the bent-knee "Traction Dog" position, and exhale back out to "High Dog." Do three or four of these "Traction Dog" to "High Dog" movements, and then come back onto your hands and knees. Remember, it is not what you do, but how you breathe while you do it that is most important. If you are losing your natural spinal alignment, keep your knees deeply bent and/or stand with your legs in a very wide stance.

When doing "Traction Dog" it is important that you do not hang from your shoulder and sacral ligaments by pressing the head and chest downwards. This will weaken the integrity of the shoulder and knee joints as you strain and compress your entire spine.

Since downward facing dog is a cornerstone of most asana practice, it is imperative that you learn to use muscular effort in this pose and do not hang from your ligament structures by locking out your knees or pushing your shoulders toward the floor.

POSITION #30 — CORE DOG

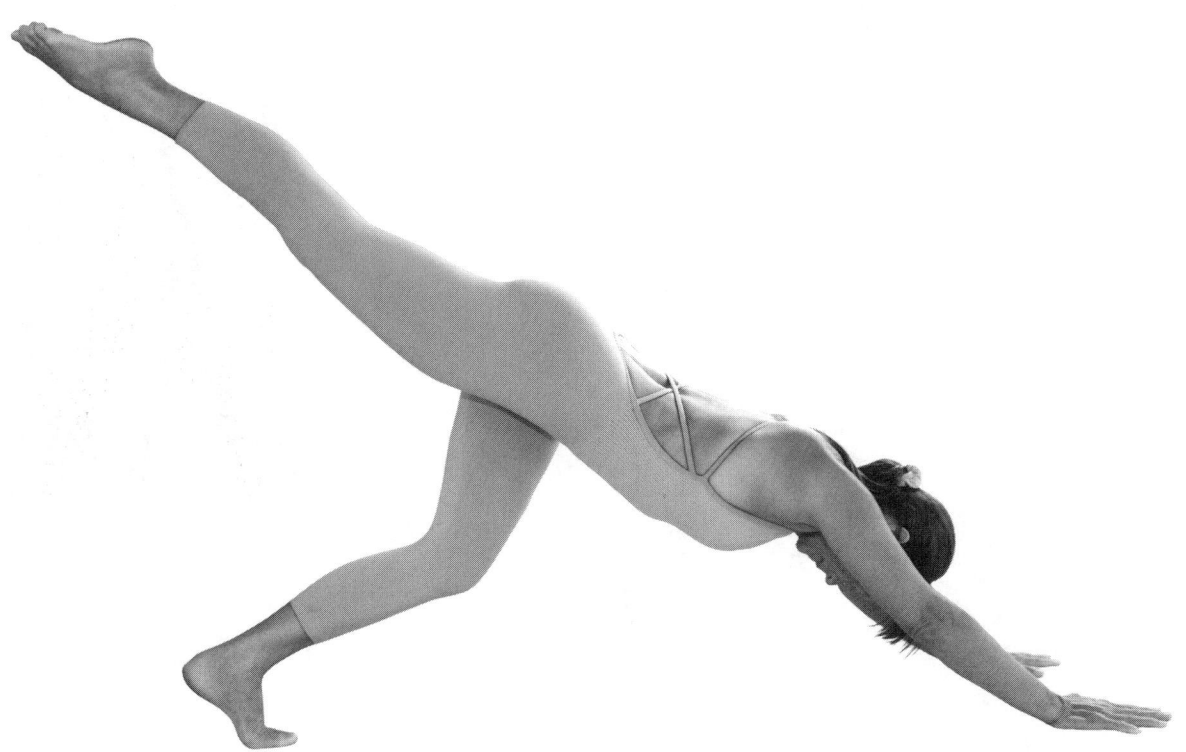

Fig. 30 – Core Dog

From being on your hands and knees on the mat, go back into "High Dog," remembering to lift your heel on your standing foot and engage your limbs back to your center. Bend both knees to go into "Traction Dog," and slide your left foot closer to your right. Lift your right foot off of the mat, straightening your lifted leg, while pointing (or flointing) your toes. Keeping the knee bent in your standing leg, press the ball of your foot into the mat, lifting up your heel. Engage your butt muscles, and keep your hips level. Spread your fingers wide, keeping your palms pressed to the floor while drawing the forearms towards each other. Turn your head side-to-side to make sure you are not holding extra tension or muscle effort in your neck or face. Take a deep Core SIP Breath, feeling the energy of your diaphragm and psoas connecting all the way down to the toes in your foot.

POSITION #31 — PSOAS DOG

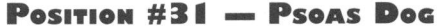

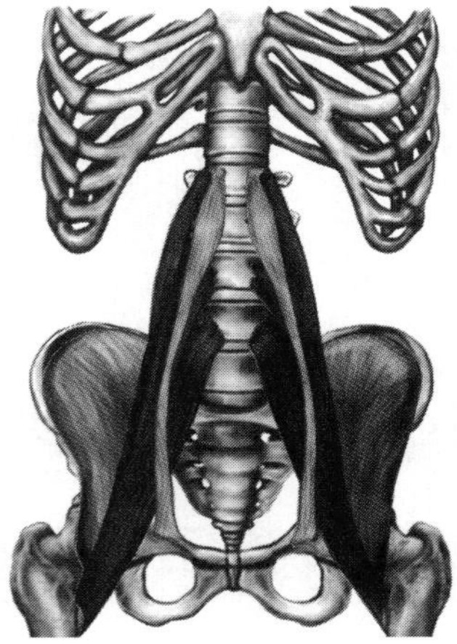

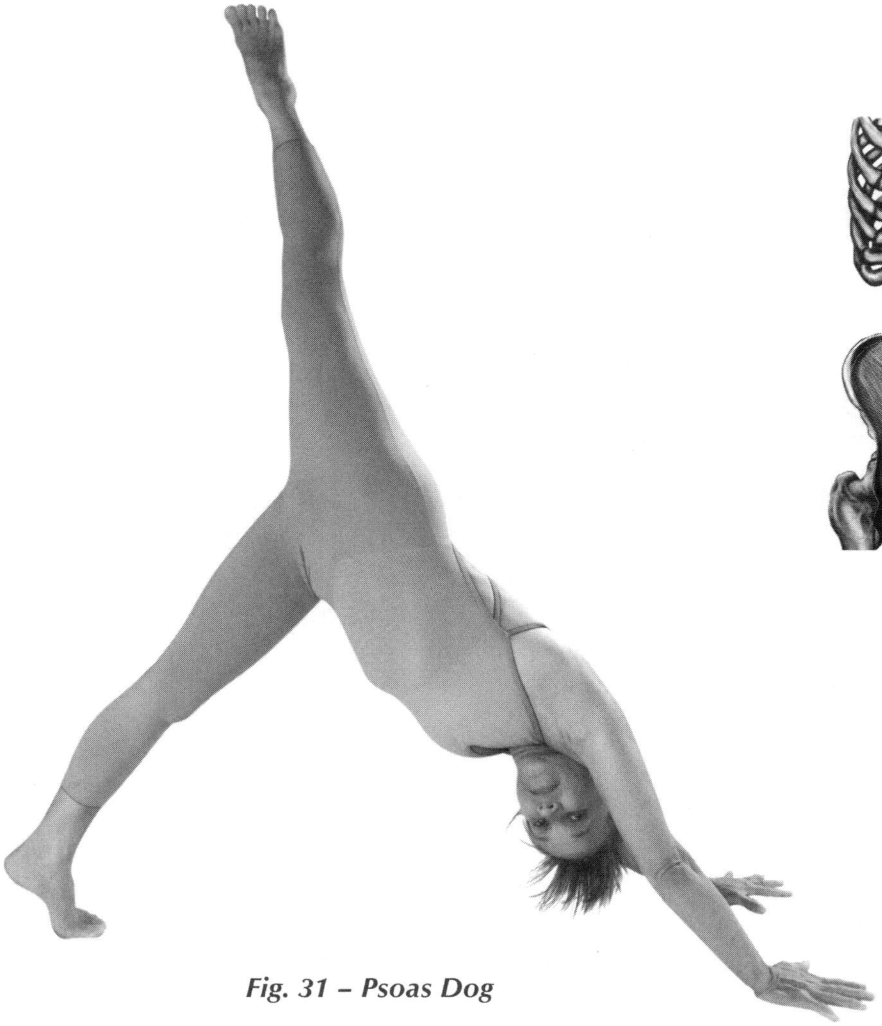

Fig. 31 – Psoas Dog

While in the "Downward Dog" position, take four or five SIP Breaths, then rotate your lifted leg out to the side of your body, at the same time rotating both hips out to the opening side. Reach your foot to the ceiling, keeping your toes spread. Rotate the inner thigh of your lifted leg up towards the ceiling. Straighten your standing leg, but keep your heel lifted, continuing to activate your arch. Inhale a SIP Breath and squeeze your leg and gluteal muscles. Your hip is now lifted, and your body is turned sideways. Feel your breathing activate your entire leg, from diaphragm to foot, through the path of the deep core fascia line. Let your head hang, releasing your neck muscles but keep your arms firmly connected into the socket, engaging your lats and functional core. Exhale with mouth wide open and tongue out, to extend the entire core line of fascia. Remain connected as long as you are comfortable, then proceed to the next pose, to keep the sequence moving.

THE PIGEON SERIES

POSITION #32 — COBRA PIGEON

"Cobra Pigeon" is a powerful opener of the superficial front line, especially when practiced with strong action in the back foot. This pose also tones your hips, releasing deep tension in the gluteal muscles and pelvic floor. By staying active in the pose, you will gain balanced actions between the inner and outer hip rotators.

> **Caution:** If you have knee pain—and particularly if you have had knee surgery—then this pose may not be appropriate for you. See Position #34, "Reclining Pigeon" for a safer pose that offers similar benefits.

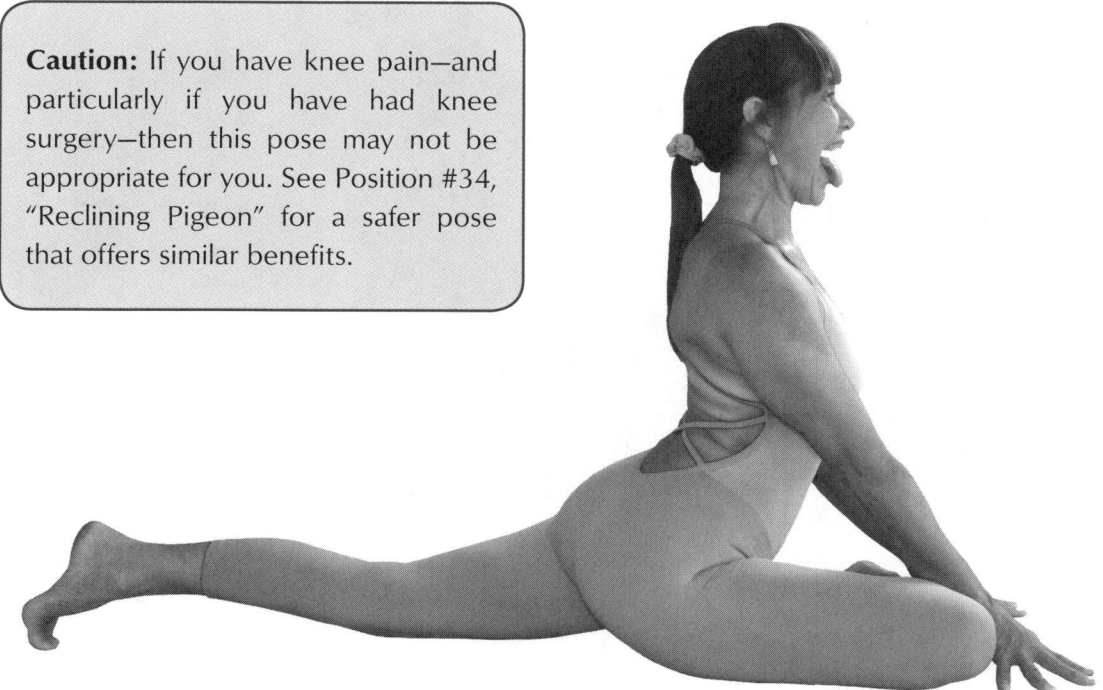

Fig. 32A – Cobra Pigeon

From "Psoas Dog," swing your lifted leg forward into a bent knee position. Press your hands and fingertips into the floor and use your breath to activate the lifting of your trunk. If you have any sharp pain around your knee, stop immediately and do the reclining version of this pose (Position #34 – "Reclining Pigeon"). Level your hips so that your sacrum and hips are aligned. If necessary, use a block or pillow under the hip of your bent-knee side to bring your hips level.

Do a Core SIP Breath to extend and lift your trunk into a position perpendicular with the floor (like a cobra). Draw your shoulder blades down and keep your head neutral. Press the top of your extended foot into the floor, pointing like a dancer, or come up onto the ball of your foot with your toes tucked under, as shown in the photo (**Fig. 32A**). Press evenly into the ball of your back foot while lifting your inner thigh towards the ceiling. Be sure that your back foot lies straight back and does not turn and "sickle" to one side. To lift higher, or to keep the upper body more perpendicular, use blocks under your hands, and practice core breathing. Notice the stretch of the outer belly and the entire superficial frontline created by your deep inhalation.

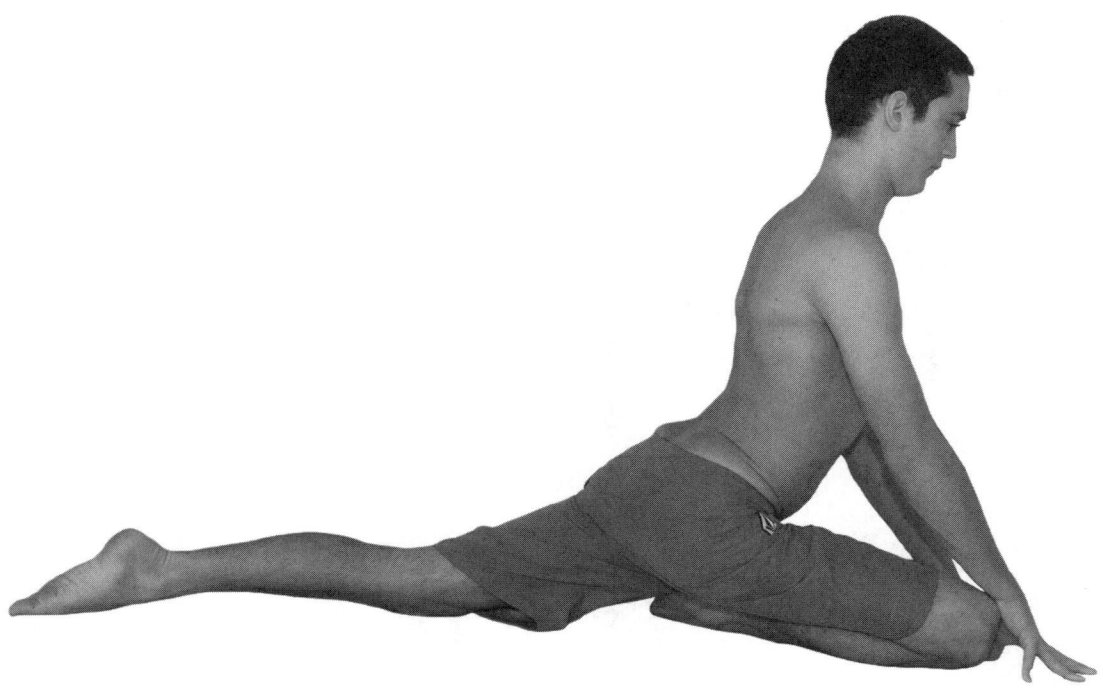

Fig. 32B – Zack in "Cobra Pigeon" stretching the muscle/fascia pathways of the superficial front line.

Now, point the toes of your extended foot like a dancer, and press the top of your foot into the mat **(Fig. 32B)** while you actively spiral your inner back thigh towards the ceiling. Take several deep SIP Breaths, exhaling forcefully through a wide mouth with your tongue extended like a cobra. Feel the tension leaving your body from your pelvic floor, belly, and jaw. Upon inhaling, visualize your psoas assisting your breath, supporting your spine, and adding length to your leg. Feel the fascia and outer belly muscles stretching as you inhale. Draw them in tightly when you exhale and hold for a moment. Take a deep breath and tighten what feels tight by squeezing your gluteals and leg muscles for several seconds. Focus on what's contracted and "tighten into tightness." Hold a few more seconds; when you exhale, release the accentuated tightness but stay lifted and engaged in the pose.

Essential YogAlign Poses

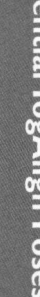

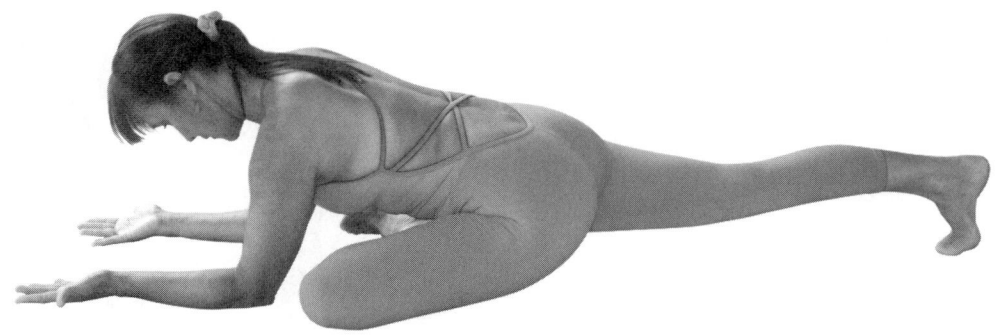

Fig. 32C – CORRECT: Active Pigeon

To do the active version of the Pigeon as shown in **Fig. 32C**, come down onto your forearms with your palms facing the ceiling. Spread your fingers wide. Check that your elbows are in line with your shoulders, and tuck the toes of your back foot under, balancing on the ball of your foot. Lift the knee of your extended leg (if possible) and "rudder" your back foot side-to-side, pushing it further back along the floor.

Breathe deeply, opening the superficial front line and supporting the curves in your spine. Do NOT let the upper back become rounded. Instead, focus on lengthening through the front with breathing. Use a mirror and ask yourself, "Is my spine in good standing posture?" By doing this, you will be sharpening your sense of proprioception, the essential awareness of your body's positioning.

Doing a "Slouching Pigeon" can also contribute to knee ligament damage, due to the unsupported weight over your knee. Proper alignment, muscular engagement and support is imperative in this pose.

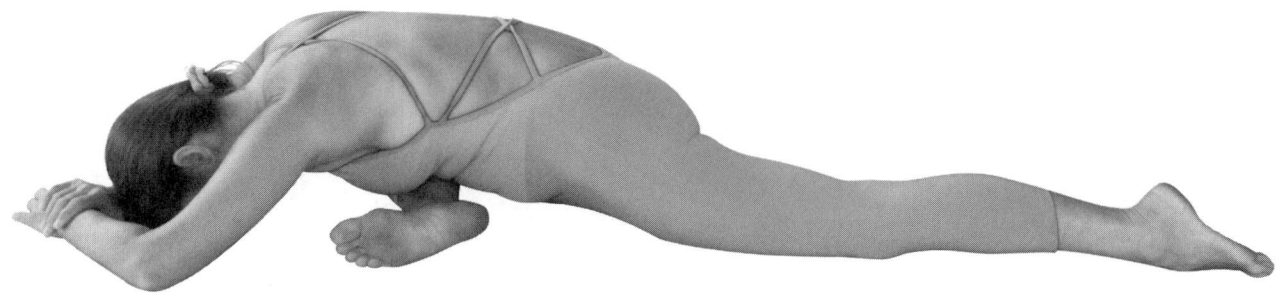

Fig. 32D – INCORRECT: Slouching Pigeon

POSITION #33 — TWISTING PIGEON

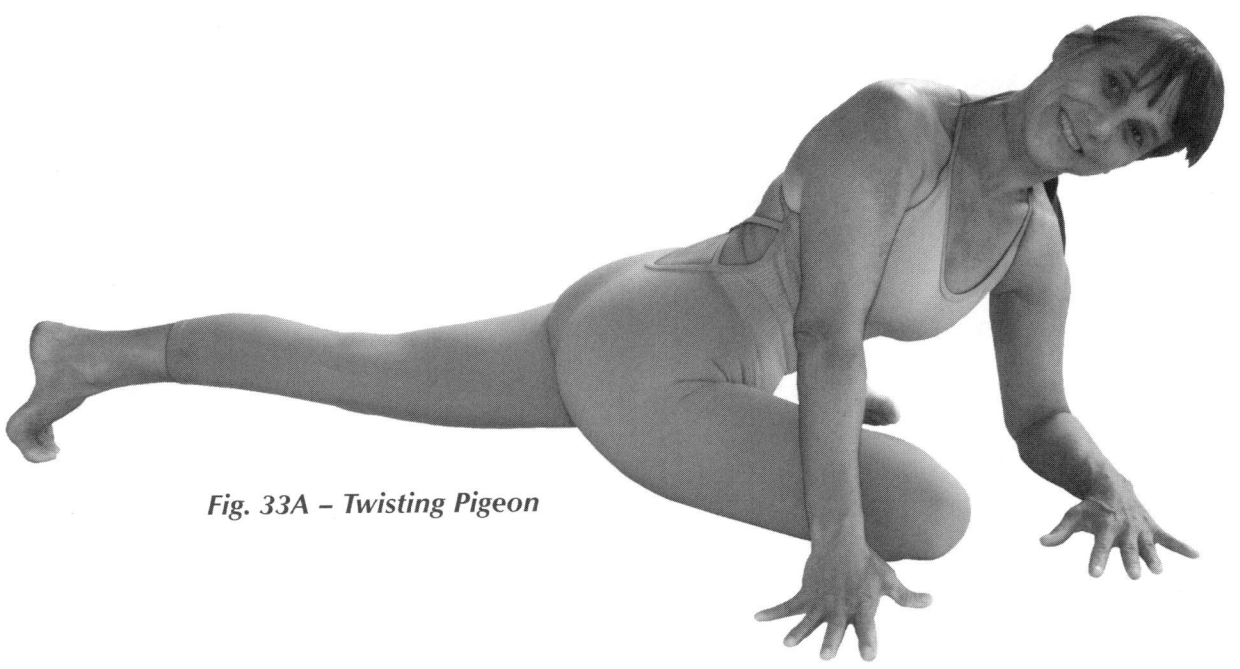

Fig. 33A – Twisting Pigeon

If your right leg is forward, turn your left arm sideways with your elbow directly below (and in-line with) your shoulder. Place your forearm on a block if you sense sagging in your spine. Tuck your toes in and balance upon the ball of your back foot. Inhale and, if possible, bring your right hand onto your hip or sacrum. Pull in towards the core and lift up towards the sky. Be sure to keep the tilt in your pelvis and maintain the curve in your lower back. Pull your shoulder blades down and draw your arms into the shoulder socket. Extend naturally through your spine, feeling movement initiate with the breath.

If your body is ready, you can now slide your right hand down and grab the ball of your right foot to accentuate the twist. Do not try to grab your foot if the movement hurts your shoulder, or if you have to round your upper back or compress your spine to get there. The ideal positioning is to keep your spine in natural alignment and feel no discomfort; the value of this pose has nothing to do with how far you can twist.

Breathe in deeply and hold for five to ten seconds while twisting further, tightening what is tight. Squeeze your trunk muscles while you hold in the breath. When you exhale, release the conscious tightening while twisting

Caution: If you are uncomfortable in this pose, or have any knee pain at all, go back to "Cobra Pigeon" (Position #32) or switch to "Reclining Pigeon" (Position #34). Do not bend forward and round your back, as this can cause pain or excessive stretching around your knee. Keep natural spine alignment. Avoid overstretching your sacrum and creating compression in your spinal discs.

further. Feel your trunk lengthen. Pull down with the shoulder blades while lengthening the spine on all sides.

Inhale and slowly unwind from the twist, coming back into the "Cobra Pigeon" pose. Inhale a Core SIP Breath and slide back onto the top of your back foot. Press your foot to the floor as you inhale, engaging the psoas, stretching the outer belly and expanding the ribs when you breathe. Exhale, opening your mouth as

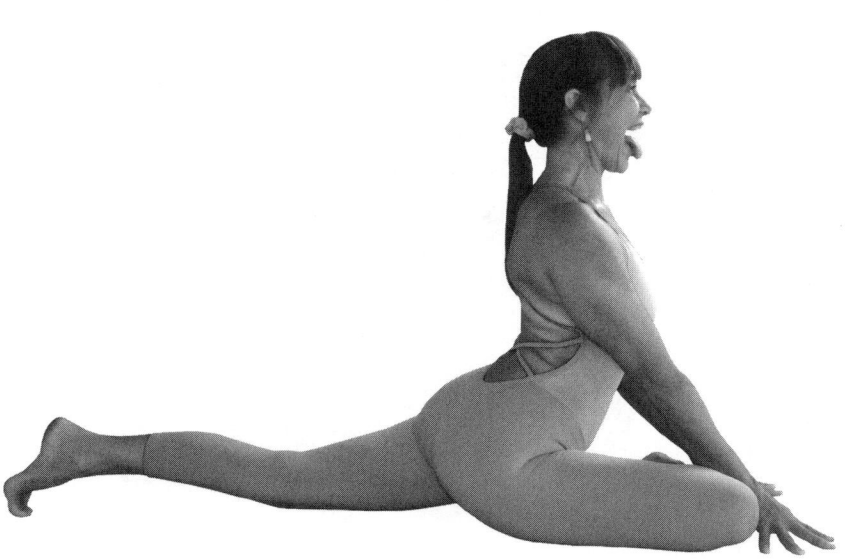

Fig. 33B – Cobra Pigeon

widely as you can, sticking out your tongue as far as it will go, stretching the front body from head-to-toe. Do four or five breaths in through the nose and out through the mouth as you stick your tongue out as far as you can. Finally you get to stick your tongue out and nobody will put you in the corner!

Coming out of the pose, do a few "Rotator Rolls" (Position #20) to massage your butt on the right side, and then come onto your hands and knees. Now repeat the entire sequence on the other side.

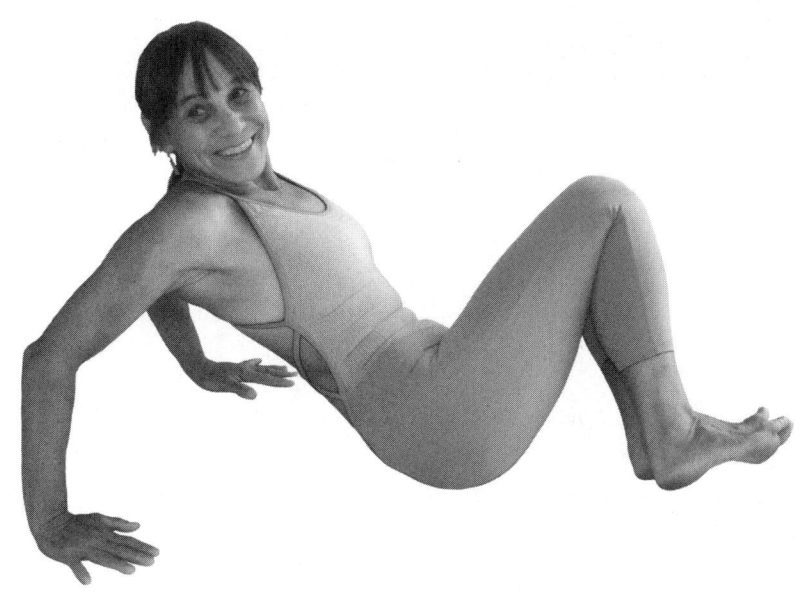

Fig. 33C – Rotator Rolls (Position #20)

POSITION #34 — RECLINING PIGEON (ALTERNATE)

"Reclining Pigeon" is a good substitute for "Cobra Pigeon" and "Active Pigeon," and gives you similar benefits without any pain or knee strain. To begin, lie on your back and cross your left foot over your right thigh so that your ankle rests upon your thigh. Reach your left hand through the space between your thighs. Interlace your fingers around either your shin, or the back of your thigh. Inhale while lifting and lengthening so that the natural curve is evident in your lower back. Draw your shoulders down away from your ears keeping your collarbones wide. Your neck should also retain its natural curve.

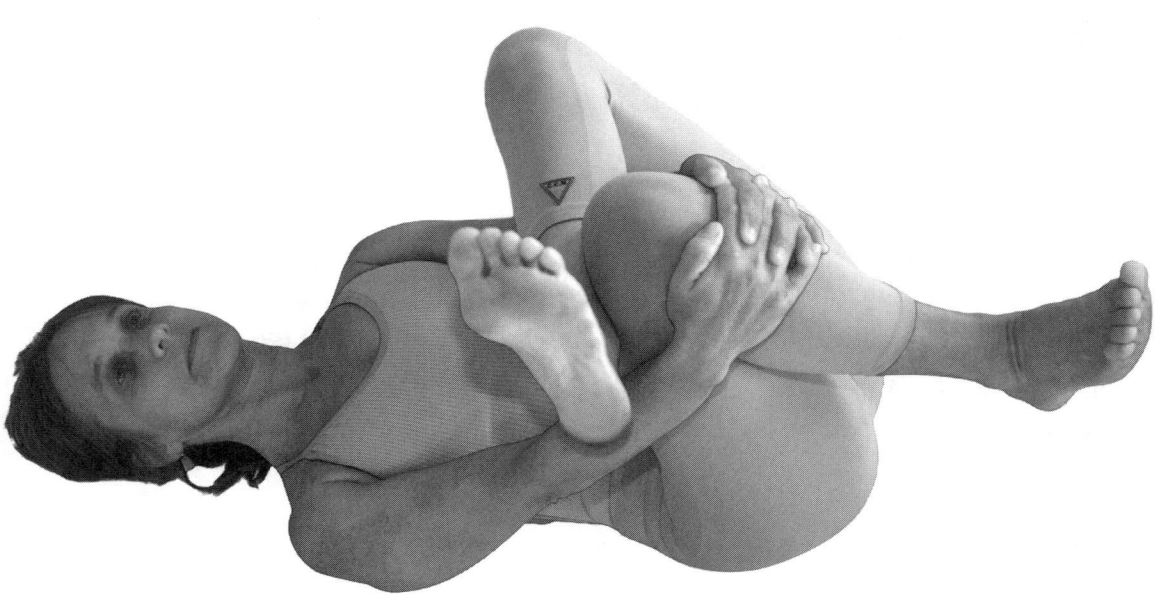

Fig. 34 – Reclining Pigeon (Alternate)

Keep your toes spread and feet level, pressing as though you were standing on the floor. Add the "PNF Hip Recalibrator" (the "wrestling match" from Position #3). Inhale while squeezing your butt, thighs and pelvic floor muscles for 15 –20 seconds. As you exhale, release the resistance and gently press your left elbow into your thigh, away from your head.

Imagine warm honey flowing through your hip and groin. Visualize tension turning to liquid, and flowing out like a river. Now repeat the position on the other side.

POSITION #35 — OPEN BOAT (ADVANCED)

This pose elevates awareness and strengthens the role of your breathing tube as a posture muscle that supports the front of your body.

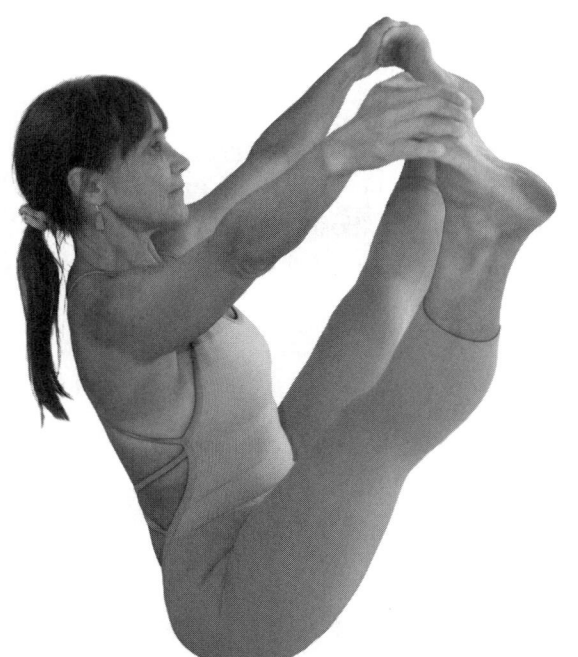

Fig. 35A – CORRECT: Open Boat

To do the "Open Boat" pose, first lie back on your mat and stretch your entire body with arms up and legs pointed down. Rock into several "Spinal Rolls," inhaling as you roll up, engaging your spinal curves, and balancing on your sit bones for a moment, before exhaling as you roll back with your spine in a C-shape. Keep your sacrum in a natural lift and tilt when you roll up, as you keep your knees apart. Each time you exhale roll back and massage your spinal and back muscles.

Feel the muscular ring of support created by the engagement of your breathing tube when you SIP deeply. Focus on the feeling of lift in the front of your body created by the movement of inhalation and retain it through each exhalation. On your next inhale, stay up. Use the SIP Breath to stay balanced on your sit bones and lifted from your core. If you can, grab the balls of your feet and open your legs wider as you straighten the knees. Open and straighten your legs as far as possible without rounding your back. If you start to round your upper back or compress in your sacrum, bend your knees. Hold the pose for several breaths, trying to get more lift and extension in your spine by engaging core breathing. Don't hold the pose so long that you fatigue and begin to sag, compromising natural spine alignment.

Caution: Do not practice the boat pose with your feet together and legs straight. Poses in which the legs are closed together and the legs are in a right-angle to the trunk are unnatural and destabilizing to the sacral platform, according to the YogAlign method. The weight of the legs in this angle creates torque and places a heavy load on the ligaments and structure of the sacrum. As a result, the integrity of the spine and sacrum are sacrificed to do a pose that serves no natural function, because you cannot move with both of your knees held straight. Only practice positions that simulate how the body moves in real life. Always practice self-inquiry. Experiment with your own body limits, but please use a mirror when deciding whether or not you are actually in alignment. We sit in chairs for so long that spinal compression and sacrum stretching can actually feel quite "normal," so you cannot go by feeling alone.

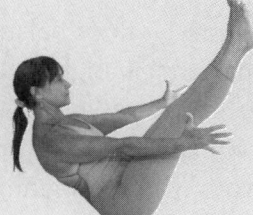

Fig. 35B – INCORRECT: Right-angled Boat

POSITION #36 — PNF HIP-BALANCER

This pose balances the action between the internal and external rotators of the hips and the functional fascia lines. Practicing this pose for several weeks releases deep tension patterns, freeing dormant energy in your pelvis. This pose will change tight hip patterns that have persisted for years when used with PNF neuromuscular recoding techniques.

The PNF Hip-Balancer Sequence

In this series, start with the position shown in **Fig. 36A**. If you are comfortable in this pose, continue with the variations in the order shown below. While it is not necessary to practice this pose in the sequence shown below, if you are going to add "Twisting Hip-Balancer" (**Fig. 36B**) and "Forward Bend Hip-Balancer" (**Fig. 36C**) to the initial pose, it is best to do them in this sequence, as it garners the best results. Each of the variations is described below.

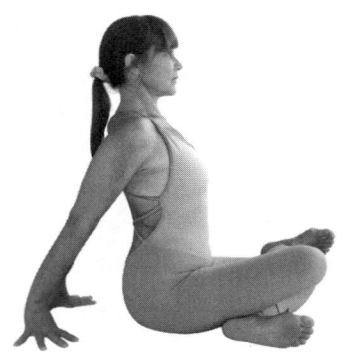

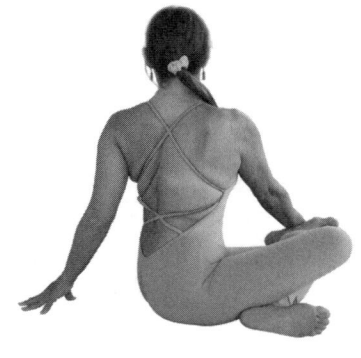

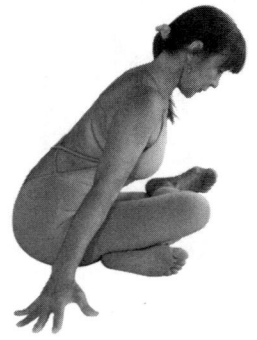

Fig. 36A –
Deep Arm Lines

Fig. 36B –
Twisting Hip-Balancer

Fig. 36C –
Forward Bend Hip-Balancer

Sit on the floor balancing on your sit bones, and place your right foot on top of your left thigh. Bring the shins in line, right over left. If you feel tension in your knees or groin area place a pillow under your hips to get them level. Maintain extension in your trunk and keep the curve in your lower back. Don't be concerned if your right thigh and knee are lifted higher on one side. The second part of this exercise will work with reprogramming nerve signals to relax your outer rotators and groin, aligning your knee action from the hip.

Keep your left shin parallel to the front of your mat and your left knee in a straight line with your hip. Keep your shins stacked in parallel, one on top of the other, with toes extended open while pressing through the ball of your foot. Keep the edges of your feet level as though you were standing firmly on the ground. If you feel that you cannot get into the basic position, you may try this pose with your legs in a simple cross-legged position. Another variation is to extend your bottom leg out, which takes further pressure off the hips. You can also lie down on your back and bring your legs up a wall practicing the pose in an inverted position.

Balance on your fingertips as you point them back towards your hips. Your shoulder blades should be down, your lower back curve and sacral tilt present, and your head should simply rest on top of your spine. If your hands don't reach the floor, balance on your fingertips, use blocks, or move your hands closer in toward your body. If you have very long arms, you may have to move your hands further back. Using a mirror, check your alignment. Is your sacrum naturally-aligned without tension in the lower back region? There is a tendency in this pose to thrust the lower rib cage too far forward, so make sure that your rib cage stays aligned above your hips. You can use the movement of the SIP Breath to bring the ribs into alignment.

PNF Exercise

Place your right hand on top of your right thigh. Keep your foot active by pressing through the ball of the foot with your toes wide-open. Inhale, tighten the muscles in your hip and leg, and press the leg upwards in resistance against your hand. Hold your breath gently for several seconds, intensifying the actions of your muscles. Consciously exaggerate this resistance, and add pelvic floor tightening. On the exhale, slowly relax the resisting action in the hip and leg while keeping your toes active. Press down gently with your hands, using extra caution to avoid pushing on or near your knee. As you relax the resistance, blood flow rushes into your leg, and the nervous system signals the engaged muscles to reset to a longer length, increasing flexibility. Imagine that there is wide open space or running water in your hip area, and remember that muscles are mostly water. Breathe in, hold and practice resistance again. Sense the length of your spine and stay balanced on your sit bones, while feeling the release in your hips.

Twisting Hip-Balancer

This is my favorite twist, as it takes all of the tension out of my hip rotator muscles, balancing the inner and outer rotation actions of the hip joint. This pose helps to

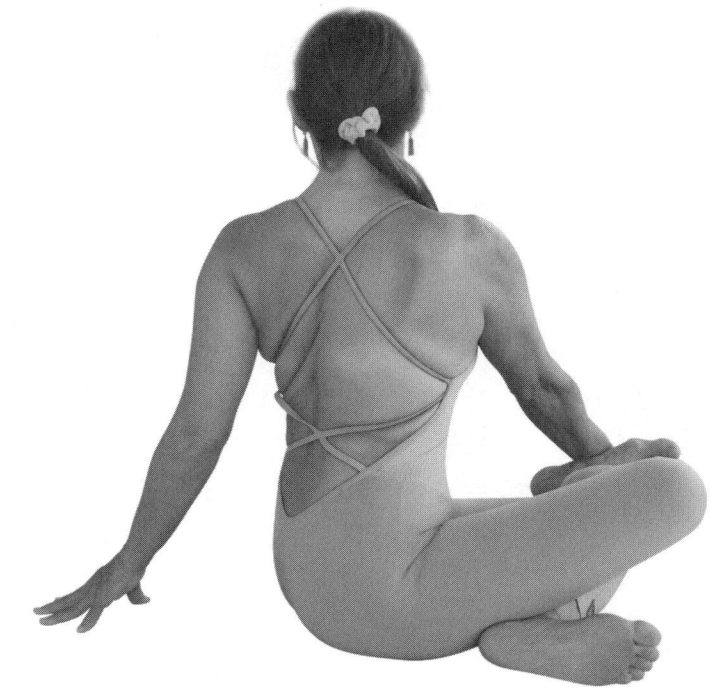

Fig. 36D – Twisting Hip-Balancer

balance the lines of pull in the spiral fascia lines and connects my movements from my inner core.

Inhale, and focus on using the movements of breath to create extension in your spine. Twisting from your abdominal area, turn to the left, holding your right foot with your right hand. Exhale while maintaining length in the waist and neck area. Inhale and hold the breath, as you keep twisting and intensifying the muscle engagements you feel to do this. Hold for several seconds accentuating the muscle forces you feel, and then exhale through a wide open mouth with your tongue extended. As you exhale, continue to twist but back off on the added tension you have been holding and focus on keeping length as you exhale. Do not lead with your head, but rather move from your abdomen and focus on keeping the curves in your spine and the length in your waist when both inhaling and exhaling. The weight of your head should simply rest atop the spine with your eyes in a soft and wide-focused gaze. Continue twisting with two more rounds of breathing. Come back to center, and sense how your entire body feels. If you feel uncomfortable at any time, continue the exercise in a simple cross-legged position. **Note:** It's very important to keep your feet engaged by spreading open your toes and extending through the ball of your foot. Make sure that your ankle is straight and not getting overstretched on one side.

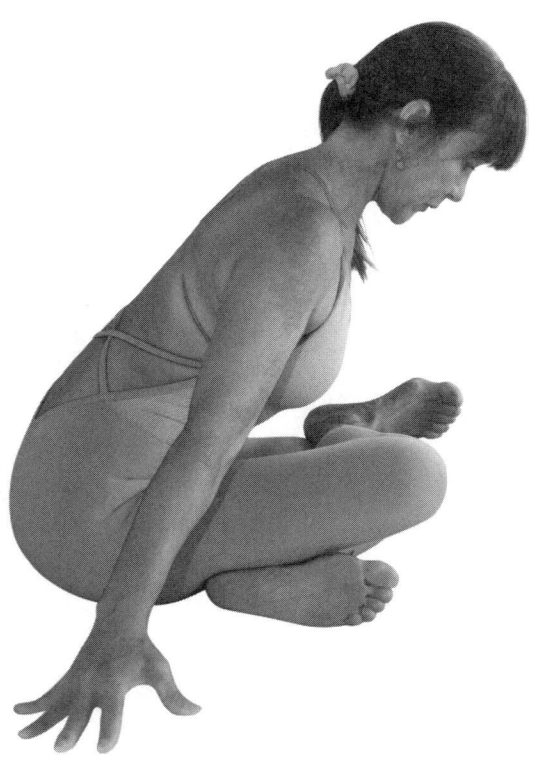

Fig. 36E – CORRECT:
PNF Forward Bend Hip-Balancer

PNF Forward Bend Hip-Balancer (Advanced)

If you can keep natural spine alignment and want to stretch more deeply, you can begin to lean forward as shown in **Fig. 36C**. Take your hands out to the sides of your body, placing your fingertips on the floor. Take a deep breath as you keep your entire spine lifted and aligned. Hold the breath for a few seconds, intensifying the muscle contractions required to do the action. As you exhale, slowly lean forward, and release the added muscle actions while lengthening the front body, in order to stay in natural alignment. Stop if you feel any strain or discomfort. Take another breath in and hold it, squeezing your buttock and thigh muscles, tightening muscles that create the action. Exhale and release the added contractions, as you continue to lengthen forward.

Finally, bring your hands out in front of you. As you exhale, slowly lean forward more. Avoid rounding your upper back or losing your sacral tilt. The best way to align your spine is to breathe into position with the core breathing technique. Feel how your body elongates during a core breathing inhale.

Maintain the lift as you exhale. Spread your toes and press through the ball of your foot; this engages leg muscles that will protect you from overstretching your knee ligaments. Keep length in your spine as you practice spiraling the inner thigh towards the floor, in order to engage your deep core line and internal rotators. This will balance the actions of internal and external rotation of the hip joint, protecting the ligaments of the sacral platform and balancing the hip rotators. Use a mirror to check that you are in natural spine alignment and staying in good postural alignment. Come out of the pose, shake out your legs, relax, and continue with the other side. When you complete this pose, do a "Full Body Stretch" on your mat, noticing the openness in your hips and legs. Do a few "Spinal Rolls" and then come up to standing.

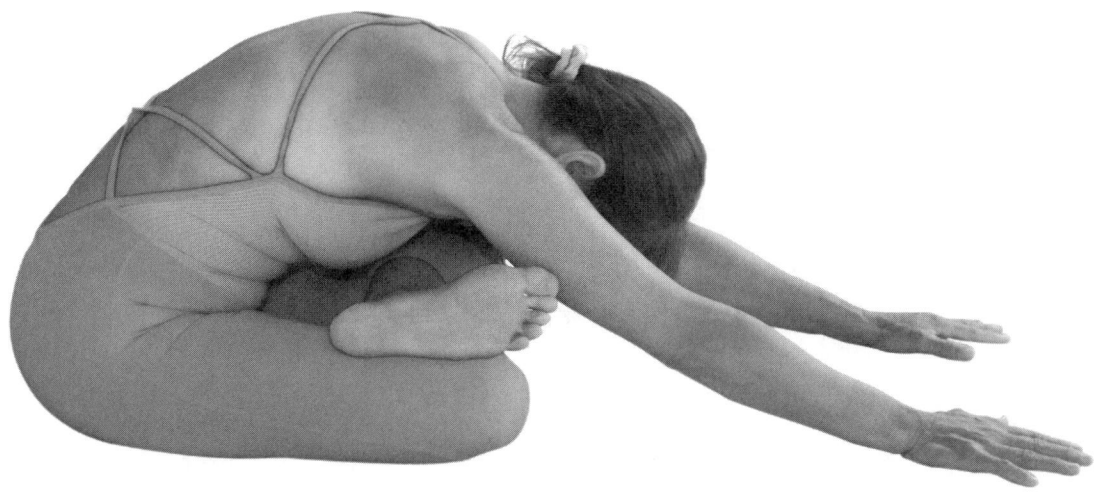

Fig. 36F – INCORRECT: Forward Bend

Caution: If you cannot keep the curves in your spine, lean back on your hands and focus on opening the front of your body before trying to bend forward. It can be dangerous to lean forward without proper spinal alignment, and the hip joint and spinal discs can be injured if you do not have good spinal support when practicing this pose. The incorrect version is shown in **Fig. 36F**, showing upper-back rounding. Rounding the upper back will overstretch your sacral ligaments, compress discs in your lumbar spine and contribute to kyphosis, which is a rounded upper-back postural patterning. All of these actions inhibit the deep movement of breath and compress your infrastructure, leading to chronic pain and premature aging. To avoid rounding the upper back, lean backward on your hands to extend the spine, or stay more vertical to maintain good spine alignment, as shown in **Fig. 36E**.

POSITION #37 — TREE (WITH A BRANCH)

A sense of well being, confidence and light-heartedness is enhanced if you regularly practice the "Tree with a Branch." Use this pose to hone alignment and balance, and to cultivate self-awareness that leads you to a sweet union of your body, mind, and spirit. The "Tree" pose develops personal power, and is an essential tool in the practice of yoga. Balance the tensile dance between the superficial front, lateral, and back lines of fascia. As you practice the pose, consider how a tree stays balanced and upright despite the wind and rain. The tree accomplishes this by producing rooting energy from the deep core line that connects it to the earth, and ascending energy which engages the trunk to lift dynamically towards the sky. The combination of these two opposing dynamic forces holds the tree in a state of balance. We are very much like the tree in that our balance is not static, and it depends upon the balance of the actions of extension and rooting. Balance is an ever-shifting event occurring in the moment. Oftentimes when we fall or lose balance, it is because we lose the connection to our whole body in the present, and dismiss the rooting actions of our legs and feet as well as the extension forces in our spine.

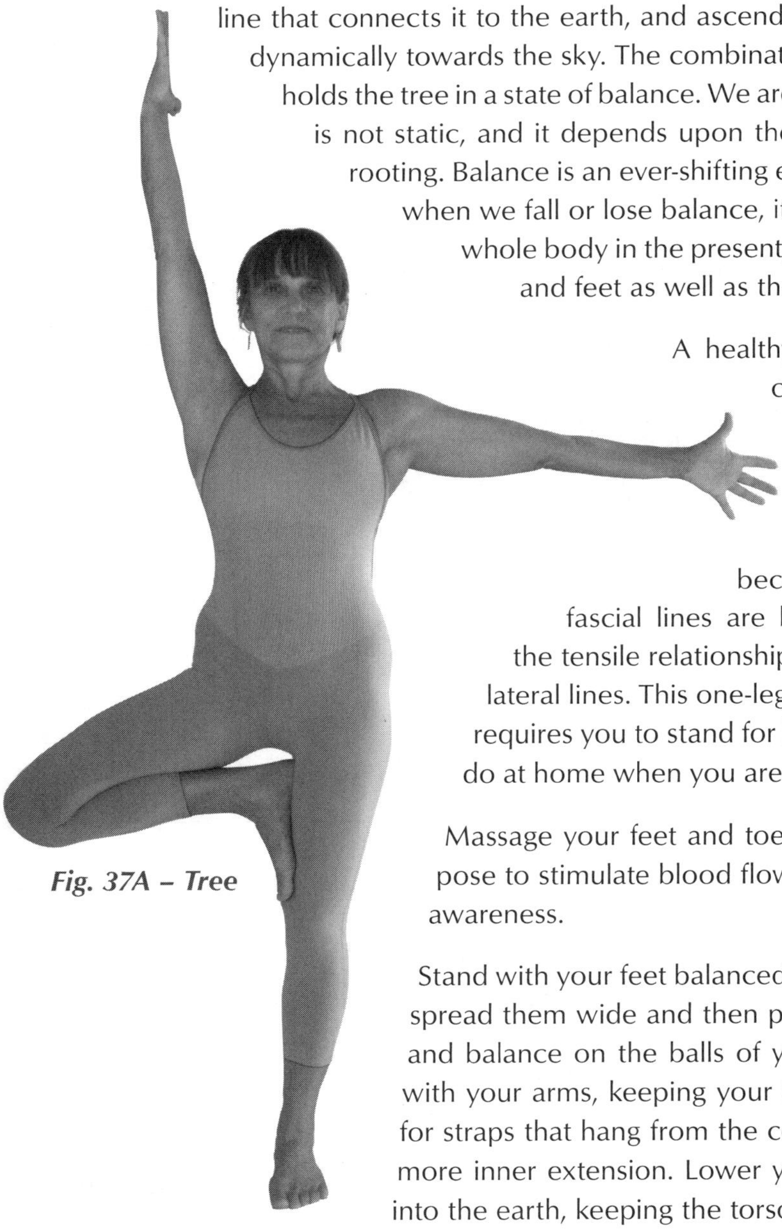

A healthy vestibular (or balance) system requires clear communication between your hearing, eyesight, and proprioceptive senses. The "Tree" pose sharpens your vestibular system, connecting your entire body to your inner core. Your feet, legs and arms become shapely and pain-free. All of your fascial lines are balanced in dynamic tension, particularly the tensile relationship between your superficial front, back, and lateral lines. This one-legged balance is recommended if your work requires you to stand for long periods of time. This is a great pose to do at home when you are standing in front of your sink doing dishes.

Fig. 37A – Tree

Massage your feet and toes for a few moments before you start the pose to stimulate blood flow, encourage suppleness, and develop foot awareness.

Stand with your feet balanced and grounded to the floor. Lift all ten toes, spread them wide and then press them into the floor. Lift your heels up and balance on the balls of your feet with your toes spread. Reach up with your arms, keeping your fingers spread as though you are reaching for straps that hang from the ceiling. Practice a Core SIP Breath to create more inner extension. Lower your heels to the floor and press your feet into the earth, keeping the torso lengthened to create dynamic tension.

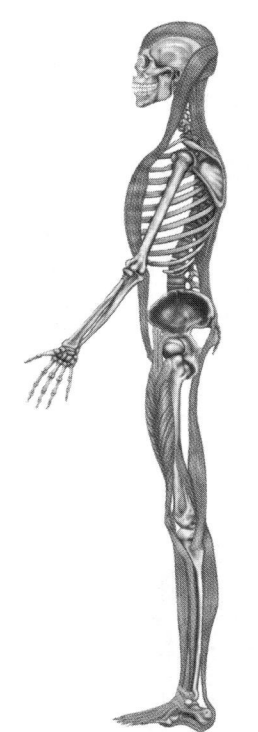

Lift all ten toes, but this time press your big toes down, keeping the other ones spread and lifted. Now try to press your pinky toes into the floor along with the big toes, keeping the other three toes lifted and spread apart. Bravo to you if you can do this, but if you can't, keep practicing the "Toe Weave" and "Foot Shake" pose (Position #5) to help you gain kid-like dexterity in your feet. Bring all of your toes to the floor, rooting down with your leg and foot energy while you practice growing and lengthening with your trunk.

To start the "Tree" pose, shift your weight to your right leg. Bring your left foot up into the inside of your right thigh. Press your foot and inner thigh towards one another, anchoring your standing leg firmly to the floor without locking back on

> **Note:** If you have difficulty balancing, stand near a wall so that you can use your hand to anchor yourself.

your knee. There should be a feeling of energy traveling all the way to your feet without stopping at the back of your knees. Bring your hands together in "Namaste" at your heart center. Set your intention to be present and aware in your mind and body.

Spread your fingers wide and press your hands firmly together. Notice how your mid-back muscles engage to stabilize your shoulder blades. Allow your shoulder

blades to sink down your back as you extend your arms up, shoulder-width apart. Keep your fingers spread wide as you reach up from the center of your body, connecting your arms to your core while using only the necessary effort.

YogAlign is about doing less, turning off the extra muscles, and feeling free in your body. If you feel your arms pulling away from your upper shoulders, exaggerate the dysfunction by lifting your shoulders towards your ears. Accentuate the muscle action created when doing this. Hold for a moment and then let go, releasing the extra effort while you keep extending your arms. Let the shoulders drop and your arms set into their sockets. Sense the root of each of your arms,

> **Note:** Keep your arms shoulder-width or wider, and focus on dropping your shoulders away from your ears. Do not try and put your hands together overhead. Doing this pushes the head forward and overengages the upper trapezius muscles, destabilizing your shoulder joint by overstretching important stabilizing ligaments.

back to your chest, down through your ribs, the sides of your body, your spine, then into your hips; feel the connection from this base of your arms expanding out to the ends of your fingers.

Now exhale, and drop your right arm to shoulder-height, creating a branch. Keep the fingers in both hands wide, with your arms and legs connecting back to center. Avoid locking your knees, and check in the mirror that you are in natural alignment. Feel the weight of your head floating atop your spine. Notice your rib cage balanced above your hips. Focus on deep core breathing through your nose or mouth. Imagine the way a tree reaches down with its roots and lengthens up with its trunk and branches to stay in

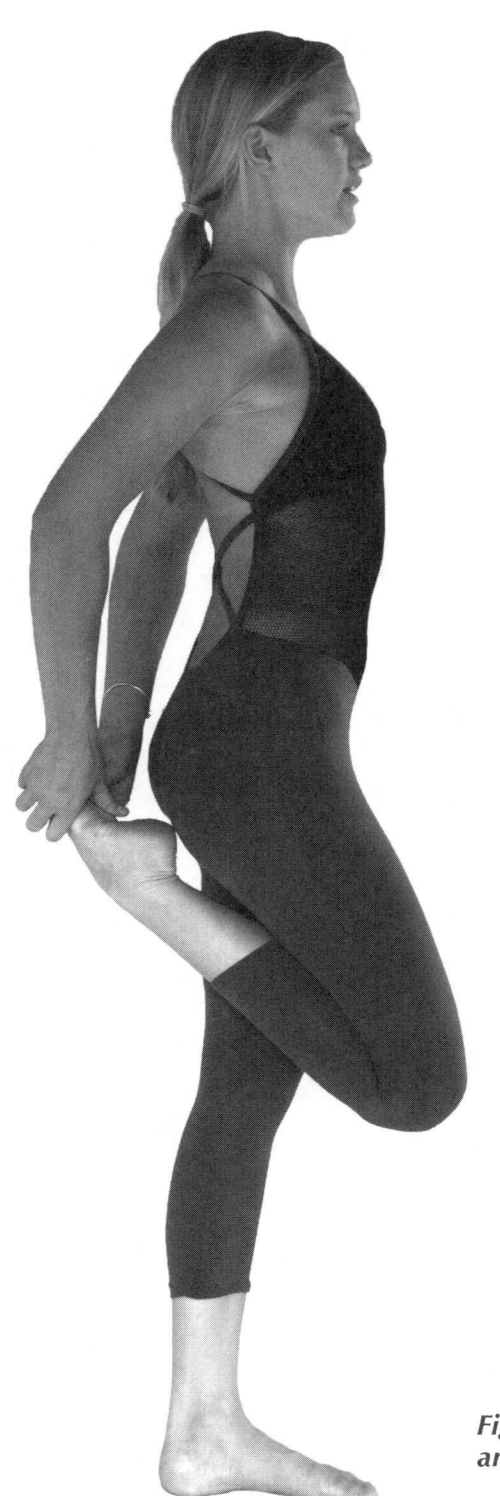

perfect balance. Sense your body in its entirety. Soften your face and eyes. Ground and extend your toes. Make sure you have natural curves in your spine and that you are not pulling your front rib cage too far forward, locking out your knees, or tucking your tail and compressing your sacrum.

For the last part of the pose, see if you can lift the heel of your right foot very slightly and continue to balance by pressing into the ball of your foot. Maintain the effort to pull your limbs to your center and focus on using the breathing process to root and extend. Come down slowly and notice the difference in the two sides. Repeat the entire pose on the other leg.

After completing the pose, take a moment to walk around with the same actions you created in tree-rooting your legs with your trunk extended. Notice how light your steps feel, and how effortless movement can be. Let this awareness go deep into your being, and imagine that you are setting up new codes in your brain to make this extended natural alignment your everyday posture.

For multi-tasking at its best — and a great way to do a one leg balance, get a foot massage and tone and open the chest and arm lines at the same time — come into the tree pose on your right leg as described above. Lift your left leg and reach behind your back with your arms and hold your foot with your hands. Keep your chest lifted and open by using the movements of breathing while engaging the scapula down the back. Deeply massage your toes and your foot while staying present in the actions of the tree pose. Keep your hips level, stay lifted and do not push back on the ligaments of your standing foot. When you come out of the pose, stand with both feet on the ground and notice how massaging your left foot has changed the feeling of your entire left side. Repeat on the other side.

Fig. 37B – Standing Foot Massage. Rayna, college student, surfer and paraglider enjoys this unique way of self-massaging her foot while balancing and engaging her inner core.

POSITION #38 — TREE STAR (ADVANCED)

"Tree Star" is a standing version of the reclining floor-pose "Star" (Position #13), that adds in balance practice. This dynamic pose gives you powerful, youthful legs and provides you with a warranty to balance safely on any terrain. A must for athletes and dancers, this pose will keep you nimble, youthful and graceful. You will develop a stronger will, determination, and courage to face the difficulties that arise in every-day living.

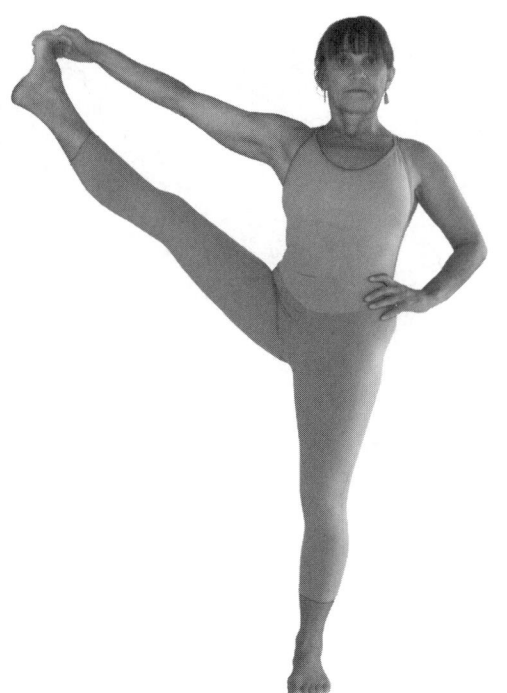

Fig. 38A – Front view

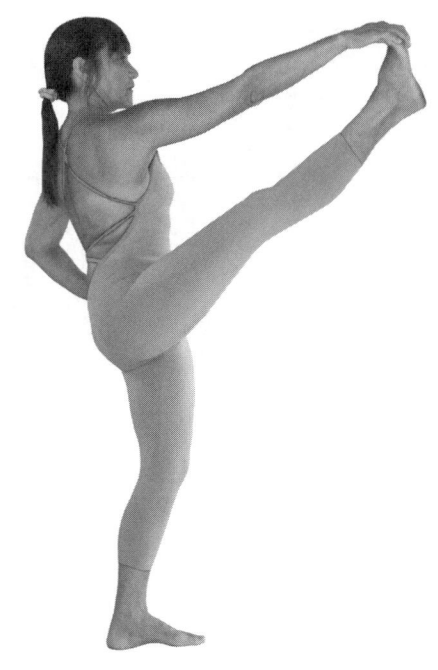

Fig. 38B – Side view

If you can easily grab your foot lying on the mat in "Star," you should try this pose. You may also try this pose using a strap on the ball of your foot.

From "Tree," bend your standing knee and hold the ball of the foot on your folded leg as you extend your leg forward. Keep reaching through the ball of your foot using the gas pedal or floint position. (**Note:** If you can't make this movement while maintaining the curve in your lower back, use a strap, but always keep the standing knee bent at first.) Inhale, swing your leg out to the side and roll your thigh inward and up, in order to keep your hips level.

For optimal balance, press firmly through your standing foot while using the SIP Breath to create extension in your trunk. Engage your limbs back towards the center with the tips of the shoulder blades drawing down your back with just the right amount of effort. Soften your face and eyes. Your head should feel light on your spine, your upper shoulders relaxed and easy. Sense your body in its entirety like a vibrant tree and a radiant star, shining in all directions from your powerful core.

Keep your front fascia line long and open, while staying in the core and balancing from front to back. Use core breathing to feel the internal muscular ring of support that effortlessly provides balanced support from the inside out.

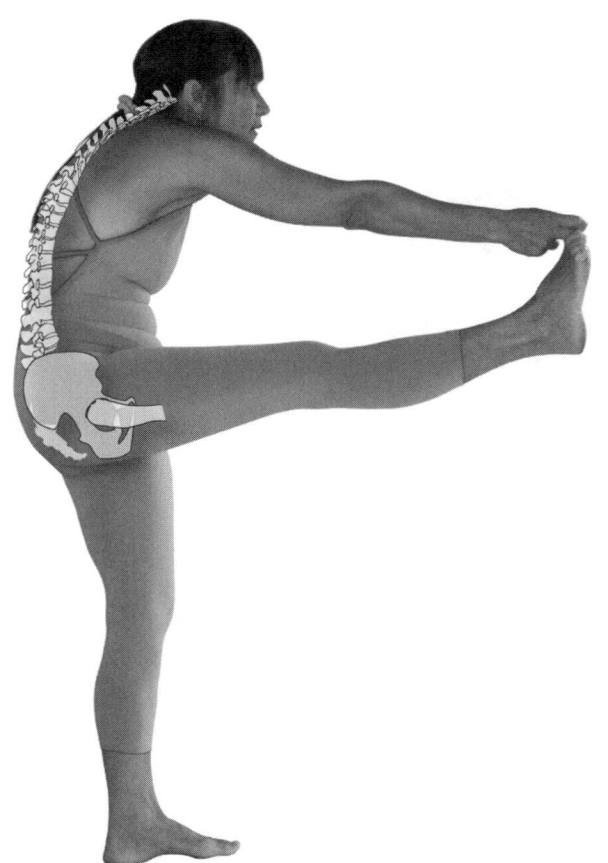

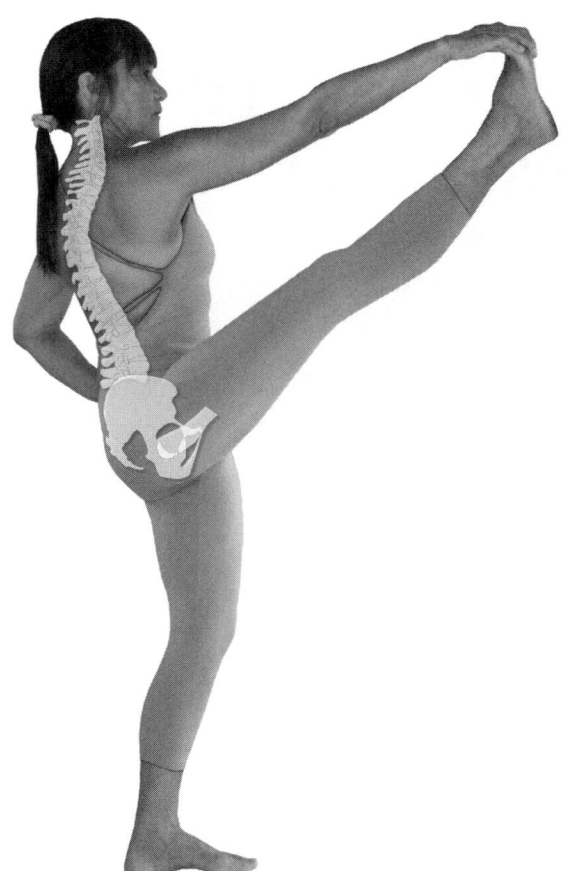

Fig. 38C – INCORRECT: Misaligned, spine compressed.

Fig. 38D – CORRECT: Aligned, natural spine.

For a more advanced position, as you extend your lifted leg, slowly move it back and forth, staying fluid and connecting to the breath. Find an effortless place in the pose, grounding in the standing leg, growing from the trunk, exhibiting perfect balance in opposing actions. Sense your entire body. Feel your breath. Stay focused on being present with less effort. Bring your extended leg back to the floor and return to standing with both feet on the floor. Sense your body and feel how the pose has affected you.

POSITION #39 — TWISTING TREE (ADVANCED)

The "Twisting Tree" gives you a toned core that creates a synergestic balance of the muscular/fascial forces that stabilize your spine as you move. You develop balance, power, grace, and fluidity when practicing these Tree poses. When the basic "Tree" and "Twisting Tree" are done in a flow, your practice becomes a series of balancing poses dynamically linked together. "Twisting Tree" strengthens the spinal muscles that give you deep postural support from the inside out. The lateral, spiral and functional lines become tuned and balanced, bringing relief from chronic neck, mid-back, knee and hip pains.

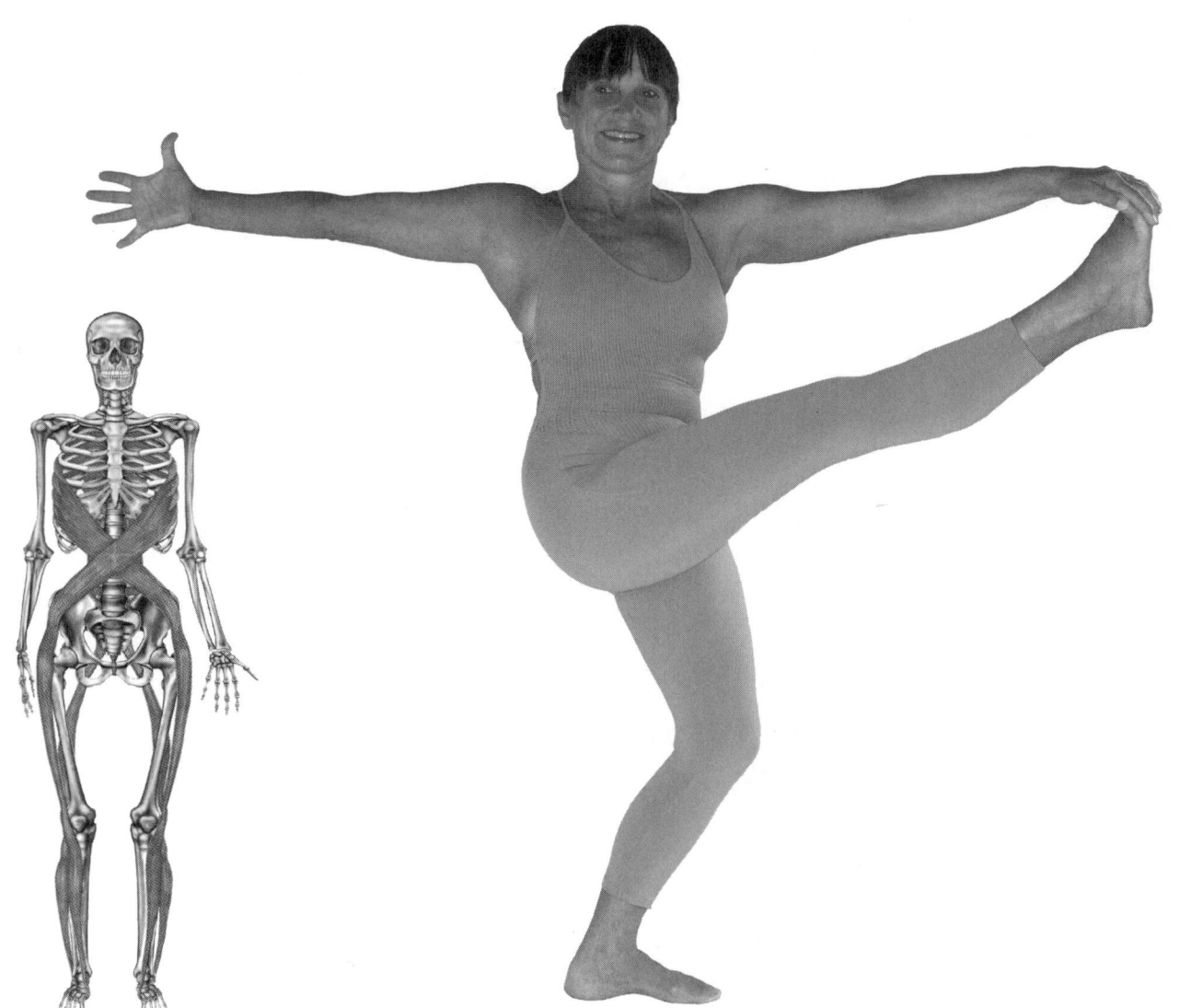

The spiral line of fascia.   *Fig. 39 – Twisting Tree (Advanced)*

To move from "Tree Star" to "Twisting Tree," bring your raised foot to the front and switch hands, reaching your opposite arm across the body to grab the ball of the raised foot. Take a deep breath and bend your standing knee while you open your free hand out to the side. If you are having trouble, you can do this pose with a strap or bend both your standing and extended knees. Open your fingers wide and feel the lateral and spiral extension from heel, to rib cage, and out to the fingertips. When doing the "Twisting Tree," you strongly engage the actions of the functional and spiral lines.

Keep your hips and foot level as you draw your upper inner-thighs towards each other. Feel the body in its entirety. Make sure you bend your standing knee, and maintain the natural curves in your spine to prevent overstretching of sacral ligaments. You can also practice this pose using PNF techniques by accentuating all of the muscle actions you are using, then releasing the extra tension as you hold the pose with only the necessary effort. Keep the same energy line directions as in the basic "Tree" pose.

Now repeat the entire "Tree" sequence on your opposite leg.

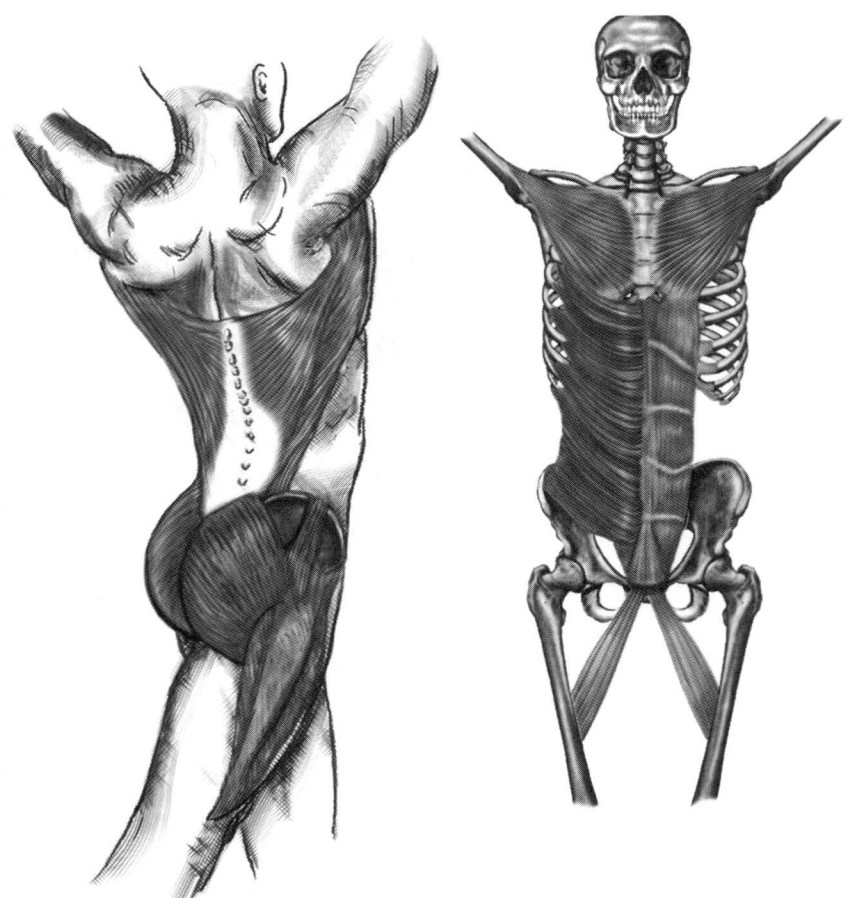

Anterior and posterior functional fascia lines.

POSITION #40 — LIGHTNING BOLT

The "Lightning Bolt" pose strengthens and tones your legs, develops inner core strength, and corrects poor posture. Learning to sit with an active trunk develops the functional muscle patterning needed to maintain good posture when sitting or driving for extended periods of time.

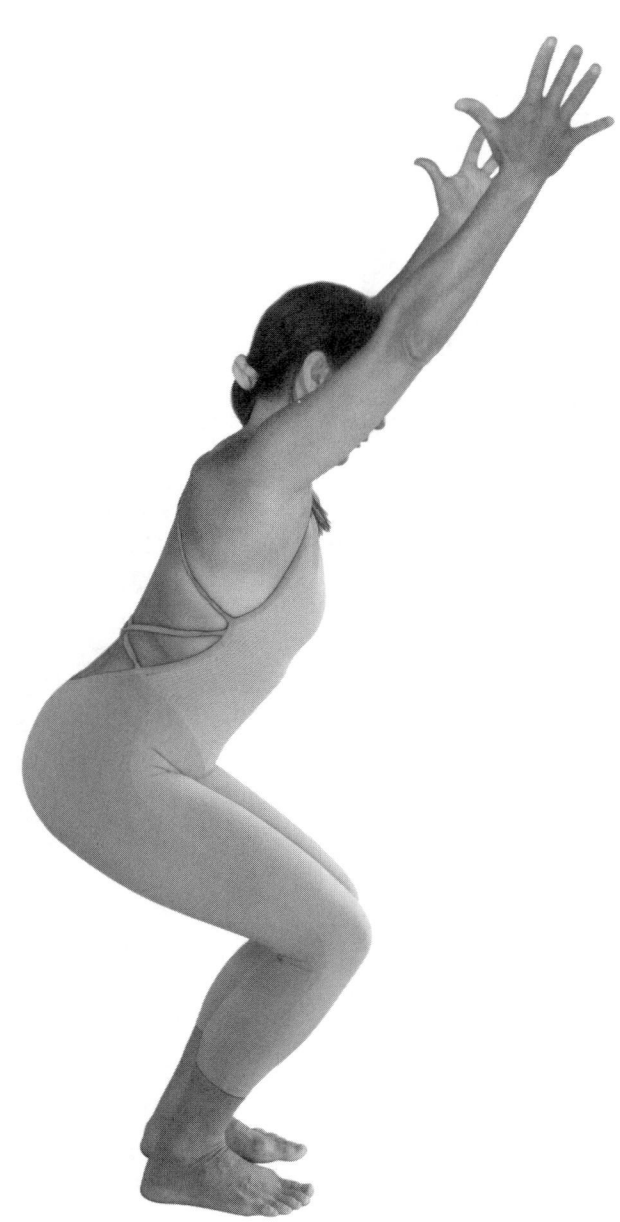

Fig. 40A –— CORRECT: Neck aligned.

Start with your feet hip-width apart and your arms by your sides. Take a deep breath as you bend your knees and raise your arms with your fingers spread wide. Make sure to engage your arms from the fingertips right into the arm socket and back to your hips as you lift them. Deepen your knee bend as if you are about to sit in a chair. Keep extending your arms upward with spread fingers, maintaining a neutrally-aligned neck and spine. This is the "Lightning Bolt" position. Practice breathing deeply through your nose and stay focused on your body in its entirety. Keep your shoulder blades drawn down and your chin level, and align your ribs directly over your hips.

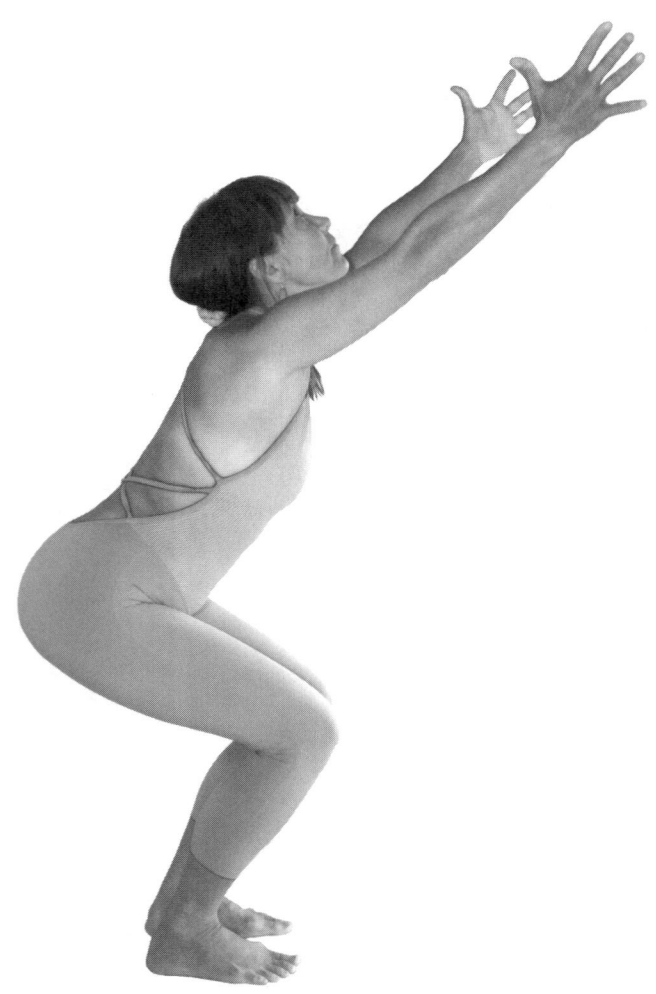

Fig. 40B — INCORRECT: Chin lifted.

Hold this position for several deep core breaths. Return to standing, circling your arms back down to your sides and then raise them as before. With your arms still raised, breathe in deeply, lift your heels from the standing position, and balance on the balls of your feet for a moment. As you exhale, lower your heels, bending your knees, and circle your arms to the back and then forward again as you drop back into the "Lightning Bolt" pose. Continue for several cycles and then stand with your feet hip-distance apart, with your arms by your side. Observe the energy shift from within.

Your spine is a flexible rod and compressing any part of it will affect the whole spine and reverberate throughout your body. When you lift or lead with your chin, the neck spine is compressed, as in **Fig. 40B**. In this alignment, the lower back curve holds the same energy as the neck and it will hold the same compression. Check your alignment by standing sideways to a mirror. As you perform "Lightening Bolt," stay long and extended in your trunk and remain grounded into your feet. Sense your body and notice where you are making the effort to move. Remember to draw into your center and move from your core.

POSITION #41 — PNF SUMO WRESTLER

The "Sumo Wrestler" pose looks much like the starting stance of a sumo wrestler. In the "Sumo Wrestler," PNF exercises are used to recalibrate muscle tension in the pelvic floor and adductor (inner thigh) regions. This pose uses the deep core line as the generator for spine extension. The objective is to attain your alignment, tone and flexibility from the inside out and release unnecessary tension in the pelvic floor and inner thigh area. The functional line gets tuned in harmony with the deep core line, and movement becomes effortless, powerful, and stable from the center of your body. Practicing "Sumo Wrestler" will also facilitate a toning and lifting of the bladder, flaccid with age, as well as with too much time spent sitting in chairs.

Your pelvic floor and the six-pack are wired together in fascia lines that dictate movement all over your body. Tightness in the pelvic floor is common in athletes who have strengthened their six-pack muscles with strong flexion exercises, unaware that the pelvic floor and abs are connected. A tight pelvic floor is the underlying cause of leg and hip tightness as well as knee pain and injuries. Take a stroll around the room with tightened pee muscles and you will have an experience of how chronically over-contracted pelvic floor muscles serve no function and lead to these injuries and pain. The "Sumo Wrestler" pose will help alleviate this excess tension. Alternatively, people with weak pelvic floors can gain strength and tone with this pose.

Throughout this pose, use the SIP Breath to add internal length to your spine and front body.

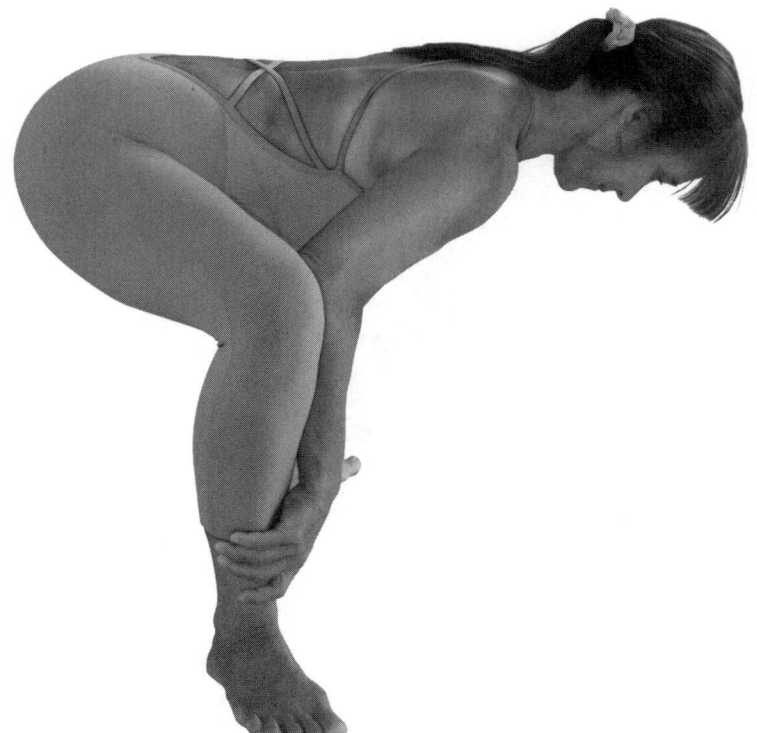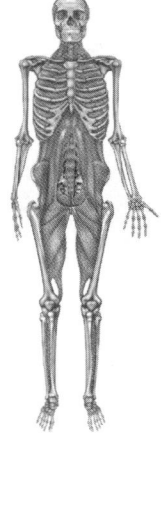

Fig. 41A – PNF Sumo Wrestler

To begin, take a wide stance, with your feet turned slightly out and your ankles aligned with your knees. Place your hands on your thighs and inhale forward, elongating the spine by using the movements of inhalation together with your proprioceptive alignment receptors. Keep your neck in neutral alignment (turn side to side to check for unconscious neck tension). Check for the curve in your lower back. Inhale and "feel" your alignment; your head, rib cage, and hips should be lined up as when you are standing well.

Slide your forearms or elbows into your inner thighs above your knees. Grab your ankles. (Note: If you can't hold your ankles without maintaining good posture, move your hands back up your leg until your spine has its natural curves and breathing is unrestricted. You can also sit on the edge of a chair.)

Press your arms or elbows against your inner thighs, tightening your muscles in the groin and pelvic floor. Inhale, hold for a moment, exhale, and release the inner resistance of your thighs and pelvic floor while you continue to press your thighs open with your elbows or forearms.

> **CAUTION:** If you have a "pull" or pain in the groin, proceed with caution. You can alternatively bend halfway over, supporting yourself with your hands on the hips or elbows on the thighs.

Stay grounded in your feet. Inhale and release tension in the pelvic floor. As you exhale, resist strongly with

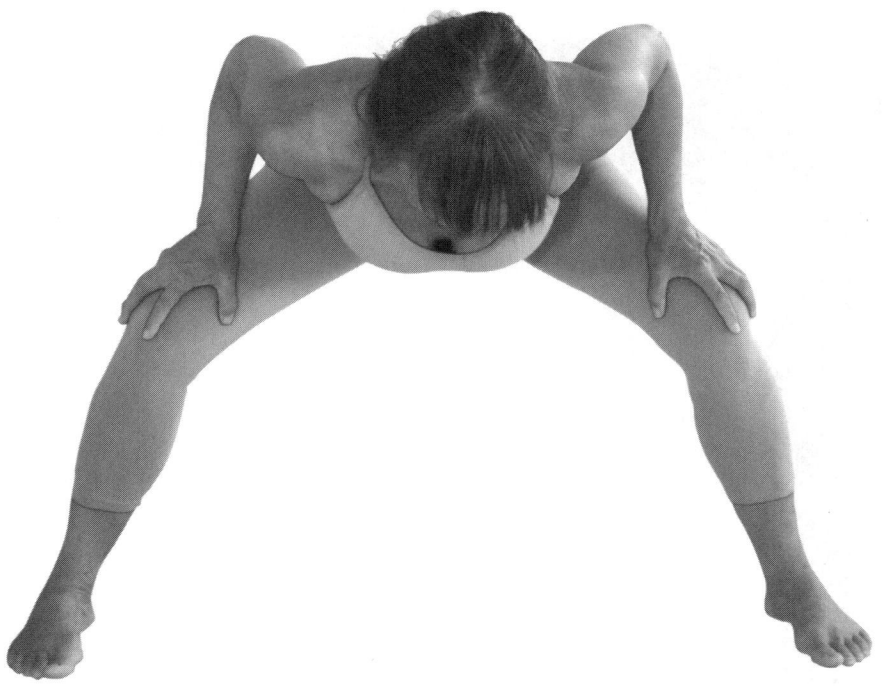

Fig. 41B – Elbows resist the pressing out of the inner thighs.
Maintain your sacral tilt and lower back curve.

your arms and tighten the thigh and pelvic floor region again. As you inhale, release the pelvic floor and inner thigh resistance, allowing the pelvic floor to open and expand. Practice sideways to a mirror so you can check that your belly is parallel to the floor, and that you are maintaining your natural spinal curves. Keep length in your front body, and protect your knees by keeping them over your ankles with your feet and leg muscles active.

Use a mirror to see if your spine is in natural alignment. Remember that what is abnormal in posture can feel normal, and you may need to do a visual check to determine what your body actually looks like; you can then find neutral with the aid of a mirror. In case you have difficulty discerning if you are in functional alignment, practice a SIP Breath to feel if your infrastructure is being compressed by poor alignment biomechanics or by unnecessary tightness or effort.

We tend to be a goal-oriented culture, looking for results and numbers. Many folks push themselves too hard, exercising with determination and focusing on goals that "must" be met in order for them to feel like they have accomplished something. In YogAlign we focus on doing less and using just the right amount of effort to attain a feeling of balance and alignment that happens almost effortlessly, with our bodies aligned through the movements of breathing. The desire to be better, look better and be fit can override the communication signals from your body saying "Ouch!" Oftentimes we don't hear the body until it is screaming, whining, and pleading with us to change positions. Many fitness classes even use loud music, distracting us from hearing the subtle language of our body. This is a double whammy because loud music causes a stress response from the nervous system: digestion slows, blood pressure rises, adrenalin is released, and muscles tense, leaving us stressed and sore.

If possible, practice these poses among the sounds of nature, do lots of self-massage and pay attention to what you are feeling. You can gain the ability to hear the subtle whispers of your being, fine tune your alignment, and be truly pain-free from your inner core.

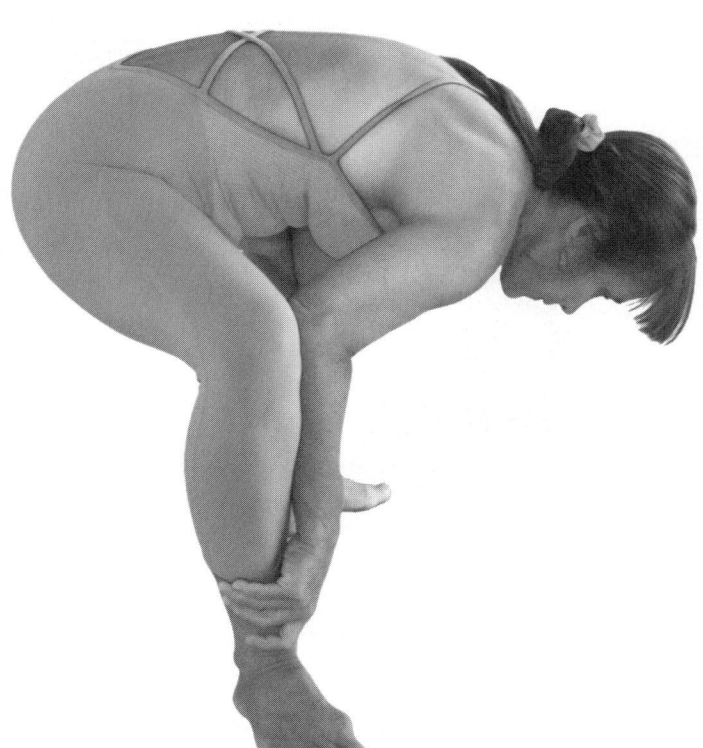

Fig. 41C – INCORRECT:
Bad Sumo with poor alignment.

POSITION #42 — SURFER STRETCH AND BEACH TWIST

These poses train your nervous system to let go of habitual tension in your lateral and spiral fascia lines and musculature. This facilitates the ability to breathe and rotate with power, ease, and kid-like flexibility. The lymphatic flow is greatly increased, supercharging your immune system. This pose also greatly benefits the entire body, increasing pulmonary elasticity and creating tone and flexibility in your legs, hips, and groin.

For surfers, these poses are a panacea for shortened lateral "paddling" muscles that connect the hip to the fingertips. In addition, golfers, paddlers, swimmers, (and anyone who wants to be able to drive a car at age 100) acquire youthful twisting abilities.

Increasing the extension and flexibility of the lats and the rib cage's breathing muscles also dramatically increases space for your internal organs. The pose also gifts the bonus of a toned, youthful waist without liposuction.

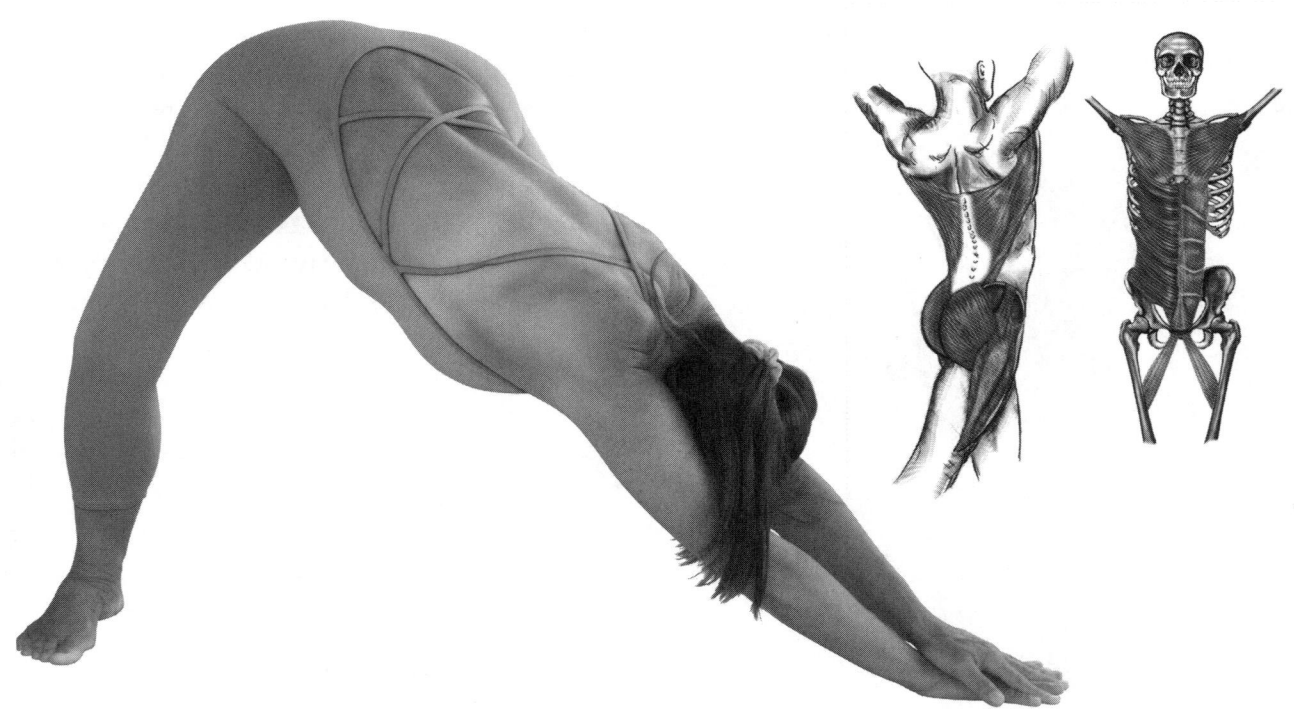

Fig. 42A – Surfer Stretch
The "Surfer Stretch" can be done while bending down to wax up a surfboard.

The Surfer Stretch

To begin, take a wide stance with your knees bent and your feet about three feet apart. Begin inhaling as you bend forward with your knees bent, placing your fingertips on the floor in line with your head and shoulders. (**Note:** If you are tall or have strong hamstring muscles, use a block or stool under your hands to lift your torso higher and protect your spine and back muscles.) Keep the bend in your knees, and lengthen your front body with the SIP inhale as you reach back with your butt while maintaining natural spine alignment. Walk the fingertips of your right hand sideways or push the block, towards—then beyond—your left foot. (Do not stress your lower body in order to do this, and remember to use a block under your hand if you feel too much tension in your legs or groin.) Rest your head on your lower arm and relax your neck and face muscles. Remember to be sustainable from within—use only the necessary effort.

Press the right hand firmly to the floor, with the palm facing down and your left hand on top of your right hand. With your arm and leg muscles activated, draw your shoulder blades down while keeping your limbs connected to the core. Initiate a SIP Breath, and gently twist your right side up towards the ceiling, stretching open your armpit. Hold your breath for a moment and intensify the muscle actions that you feel engaging (PNF). Release the breath and the extra muscle tightness as you exhale, keeping in the pose as you press your hands and stretch deeply with your muscles active. Repeat these actions two or three times using the PNF resistance techniques. As you do the SIP Breath, laterally rotate your right side back and forth up towards the ceiling. Maintain natural spine alignment in the pose and feel your body in its entirety. If you want to feel more and deepen the actions of the "Surfer Stretch," slowly straighten your bent knee on the side you are reaching towards, while keeping your hips low and your butt pulled back.

Complete this entire sequence on the opposite side, then place your hands on your thighs with both knees bent. Come up slowly, breathing through your nose, bending your knees and using the large muscles in your legs and butt to come to standing as you maintain good spine alignment without rounding the upper back.

Observe a friend in the "Surfer Stretch" and look for the outline of the "lat" muscle. If a person has skin that shows blood close to the surface, an observer can see the flow of blood through the lats, and can see the outline of the muscle from the arm, through the ribs, to the hip.

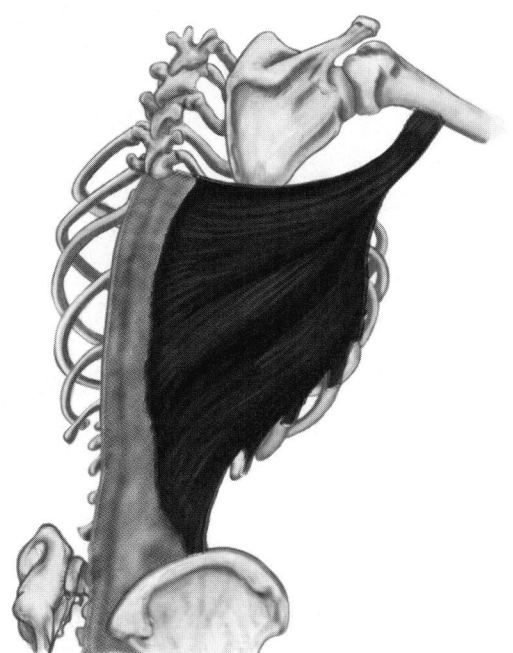

The Beach Twist

The "Beach Twist" engages the lats and the functional line while strengthening and toning your body for powerful deep movements requiring twisting and bending. The "Beach Twist" keeps you in shape for activities like surfing, volleyball, golf, skiing and dancing.

To do the "Beach Twist" stay in the same wide stance as in the "Surfer Stretch." Do the pose in front of a mirror if available. Place a block forward of your feet and place your right hand on the block. Adjust the height of the block to allow you to have your arm pit and groin pit on the same level. If you are highly flexible, you may not need a block and if so balance on your fingertips.

Keep your knees bent at all times and retain the natural curves in your spine. Place your left arm out to the side with your elbows bent as in **Fig. 42B** and act as though you are pressing a wall with your hand as you keep your shoulders pulled away from your ears. Move from your abdomen and tighten your muscles as you twist, holding the muscle actions while gently retaining an inhalation. As you need to exhale, release the tension but stay in the extension of the pose and twist deeper. If your shoulders line up, extend your arm up towards the ceiling (**Fig. 42C**) while retaining the actions of drawing your limbs back towards center. Repeat on the other side.

The "Sumo Wrestler," along with the "Surfer Stretch" and "Beach Twist," prepare the body for the "Dancing Warrior" series (beginning with Position #43) by opening the side body and bringing sensory awareness, blood flow, and muscle balance into the feet, legs, hips and groin.

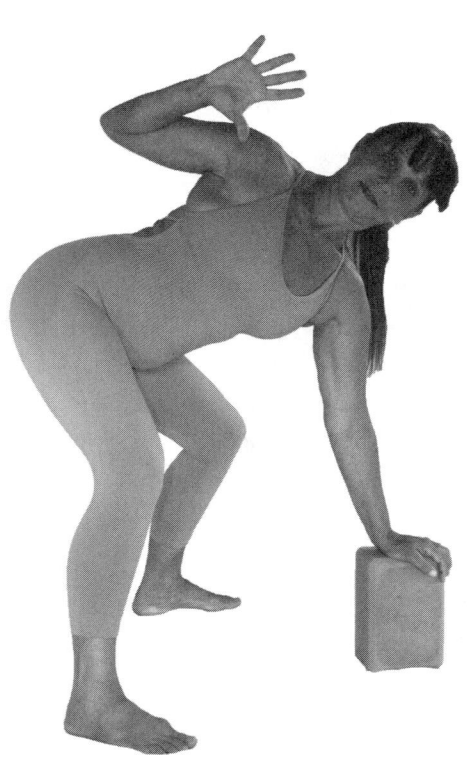

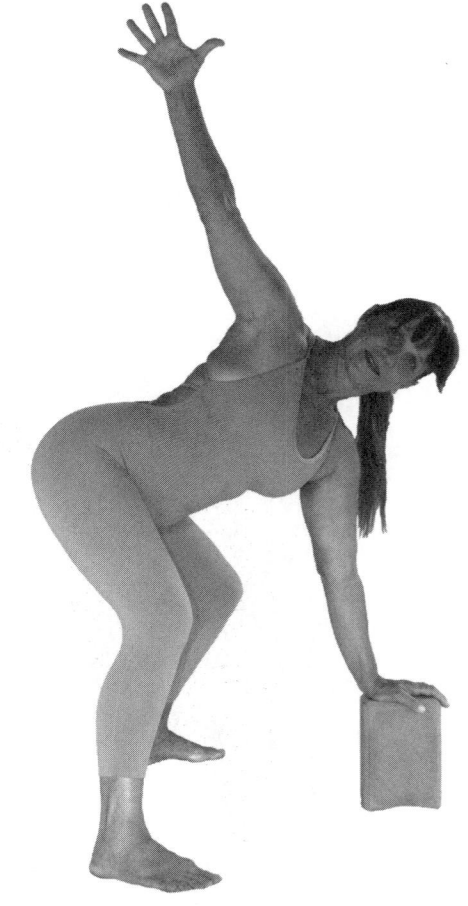

Fig. 42B – Beach Twist arm prep engages the elements of the deep core line in driving body movement from the inner core.

Fig. 42C – Drawing limbs to the core while extending energy through the fascia lines of the arm.

POSITION #43 — DANCING WARRIOR SERIES

This series links poses with the breath in a vinyasa, or "flow style" yoga, so that you are "dancing" from one pose to the next. This book's accompanying DVD will help you understand and execute the fluid movements of the powerful positions used in "Dancing Warrior." In YogAlign, there are many different variations in the movement of the arms and the bending of the knees. Once you know a few of the moves, intuitive movement is encouraged to keep your practice fresh and playful. The "Dancing Warrior" series strengthens your legs and feet, and brings flexibility to your hips and groin. The tensile forces of the fascia lines in your legs become balanced, protecting your hip, knee, and ankle joints from pain and preventing injuries associated with chronic misalignment syndromes.

The YogAlign "Warrior" focuses on keeping the four natural curves of the spine, with the feet, knees, and hips aligned to protect knee, hip, and sacral ligaments. We also add specific arm and hand movements that activate, lubricate, massage, and stabilize the shoulder joint. The "Dancing Warrior" promotes functional movement patterns that reverberate throughout your entire body. Remember that it is important to concentrate on ideal posture in every pose and with every breath, until your neuromuscular patterns automatically support optimal alignment. At the point of automation, it becomes normal and "easy" to be aligned.

Focus on these points as you practice the "Dancing Warrior":

- *Practice in front of a mirror. It is especially important for beginning practitioners to be able to observe alignment and correct habituated poor postural patterns. Many of us have become accustomed to being out of alignment, and visual cues are very beneficial for helping us see what needs to change.*

- *Use the movements of breath to support and sustain you.*

- *Engage your limbs back into the socket and feel the fascial connections as you breathe.*

- *Dance with the least amount of effort, and, in particular, keep your upper trapezius, eye, jaw, and facial muscles relaxed, using only the necessary muscle actions.*

- *Always maintain your natural spinal curves and keep the actions of rooting and extending equalized between your legs and your trunk. Spiral your inner thigh muscles back to balance the inner and outer hip rotations that are a major determinant of your pelvic angle, and avoid locking back with your knees or tucking under your tail.*

In YogAlign, we seek to create ideal posture in each pose so it is extremely important in these lunges to create a balanced and level pelvic bowl and rib cage. Inhale to create lift in the spine and expansion of the rib cage as you work through these movements. Notice and keep the lift through the exhale, drawing the shoulder blades down the back. Do not brace yourself by tucking your buttocks under, lifting your chin, or locking out your back knee. Keep your eyes in a soft gaze and notice everything without labeling or judging.

Before you begin, review the anatomy of the fascial connections in Chapter 2. Sense and feel how your arms are attached through muscular/fascia lines from the fingers to your chest in your front, and all the way to your ribs and hips in the back and side of your body. Also be sure that you have massaged your feet and toes before you begin, so that you bring sufficient blood flow and awareness to the actions of your feet.

Warrior Dance, Part 1

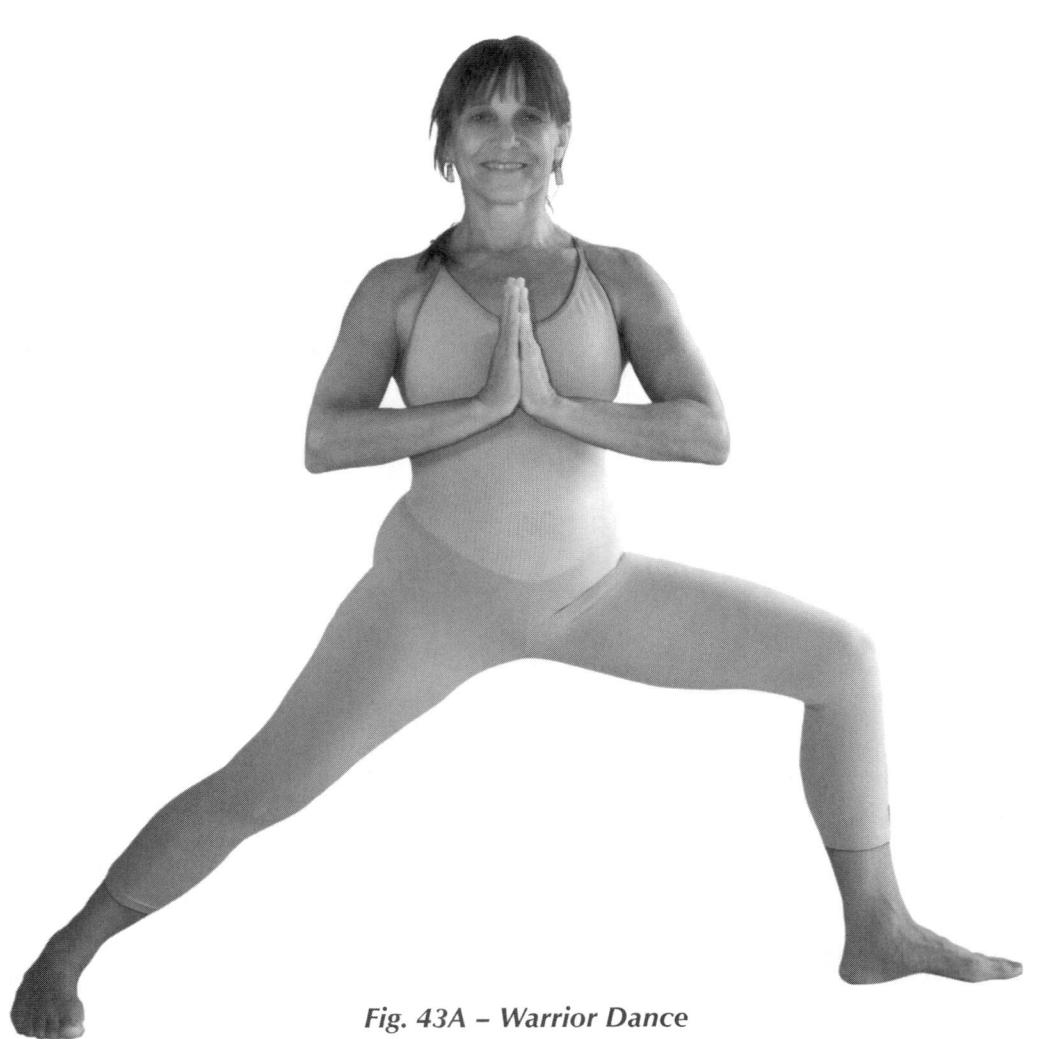

Fig. 43A – Warrior Dance

Start with the left leg in the bent knee position as in **Fig. 43A**. To begin, take a wide stance, turning your right (back) foot perpendicular to your left or (front) foot in the pose. Align the center of your front heel with middle of the arch in your back foot. (While I use the term "front foot" to represent the left foot, and "back foot" to represent the right foot throughout this narration, you may begin the dance with the right foot forward, if you prefer.)

Spread your toes wide, feeling your heel, the balls of your feet and your toes engage evenly into the mat. Place your front knee directly above your ankle, with your shin perpendicular to the mat. Keep your ankles strong and avoid rolling to the extreme outside or inside of your feet. The width of your stance will be determined by the openness in your hips and groin, so stand wide enough to create some intensity and power, but not so far apart that you lose length in your torso. Be careful to support your posture from the deep core line and avoid bracing yourself to lunge by hanging in your hip or knee ligaments. Too wide of a stance will ultimately destabilize and damage your joints.

Be careful not to reinforce dysfunctional postural habits like standing with your knees locked or hyper-extended. Do the Core SIP Breath when you are in a deep lunge to check on your infrastructure. If the breath happens easily, your stance is probably balanced. If extension and breathing are difficult when you bend the front knee, then your feet are placed too widely apart.

Many of us tend to place more pressure on the outside or inside of our foot when we walk, creating imbalances that can lead to pain and injuries in the short and long-term. These ingrained patterns can be changed at the brain level, but first one needs to be aware of their unique gait and the way they use their feet. What you can sense, you can change.

If you *pronate* (your ankle falls inward), bring your inner ankle bone towards your outer ankle to balance the foot actions. Press on your outer heel and under the mound of your big toe.

If your foot tends to *supinate* (roll outward), press on your inner heel and the ball of your foot behind the smallest toe. Observe your *samskaras*, or patterns, and begin to use these foot positions to reshape the positional patterns of your feet.

Inhale one deep SIP Breath, straightening your front leg for a moment as you focus on the lift of your arches and spinal elongation. Retain the gift of the lift as you exhale through your nose.

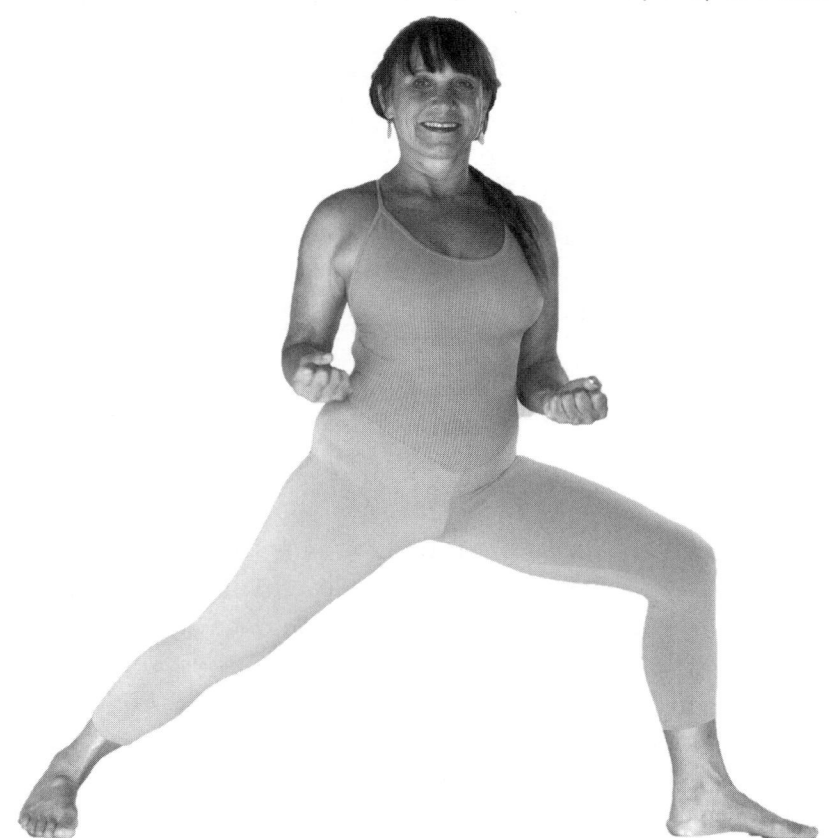

Fig. 43B

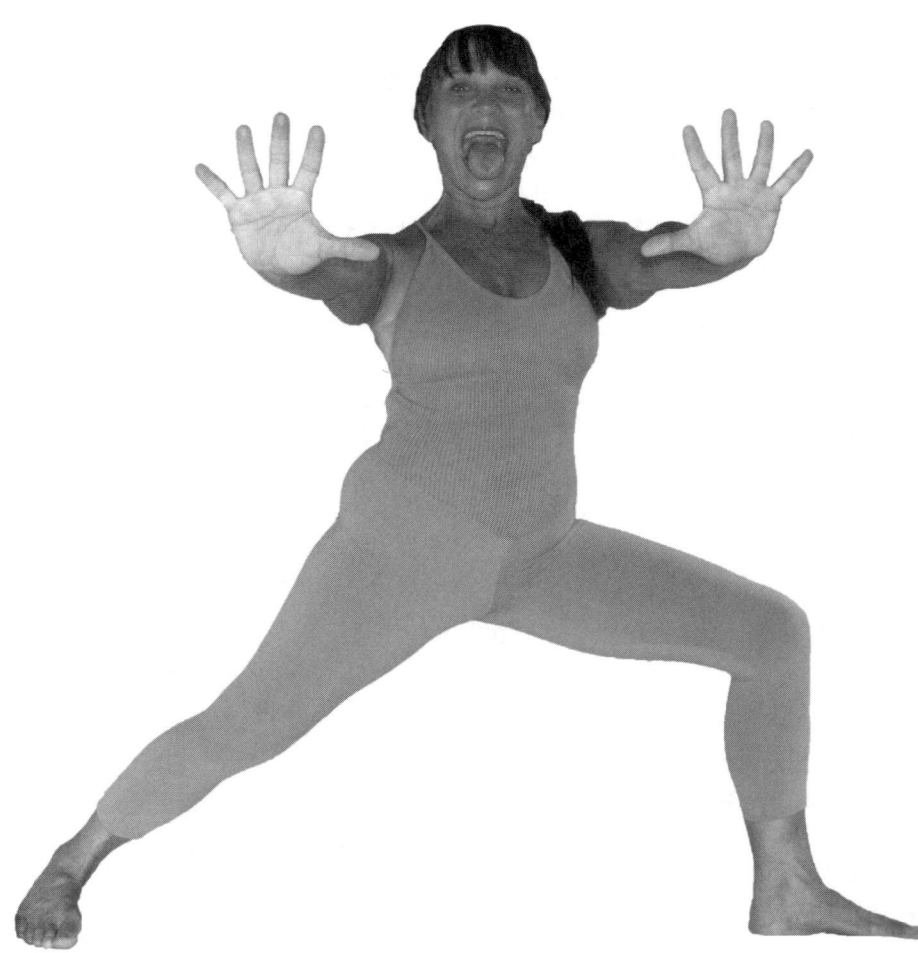

Fig. 43C – Don't be concerned about looking silly! As you exhale, open your fingers and mouth as widely as possible, while extending out your tongue.

Starting with your hands in the prayer position, inhale through your nose and lift your arms up to shoulder height. Keep your fingers wide open with your thumbs up and palms facing out, and lift your arms overhead into a Y shape. Exhale as you begin to lower your arms, bending your elbows while bringing your hands together in "Namaste" at your heart as you once again bend your front knee into a right angle. Do this movement 4 or 5 times, while breathing through your nose. Feel the fluidity of your movements as you connect your limbs back towards the center of your body. Retain lift through your arches, extension in your trunk, and natural curves in your spine. Feel the movement of breath in your entire body as you move. Add powerful affirmations on your inhaling or sustaining breath. As you inhale visualize bringing in power, love, clarity or compassion. On your cleansing or exhaling breathe, let go of any thoughts or beliefs that are not serving you in your life.

Warrior Dance, Part 2

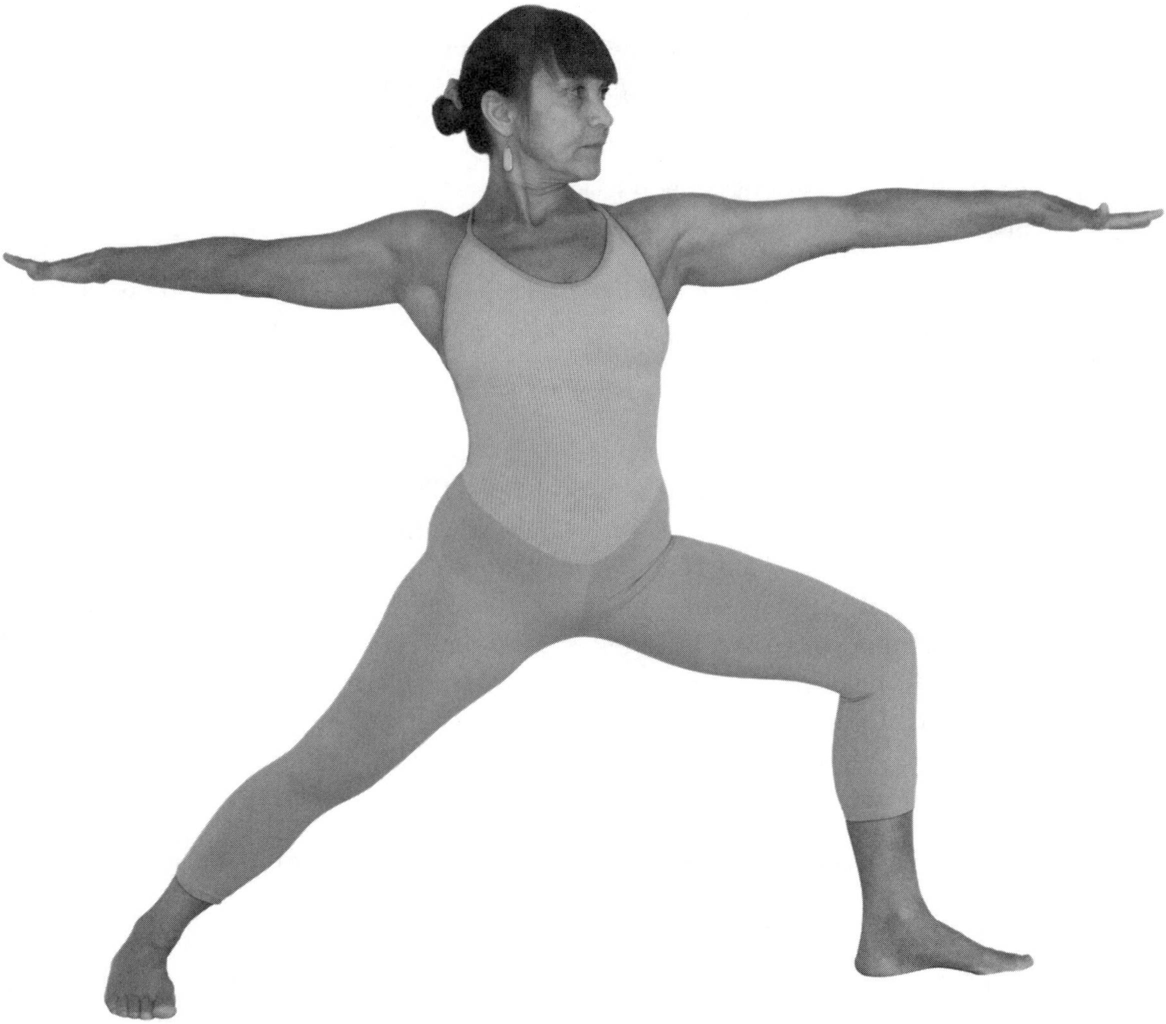

Fig. 43D

Inhale through your nose, straighten your front knee and pull your elbows alongside your waist, making fists with your hands, palms up **(Fig. 43B)**. Draw the tips of your shoulder blades gently towards your hips, opening your heart and aligning your shoulders.

As you exhale, extend your hands out in front of you, with your thumbs pointed up and your fingers spread wide, as shown in **Fig. 43C**. As you exhale, open your mouth wide, while extending your tongue as far as it will go. Say "ahhh" as you focus on the energy in the tip of your tongue.

As you do each movement, sense your body in its entirety and notice your posture and alignment as you become more present in all aspects of your breathing and body movements. Your neck is extended but relaxed, and the weight of your head rests atop the spine. Your gaze is soft and expansive. Avoid lifting the chin, looking up, or straining your eyes. Keep the neck long in the back to avoid strain in the occipital region at the base of the skull. Establish equal balance, rooting through the legs and extending through the core.

By balancing the actions of rooting and extension, you will find yourself "floating" in every pose, as though your entire body is light and spacious, or filled with helium.

Repeat the sequence, beginning with the position shown in **Fig. 43B,** four or five times, then take your arms out to the sides as shown in **Fig. 43D**, to prepare for Part 3 of the "Warrior Dance."

Warrior Dance, Part 3

From the arm position shown in **Fig. 43C**, inhale with a Core SIP Breath as you swing your arms out to the sides, looking out over your front (left) hand, as shown in **Fig. 43D**. Exhale while staying stationary in the lunge, keeping your fingers wide open, and resisting with downward pressure in your hands and feet. Maintain extension in your trunk. Initiate a SIP Breath, feeling the movements of breathing reverberating throughout your whole body. As you exhale, straighten your front knee and bring your hands shoulder-width apart, extended out in front of your chest. Do another SIP Breath as you bend your front knee, while again swinging your arms open and in line with your shoulders. This time turn your head and look out over your back (right) hand. Remain in this position for your exhale while practicing resistance with your arm and leg energy. Use the SIP Breath technique and focus on your body in its entirety. On your next exhale, straighten your front knee, and bring your hands to the front of your chest, spaced shoulder-width apart.

Turn your hands until your thumbs face up, and repeat the entire sequence of Part 3.

Warrior Dance, Part 4

PNF Variation: On the inhale, make fists of your hands and hold them out to the side for a moment. Intensify your muscle actions as you hold your breath for a moment. Looking out over your front hand, exhale and spread your hands open wide, feeling connection to your center and the release of tension in your fascial front and back arm lines.

Engage your breath with the SIP, keeping your fingers wide open and your thumbs pointed up. Exhale as you bring your arms to center, shoulder-width apart. Make your hands into fists and inhale with a SIP Breath. Now repeat Part 4, looking over your back hand instead of the front one.

After you complete this movement on each side, inhale through your nose, straighten your front knee and bring your hands to namaste at your heart center. Take a moment before you move into Position #44, "Lateral Lunge." If you feel dizzy, do not keep doing the SIP Breath; instead, breathe through your nose throughout the practice.

POSITION #44 — LATERAL LUNGE

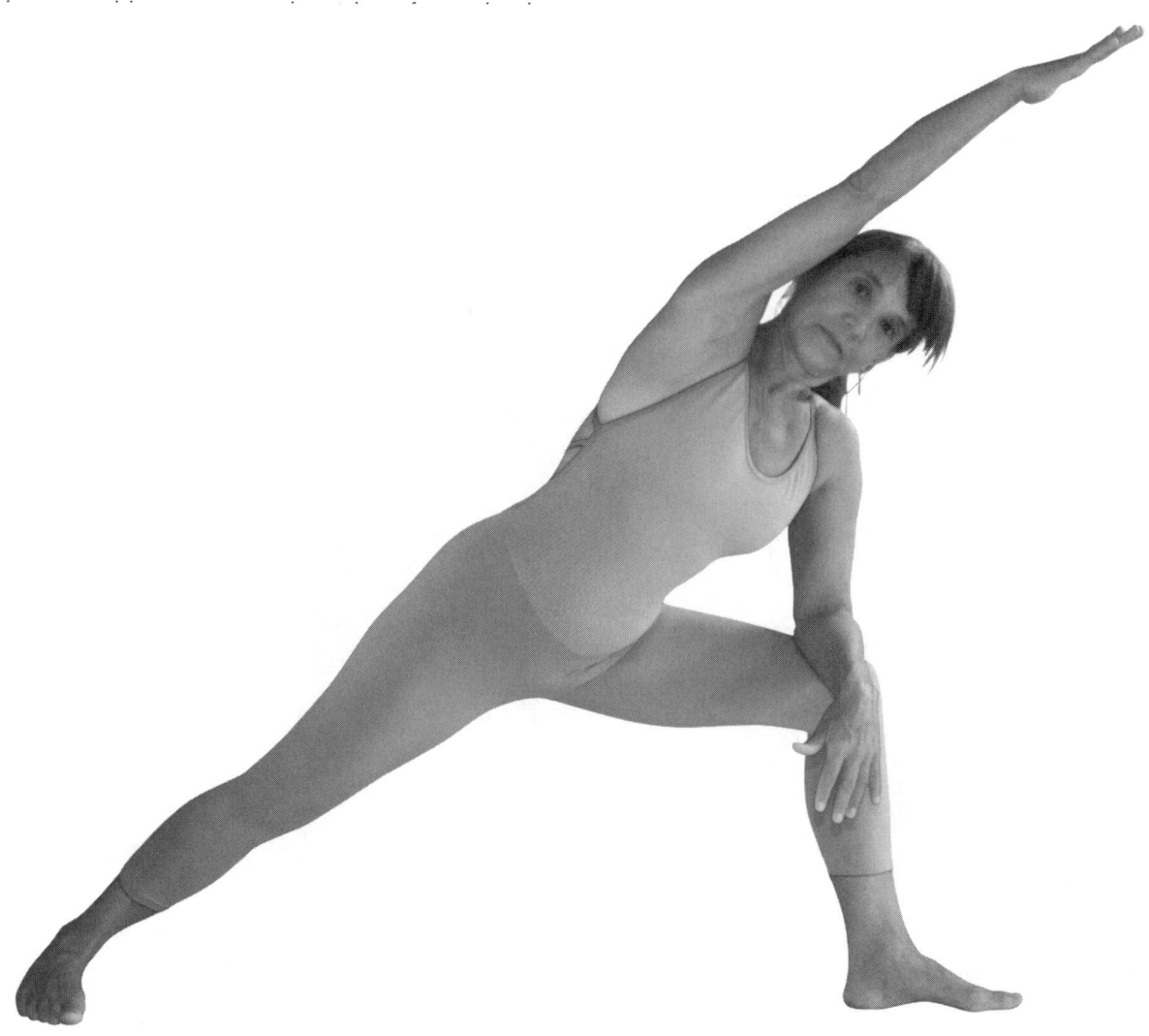

Fig. 44A

Continue the flow you started with the "Warrior Dance" and bend your front knee as you bring your forearm on the same side to rest at a right angle on your thigh. Stay grounded in your feet and extended in your spine. Balance your stance so that you feel equal weight in both legs. Inhale, and extend the opposite arm alongside your ear, reaching with wide fingertips while connecting your arm back to its foundations at the hip and breastbone. Keep both sides of your waist lengthened and your rib cage aligned with your hips as you draw the top of your inner thighs towards each other.

Never pull your arm out of the shoulder joint; instead, keep it firmly connected by drawing your arm in toward the core center of your body, engaging muscular forces that stabilize your joints. At the same time, feel how you can expand your energy outwards by radiating energy out through the fascial sheaths that surround your muscles.

For a deeper opening, slide your top hand behind your back to your thigh as shown in **Fig. 44B**. This will grant you resistance, allowing you to open your chest as you grab your thigh. (Note that the arm movement shown in **Fig. 44B** is an advanced pose, and not for everyone.)

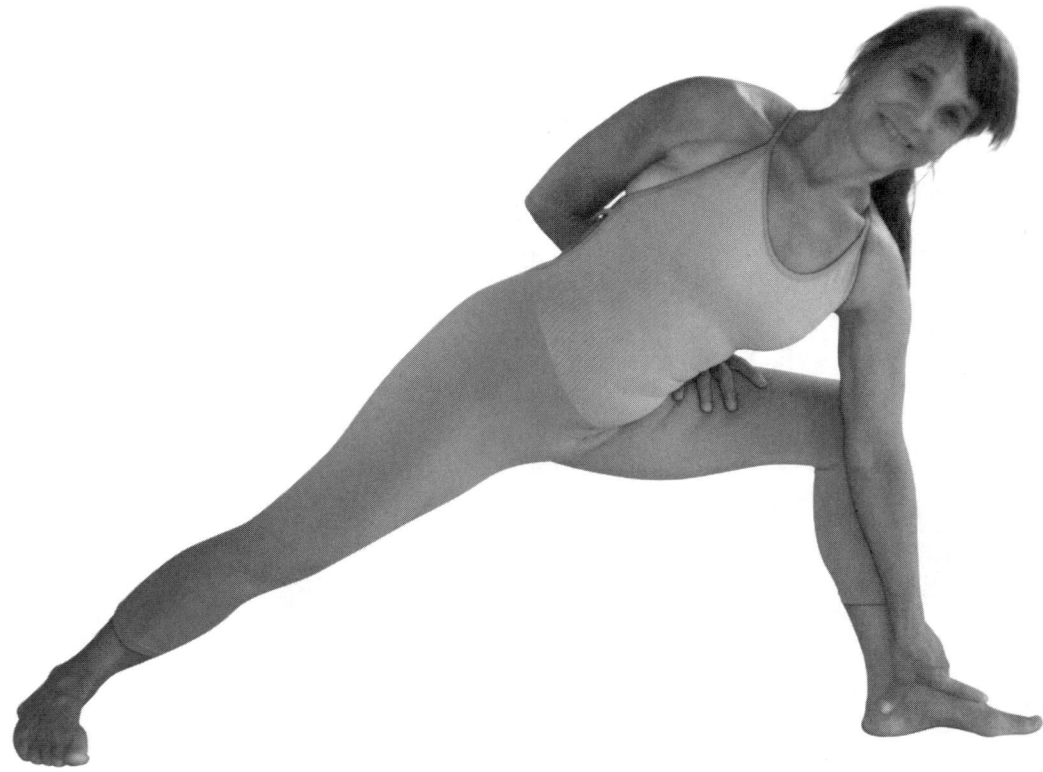

Fig. 44B

CAUTION: Make sure that as you perform this pose, you can comfortably grab your thigh. If you cannot, simply place your hand on your hip or press your palm flat on your sacrum. Focus on the opening of your chest and the downward movement of your scapula as you breathe deeply, using your rib cage muscles.

POSITION #45 — CORE TRIANGLE

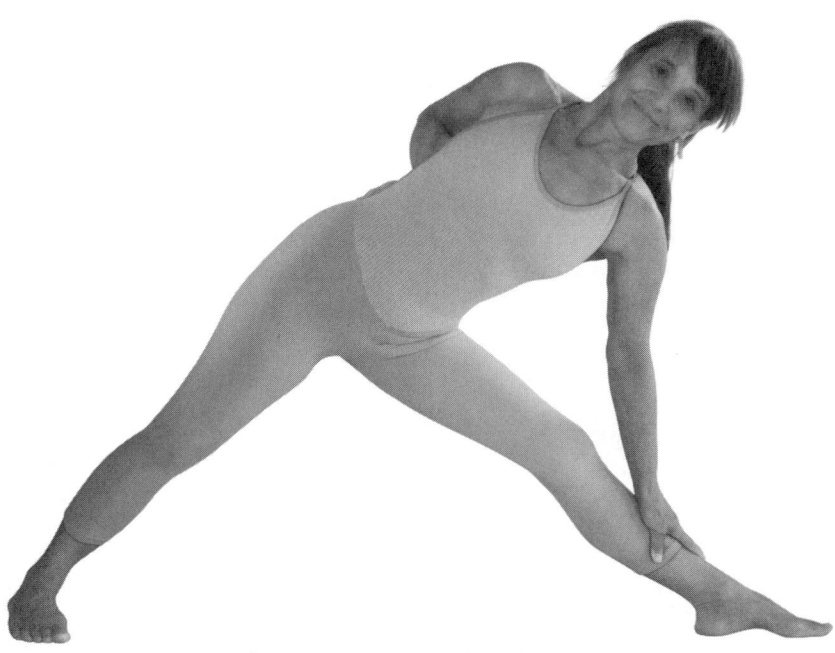

Fig. 45A – Core Triangle

From the "Lateral Lunge," you can move into the "Core Triangle." Straighten your front leg without pressing out or hyper-extending your knee joints. Slide your right hand down your leg to just below or above your knee cap, keeping your spine in its natural curves. Do not lean your trunk forward of your legs just to get down further; lower is not necessarily better for your structure. To gauge how far you should go, your head and rib cage should stay aligned with your pelvic area as it would be if you were standing well. Place your other hand on your sacrum, palm down, and draw down with the muscles that bring the shoulders and scapula away from your ears. If you cannot comfortably reach the sacral area, place your hand on your hip and practice bringing the shoulders down while keeping the spine extended. Massage the sacrum or side body for a moment, bringing blood flow and awareness to the area.

Engage your sacral tilt by pressing in and pulling up with your hand. Inhale using the SIP Breath and notice how the actions of the breath contract your core deeply, engaging the inner "ring of support" in your center. You will feel this action clearly when you do the Core SIP Breath from a sideways position such as the "Core Triangle" pose.

Once you feel supported from your center, make sure that your shoulders are aligned with each other and then bring your left arm straight up towards the ceiling. Keep your fingers wide open, and keep your shoulders moving down away from your ears while you maintain your gaze looking forward, rather than trying to look up at your hand. Practice maintaining a neutral spine in the neck and lower back region, and keep your fingers wide and radiant as you stay active in your feet, without pressing back with your knees. Lengthen both sides of your waist using breathing to support yourself from your core. Use a mirror to check your alignment.

Keep your collarbones level. Engage the lower trapezius and rhomboid muscles between your shoulder blades, ensuring that your shoulders are drawn away from your ears and are not shrugged.

Do not attempt to bring your right arm further down your leg unless you can keep your rib cage aligned with your hips. Remember that the most important part of every pose is natural spine alignment, breathing, and movement supported from your core.

Make a fist with your extended hand as though you are pulling on a rope, as shown in **Fig. 45B**. Inhale deeply, hold for a moment, and accentuate the contraction you feel in your muscles. Exhale and look up, staying in the stretch but releasing the extra muscle actions. As you look up and exhale, extend with your fingers and your tongue as seen in **Fig. 45C**.

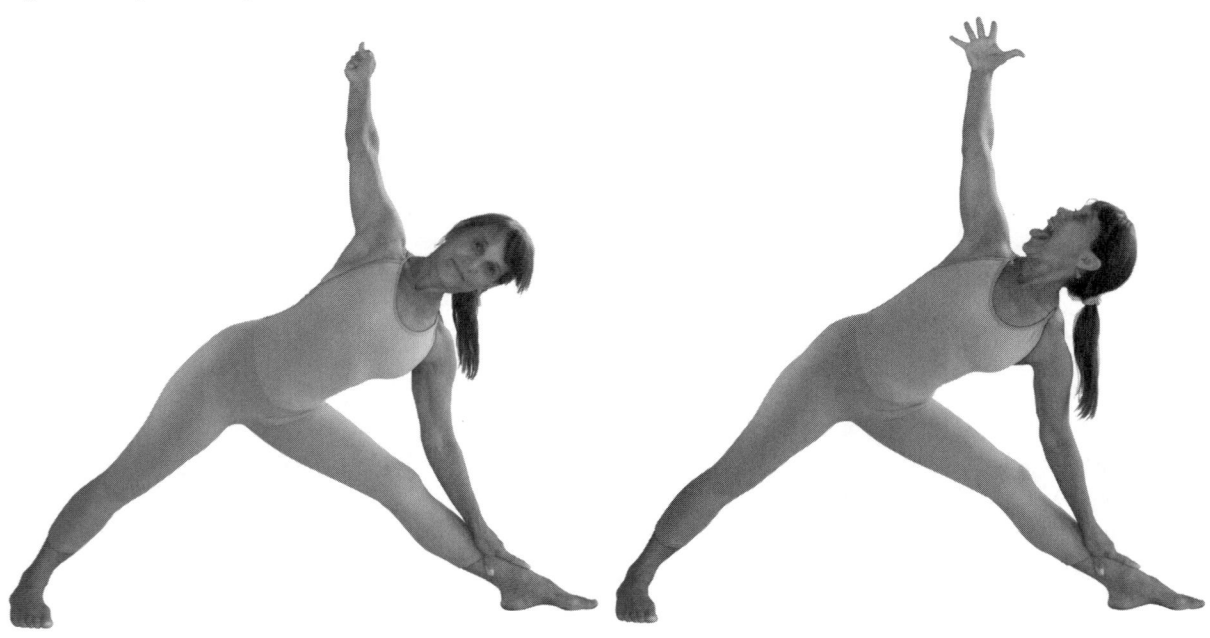

Fig. 45B   *Fig. 45C*

Repeat the "Core Triangle" several times and then go back to the previous position (#44), the "Lateral Lunge."

Keep consciously breathing as you engage your whole body in the lunge while doing several circles with you arm. Circle your arm as you inhale, coming back to a standing position and placing your hands on your hips. Notice what you are feeling, and practice being present in your breath, in your mind, and in your body.

Reverse the positions of your feet with the left foot now leading and the right foot behind. Repeat the entire sequence of Positions #43 – #45 on this other side. Be playful, have fun, and cultivate intensity and energy with these flowing movements.

Position #46 — Half Moon (Advanced)

"Half Moon" promotes confidence, will-power, and self-reliance. This posture is a full body-tuning pose that balances the fascial and muscle actions in your entire body from the inside out. This pose also gives you powerful feet, ankles, and legs while cultivating a strong connection that allows you to move from your center. You get it all by inverting, moving from your core, balancing on one leg, and overcoming fear.

"Half Moon" pose may be done immediately after the "Core Triangle," adding it to the "Warrior Dance" sequence. Or you may want to do this pose supported against a wall after you have completed "Warrior Dance" on both sides. It is recommended to use a block under the hand on the floor for safety and stability.

To come into "Half Moon" from the "Core Triangle," bend your front knee and place the fingertips of the corresponding hand on the floor (or block). Ground your standing leg and foot, being careful to avoid locking or hyper-extending your knee or collapsing in the ankle or foot. Place your back hand on your hip, lift your back leg from the floor, and come into balance using the core breath technique. If your shoulders are aligned vertically, lift your back hand from your hip and extend it towards the ceiling as though you were grabbing a strap suspended from above. Open your toes and point through the ball of your lifted foot.

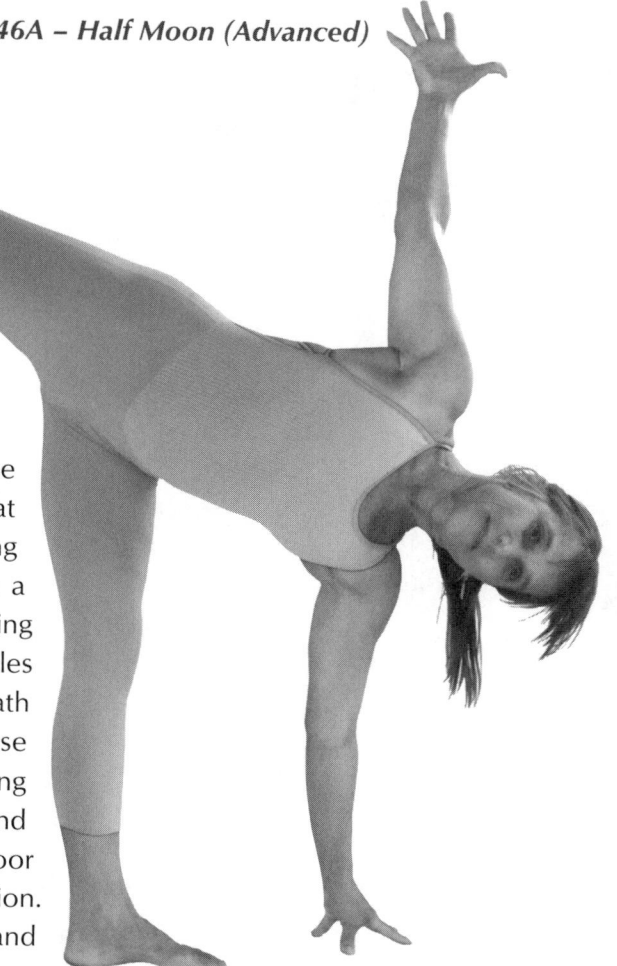

Fig. 46A – Half Moon (Advanced)

Think of the principals of natural alignment for your spine and sacrum. Pull your limbs into the center of the body at the same time that you extend from the center, radiating life force through the fascia lines. Keep your neck in a neutral position by looking straight ahead instead of trying to look up. If your neck begins to hurt, relax your muscles and look down towards the floor. Use the SIP Breath technique and let your breath inform you of how to use the forces of extension in your core. To return to standing upright, bend your standing knee, put your lifted hand on your hip and slowly bring your lifted foot to the floor while you tilt your trunk into an upright standing position. Practice coming out of the pose slowly, with precision and awareness.

Are you ready to try "Core Half Moon?" Make sure you can do "Half Moon" without putting any weight on your bottom hand. If you can do so, you are ready to try this pose. Stand next to a wall or post for extra support and safety, if needed.

From "Half Moon," slowly move your fingers from the floor, to the top of your foot or the back of your ankle. Use the SIP Breath to find the ring of support at your center as you draw your limbs into your center and radiate back from your core. Practice feeling your body in its entirety and feeling the forces of extension and grounding holding you in balance. You should feel grounded, yet floating at the same time. Look through both eyes evenly with a soft gaze. Release any unnecessary tension in the your body, relaxing the toes, neck, and face. Find a place of "effortless effort."

Come out of the pose by bending your standing leg and bringing your raised leg down to the floor. Stand with feet hip distance apart and shake your legs to release any tension. Repeat on the other side.

Fig. 46B – Core Half Moon (Very advanced)

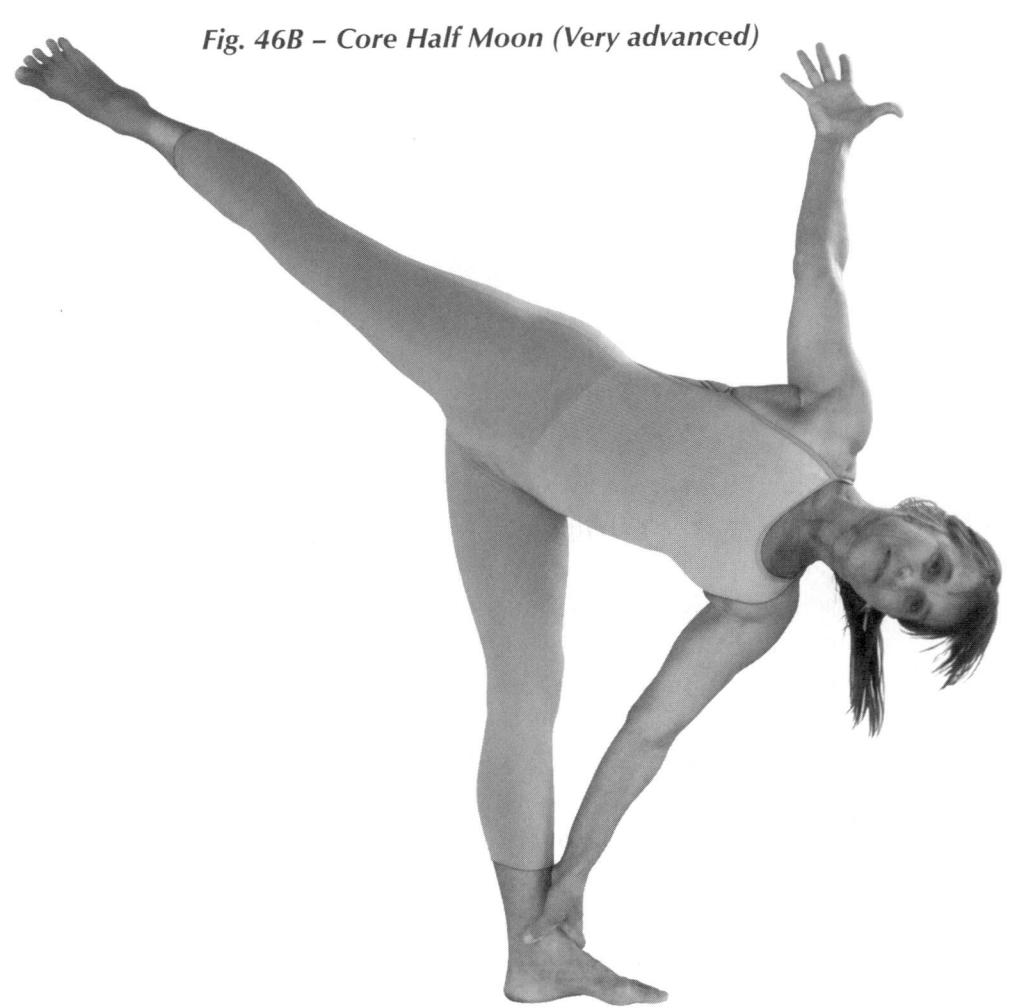

POSITION #47 — POWER LUNGE

This pose activates your deep core and awakens the connection between the psoas and the diaphragm. Done properly, it will balance tensile forces and muscle actions among your spine, hips, and groin. Your psoas is a breathing muscle, spine stabilizer, hip flexor, a shelf for your organs, and a receptacle for your emotions. Learning to activate and consciously use this muscle will greatly enhance the quality and power of your life.

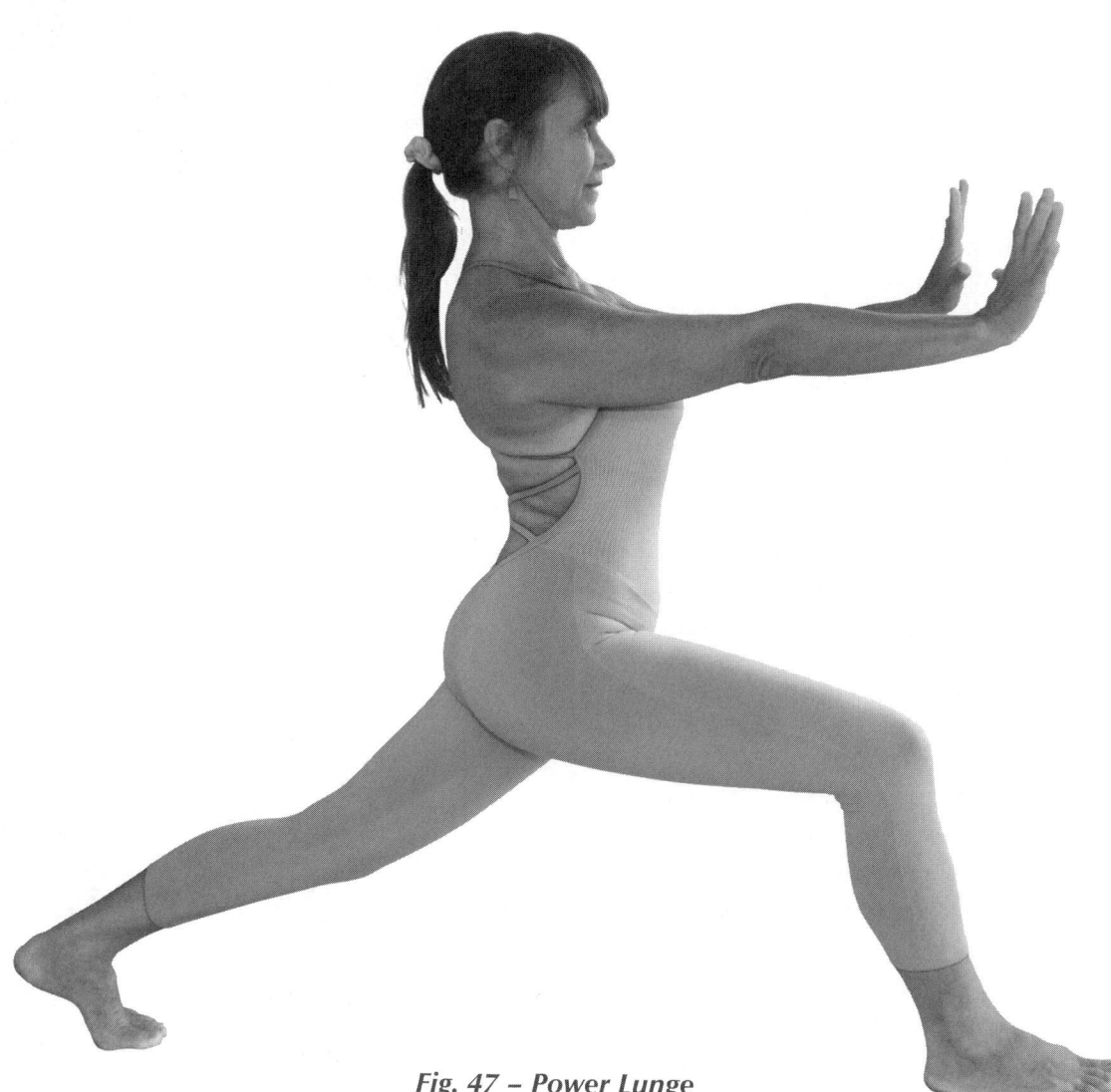

Fig. 47 – Power Lunge

Come into a lunge with your right foot forward, and your left foot back, as shown in **Fig. 47**. Lift your back heel and balance on the ball of your foot, but continue pressing evenly through your back heel. If you need help balancing, push against a wall or post, sliding your front foot so that your toes meet the wall.

Targeting the Psoas Muscle Group

One foot is now forward and the other one is back, in a wide and stable stance approximately shoulder-width apart. Your front knee should be positioned over your ankle, as you press into both feet. Maintain the curve in your lower back, a lift to your sacrum, and a slight bend in your back knee as though you were running. Avoid locking the back knee, as this puts pressure on the sacrum, flattens the lower back, and constricts the movements of breathing.

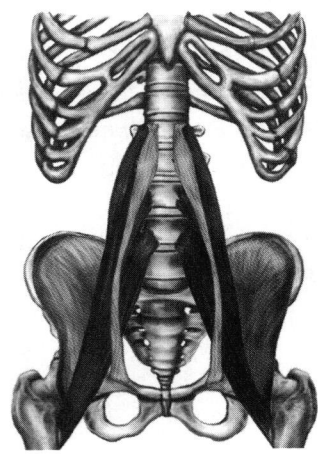

Do a SIP Breath, activating from your core and sensing the inner ring of support that brings extension. Keep your hips level and spiral your inner back thigh up towards the ceiling. Bring your hands up as though you are pushing against a wall with your shoulders pulling away from your ears and drawing your scapula down. Slightly bent elbows are OK in this pose.

Take a SIP Breath, and feel how the movements of breathing engage the psoas in the groin and inner-back thigh area of your back leg. The entire femoral triangle and groin area is being stretched and toned, deepening connections through your core and functional lines. This lunge, combined with core breathing, engages the psoas in an eccentric muscle contraction, in which it actually lengthens as it contracts.

Spread your toes, be active in your feet and hands and lightly firm your buttock muscles. Balance your front and back ribs over your hips. Feel your psoas/diaphragm connection activating your core for inner support. Be strong and light, with your head balancing effortlessly atop your spine while sensing the roots of your legs at your diaphragm/psoas connection.

Working the Functional Fascia Lines

Still in the lunge position, inhale, reaching up with your arms shoulder-width apart, and your palms facing each other. Generate movement from your center with the breath. Exhale, and circle your arms behind you (palms down) with your fingers spread wide. Now inhale, circling the arms forward and up, and then hold the breath as you make fists and tighten all of the muscles in your body that you can feel. Hold for a few seconds and then exhale, keeping your arms up, your shoulders dropped and your fingers and mouth extended wide open. Repeat this circling movement for several breaths and then place your hands on your hips to prepare for "Twisting Lunge to Half Split."

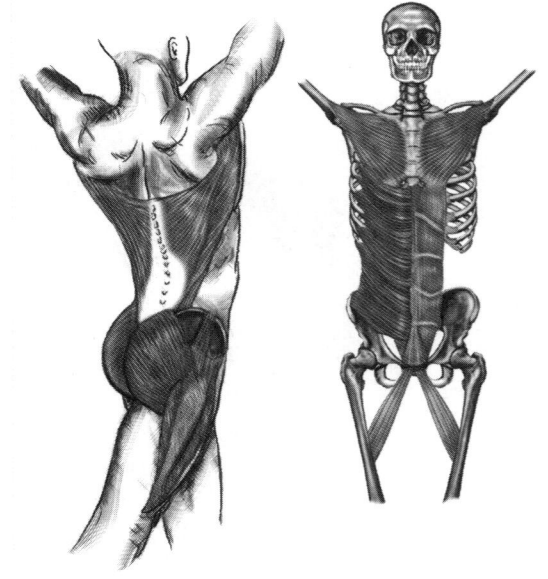

POSITION #48 — TWISTING LUNGE TO HALF SPLIT (ADVANCED)

"Twisting Lunge" gives you strong and flexible legs and trunk muscles. Core lateral strength is enhanced, enabling you to excel at sports that require balancing and twisting movements. Having flexibility and stability from the legs to the core protects you from injures and corrects misalignments that can inhibit fluid movement.

Begin in the "Power Lunge" (Position #47) from the previous pages. With your hands on your hips and your feet active, begin to twist toward the leg that is in front of you.

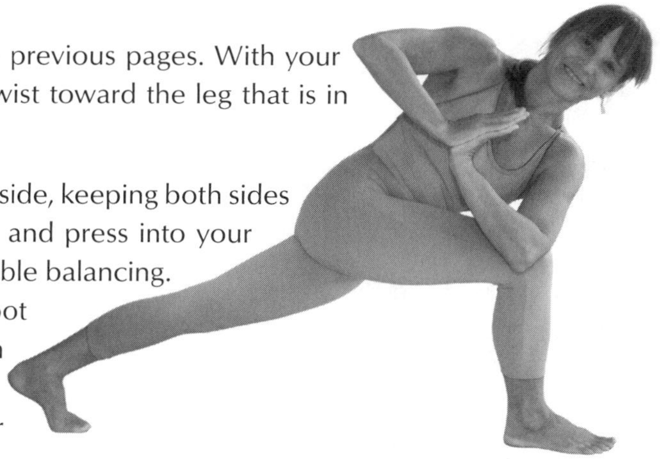

Inhale as you twist towards the right or the bent knee side, keeping both sides of your waist long. Maintain your lower back curve and press into your feet. Bring your left foot further back if you have trouble balancing. Lift your back heel and press into the ball of your foot with toes spread and active. Twist as far as you can staying upright in the trunk retaining the shape of standing well. Begin to lean forward and bring your hands together in namaste. Spiral your back thigh inward and up towards the ceiling. Breathe from

Fig. 48A – Twisting Lunge to Half Split

your center and notice the connections from your core out to your limbs. Keep your sacrum level in its natural uplifting tilt. Take your left elbow to the outside of your right knee as shown in **Fig. 48A** or extend one arm towards the floor and one towards the ceiling, as in **Fig. 48C**. Use the pressing of your arms against your leg to create more traction and practice keeping the length of the core body

Breathe into the pose and hold for a moment, contracting the engaged muscles more. As you exhale, release the added extra tension but retain the twisting action. Stay for several breaths, accentuating muscle contraction and then releasing to a deeper twist. Inhale, and with hands on your hips, come back to center. Jump or step your feet to the "Power Lunge" position on your opposite side, and repeat the sequence.

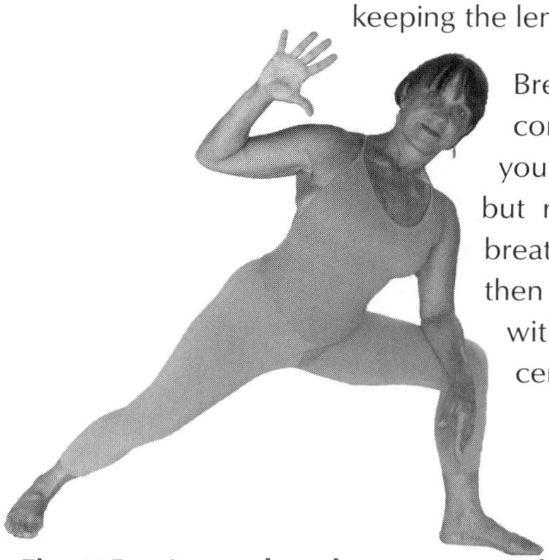

Fig. 48B – Act as though you are pressing your hands against a wall to stabilize your scapula and strengthen the muscles of your mid back.

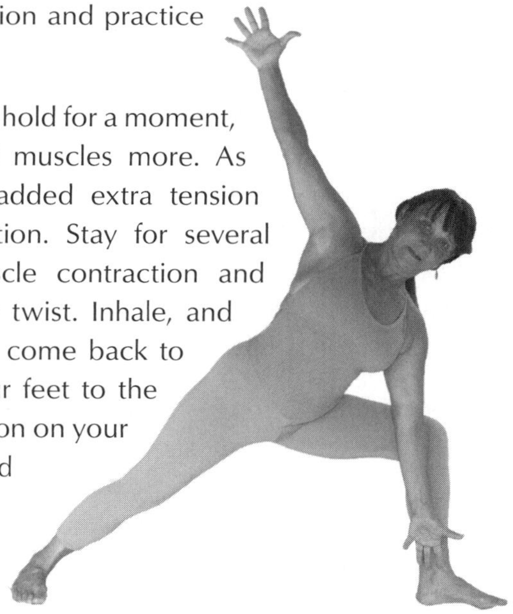

Fig. 48C – Arm variation for core strength.

POSITION #49 — HALF SPLIT

Many of us do yoga and fitness poses with unnatural spine alignment, overloading our back muscles and placing dangerous pressure on our discs. The "Half Split" is self-applied physical therapy to keep your discs healthy and back muscles tuned and toned. The "Half Split" pose actively balances tensile forces along the entire back fascia line, which runs from your eyebrows over the top of your skull, then down both sides of your spine to the bottom of your feet. Using PNF techniques in the "Half Split," you can recode muscle tension in your hamstrings and free your fascia all along the superficial back line while keeping the front body extended and supported. This allows you to move through your daily life with a core connection and a balanced fascia web of support, which serve as a warranty against injury to your spine.

From the "Power Lunge," drop your back knee to the floor and shift your hips back over the back leg, keeping a bend in your front knee. (**Note:** If your upper back is rounding and your front body shortens, put your hands on blocks to create more height, which will allow for proper spinal alignment.) Extend through the ball of your front foot using the floint position. Take a SIP Breath and hold,

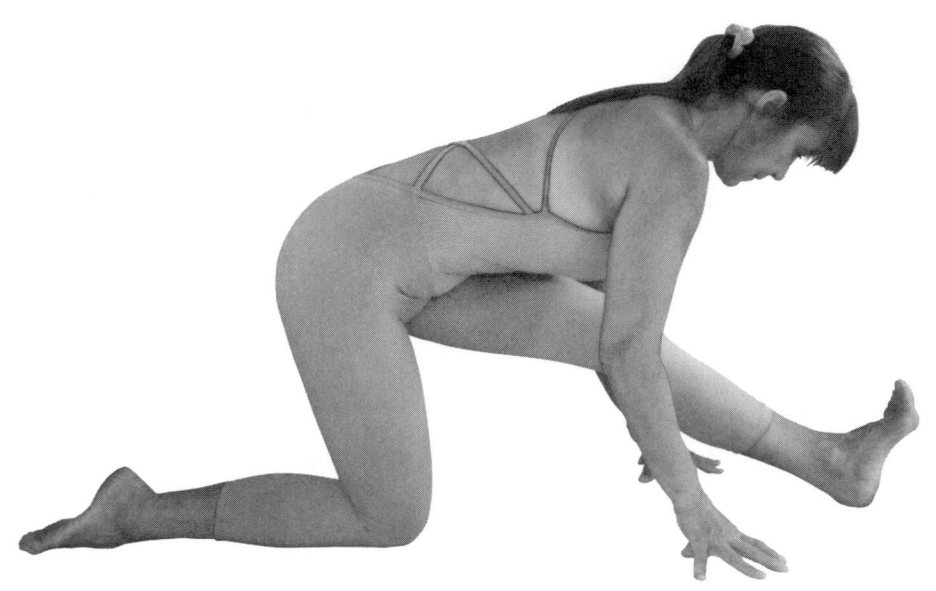

Fig. 49 – Half Split

while adding extra contraction to the hamstrings. After 5 to 10 seconds, release the extra tension but stay in the stretch as you lengthen from your core.

It is important that you keep your front knee slightly bent. If you straighten this leg, you will compress your back or overstretch your sacral ligaments. Remember that your psoas muscles attach from your inner leg up to your spine and diaphragm, and your fascia lines connect your leg muscles all the way up the back, over your skull, and to your eyebrows. You will feel strong hamstring engagement even with a bent knee, especially if you combine this move with core breathing and PNF recoding.

Stay in the "Half Split" as you shift your hips side-to-side, feeling the stretch in your gluteals and down your outer leg. Begin to shift your weight back to center in preparation for the next position.

Position #50 — Runners Lunge and Psoas Lunge

The "Runners Lunge" (Fig. 50A) develops deep core strength as it tones your legs, hips, toes and feet. Posture is greatly improved by the regular practice of the Runners and Psoas Lunges. (Fig. 50B).

To do the the "Runners Lunge," place 2 yoga blocks on the right side at the front of your mat. Get on your hands and knees and then bring your left foot forward (in line with the blocks) to step into the lunge. Position yourself in front of a mirror to observe your alignment and make sure that you are not lifting your chin or rounding your upper back. Be careful to use muscle energy and to avoid hanging in your sacral or shoulder ligaments. Your spine should be in good standing posture and your head should be aligned with the rest of your body. Lift and spread the toes of your left foot and then place them back on the mat retaining the lift of your arch. Balance on the ball of your right foot with your toes spread wide. Use the SIP Breath to align and engage your core, and then

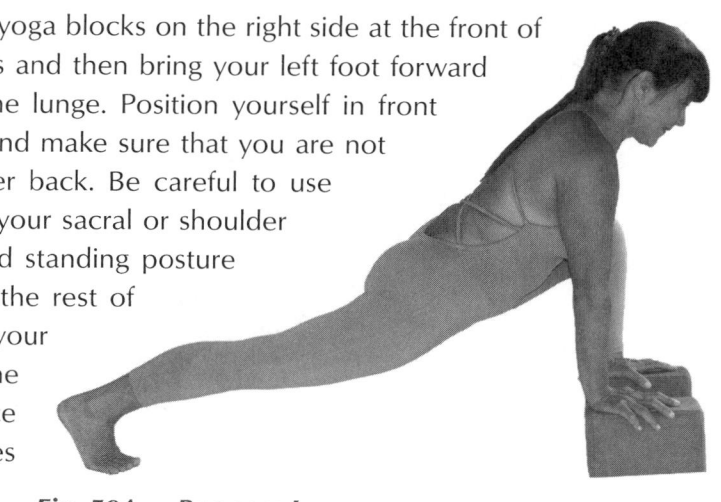

Fig. 50A — Runners Lunge

practice staying in the lift as you switch to breathing through your nostrils. Pay attention to the movements of breathing and how they affect your entire body. Stay in the pose for several breaths and then lower your right knee to the floor and proceed to the "Psoas Lunge."

The "Psoas Lunge" stretches the entire superficial front line and tones the deep core breathing line. This pose helps reduce headaches and pain in the jaw, back, and neck caused by poor postural patterning and fascial imbalance. Many people who feel tight in the hamstrings will gain a lot of relief by stretching the deep groin or "femoral triangle" that is targeted in the "Psoas Lunge."

Most hanstrings are tense, not tight

Oftentimes the tension and stiffness one feels in the hamstrings is simply an automatic contraction response by the muscles, put into effect to counteract the forces of tightness in the groin or front body. If the hamstrings or back feels tight, STRETCH YOUR FRONT!

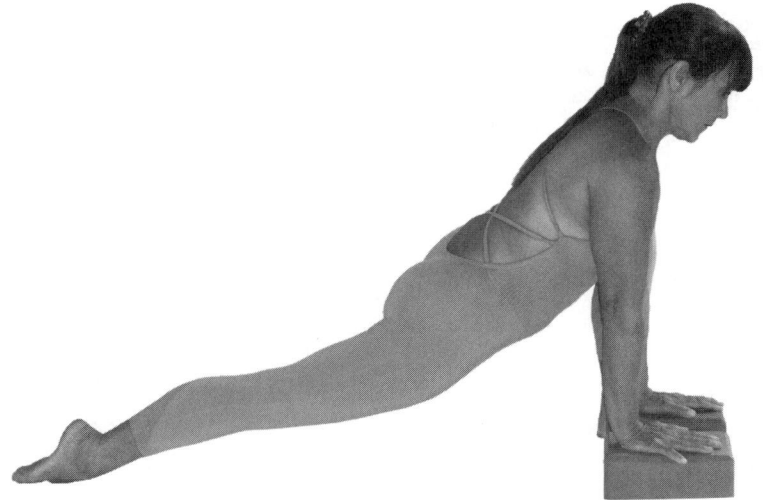

Fig. 50B – Psoas Lunge

Pay attention to your alignment.

If you have a front line that is strung tight, or if you have misaligned ribs, you may be suffering from back pain and nerve impingement caused by lumbar/sacral compression. Pay attention to your rib-to-hip alignment and also to the distance between your back ribs and your hips; a shortening in this area can cause sacral imbalance, leading to lower-back pain from nerve/disc impingement.

Your rib cage is like an upside down bucket. Tipping your ribs up in the front brings your rib cage (the bucket) lower in the back. The bottom of the entire rib cage needs to be level and aligned above your hips to be in natural alignment. Use core breathing to initiate spine elongation and functional rib cage alignment. The descent of your diaphragm on inhalation will align your ribs through the connection of the diaphragm to the entire inner surface of the ribs. There is an especially strong fascial connection on the bottom of your breastbone called the xyphoid process which helps to keep the ribs from popping out of position above the hips. Do a SIP Breath and feel how your rib cage aligns above your hips by way of the dynamic tensile forces of breathing. Ribs need to float and be free; the simple movements of deep breathing can and will keep them aligned from the inside out.

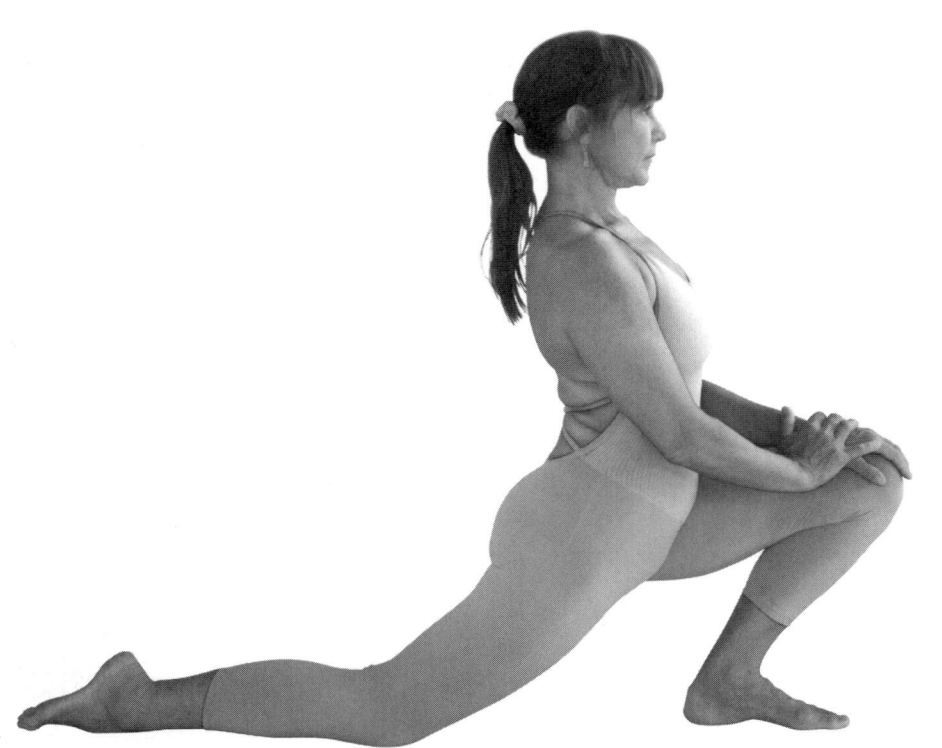

Fig. 50C – Upright Psoas Lunge

From your hands and knees, bring your right or left foot forward as in **Fig. 50A**. Shift your weight to center and place both hands on the forward thigh. Take a deep breath and lean forward, lifting through your trunk and keeping your head aligned with your spine. Press the top of your back foot towards the floor and continue to lengthen the spine using core breathing.

Breathe in and imagine a lengthening of your psoas and the whole front of your body.

Essential YogAlign Poses

You can add arm movement by lifting your arms alongside your ears or slightly in front of your head, always keeping them at least shoulder-width apart. Breathe in, retain, and make fists with your hands while squeezing your arm muscles. Then exhale deeply, open your fingers and press your back foot to the floor, elongating your spine upwards. Engage the muscles of your raised arms back toward your core, pulling them deeply into the socket. Feel your arms connected to the center of your body through your fascia lines. Feel the connections all the way from the toes and fingers to your core breathing process.

To advance the pose further, lift the back knee from the floor as shown in **Fig. 50D**. If you feel any pain at all, keep your back knee down on the floor. If you do lift your knee, press down on the top of your back foot as you do deep core breathing. Notice the fascia connection beginning at the head and continuing through the diaphragm/psoas and all the way down the thigh to the top of your foot.

As you do the "Psoas Lunge," align your rib cage with breathing and make sure that you are not sticking your chest out too far and over-lifting your front ribs. Keep your lower back and waist lengthened throughout the pose.

Keep it simple and let your breath align you from the inside out.

Repeat this entire pose with your legs reversed.

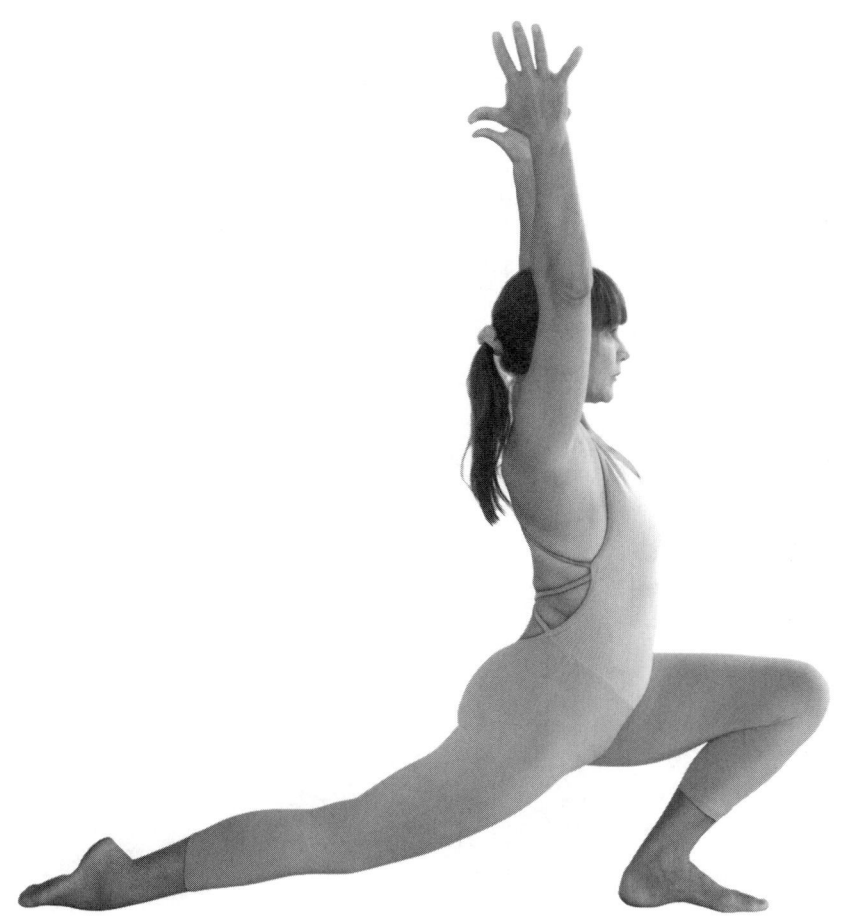

Fig. 50D – Psoas Lunge with lifted back knee.

POSITION #51 — WHOLE BODY RECALIBRATOR (ADVANCED)

This position provides an expansive tuning and balancing of your entire fascial web. Chronic foot, hip, and sacroiliac joint pain are relieved as your hips align and balance. Short leg syndrome and the pain associated with scoliosis are oftentimes alleviated by regular practice of this pose. Although this pose is considered advanced, almost everyone can do it with the aid of blocks, which will keep them safe and comfortable. This is a pose that transforms you quickly, helping you develop new neural pathways that rewire your body, allowing you to move like a kid again. The "Recalibrator" is "one-stop shopping"—effectively tuning, toning and balancing your entire being and your major fascial forces from the inside out. It's all available here.

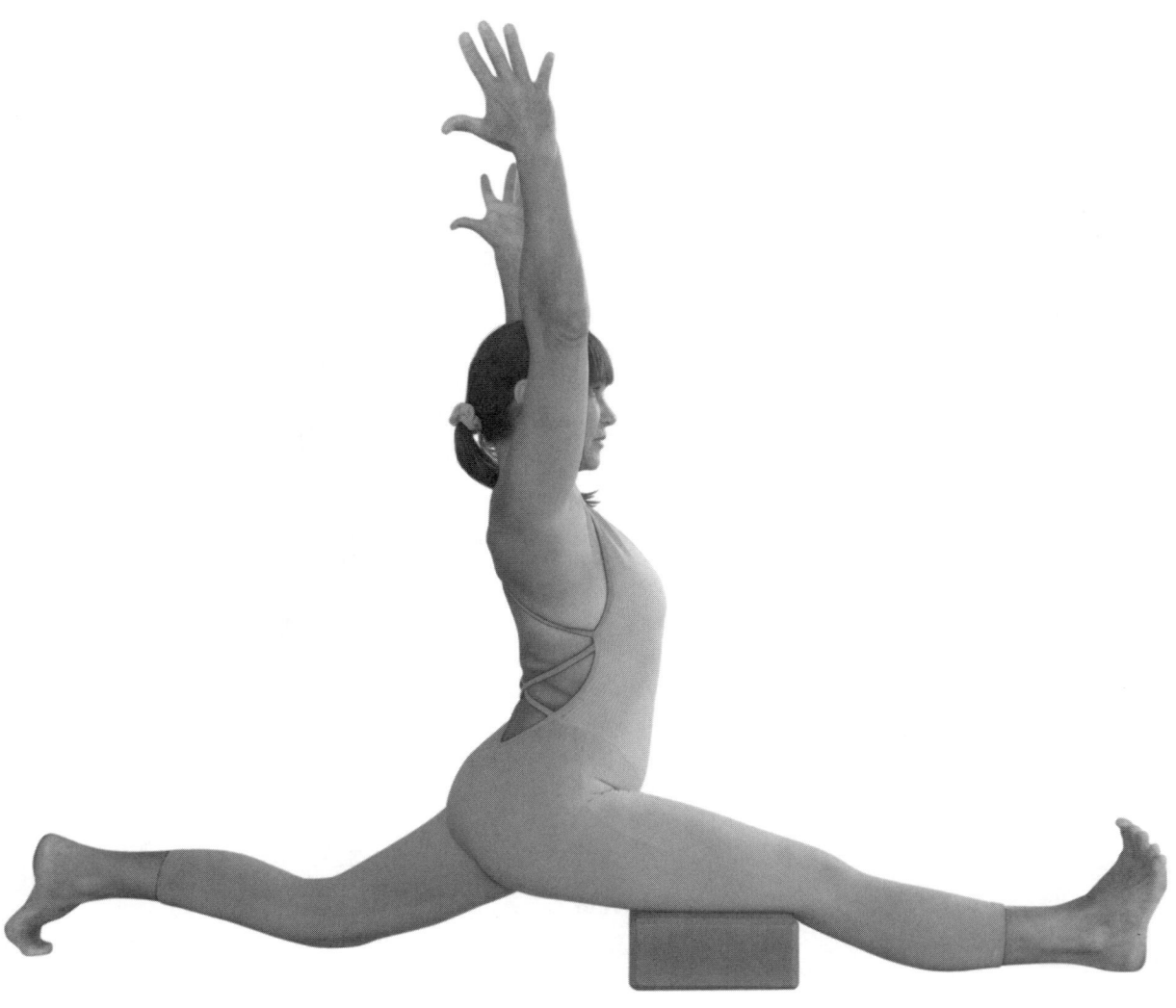

Fig. 51A – Tune your whole body at once with the Recalibrator.

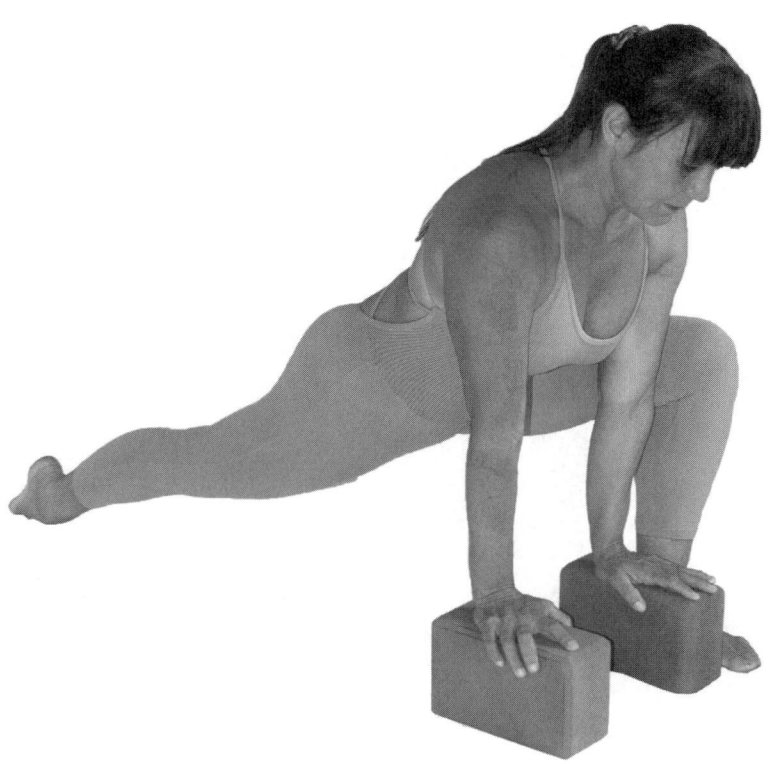

Fig. 51B – Psoas Lunge

Start from the "Psoas Lunge" with your left leg back if you are right handed and your right leg in back if you are left handed as shown in Fig. 51B. Your dominant side will be tighter so starting with the more flexible leg in the back will help you do the pose with more comfort. Keep the top of your back foot pressing down to the mat. If you are tall, place your hands on the floor or use blocks under your hands. Begin to move your front foot carefully forward, spreading your toes, and reaching through the ball of your foot in the flointing position. If your hamstring feels strained, keep your front knee in a bent position, but always stay active in the toes and ball of your foot.

Keep the deep lunge in the back leg and press your back foot firmly into the mat. When you reach the point where you can go no further with the front leg, support yourself with blocks under your front thigh near your sit bones. Keep a bend in your front knee if you feel tension, and focus on keeping length in the neck and waist and the curve in your lower back. Keep your hips level and squared, bringing the hip of your back leg level to the hip in the front leg. Stay active in both feet and hands at all times.

Inhale using the SIP Breath, finding your inner alignment and placing your hands on your hips. Can you balance comfortably while practicing core breathing and extension? If not, add another block under your leg, or stay low and keep your hands on blocks.

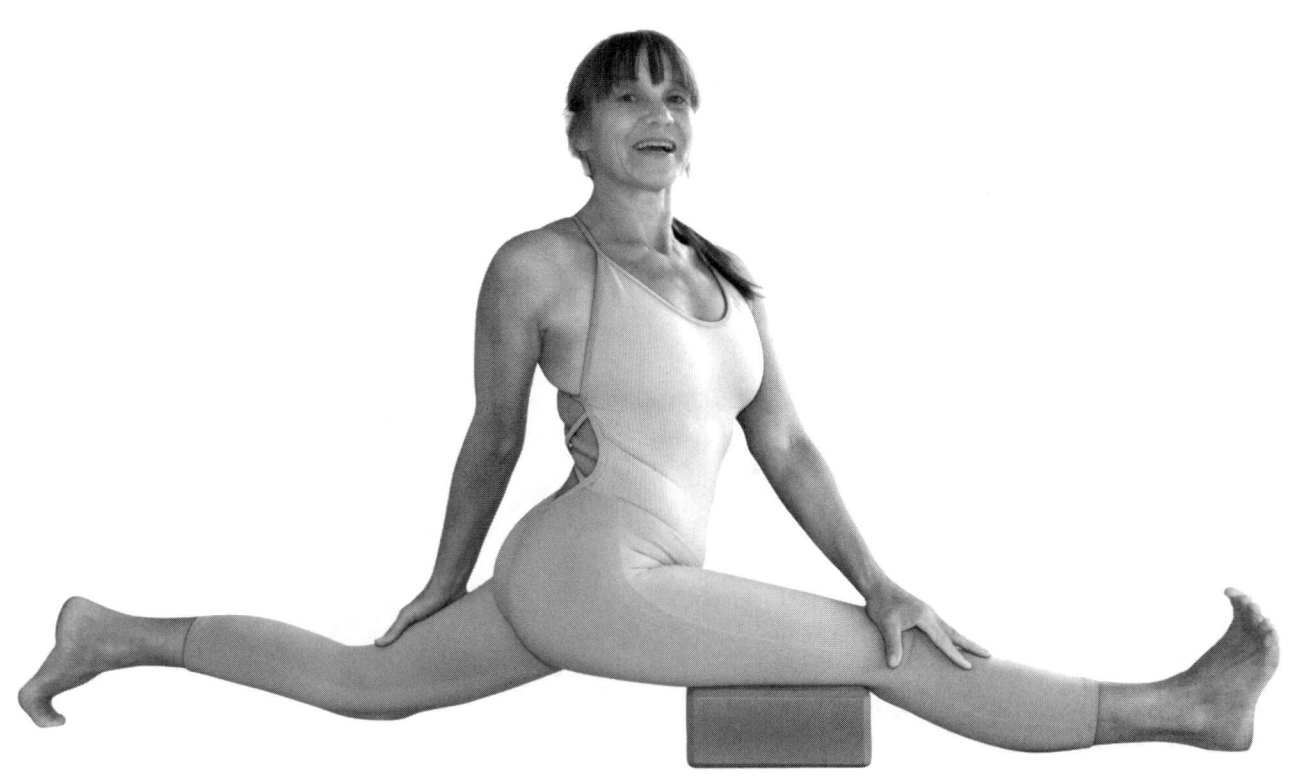

Fig. 51C – Twister

Notice the engagement of the muscles through the groin and psoas of the back leg. This action will be accentuated when you do the Core SIP Breath. If you mostly feel the action in your front leg, bend your front knee. With your hands still on your hips, squeeze the tops of your inner thighs together. Hold your breath and tighten where you feel muscle actions. Exhale and release the extra tension, but stay long in your trunk, keeping the "gift of the lift." If you feel comfortable and balanced, inhale and bring your arms up overhead. Make fists and imagine that you are pulling on straps that hang from above. As you exhale, open your fingers and mouth wide, and practice pulling in with your limbs as you radiate energy from your center.

On your next inhale, tighten all of your muscles, but this time bring special attention to your pelvic floor area. Squeeze tightly as though you are trying not to pee and exaggerate all muscle actions. Exhale with open mouth and extended tongue, and reach with open fingers. Draw your limbs in towards the center as you extend out energetically along your fascial lines. Sense and engage your body in its entirety. Come out of the pose if you feel any discomfort; otherwise you can begin to go into a twist.

Twister Variation

To add a twist **(Fig. 51C)**, first inhale, causing extension into your waist. Retain the lift as you exhale and twist to the right, placing your left hand on the outside of your right leg. Bring your right palm up to your sacrum. Inhale and then hold your breath for a moment as you stay in the twist. Notice the muscles that activate when twisting, and accentuate those actions. As you exhale, release the extra tension, making an effort to extend your body up as you consciously exhale. Remember at all times to stay grounded in your feet, keeping your toes spread and your feet active and alive.

Still in the twist, reach up with your right hand, as though pulling on a strap, and make a fist. Inhale, hold for a moment, and then exhale with open mouth and hand wide open. Keep your hips level and feet active. Come back to center. Lean forward with your hands on the floor, lengthening your spine.

Come out of the pose by coming on to your hands and knees for a moment.

Go back into the "Psoas Lunge" (Position #50) with your opposite leg now forward. Repeat the pose on this side.

After doing the "Recalibrator" on both sides, do a "Full Body Stretch" **(Fig. 51D)** noticing the openness in the front body and the deep core. Sense the change that has occurred, especially in the groin area, or femoral triangle, of the back leg.

Close your eyes, take a deep breath and notice how you feel. Try a few "Spinal Rolls," come up to standing and walk around noticing how it feels to be in your body as you move. After doing this pose, people oftentimes feel the kid body emerging.

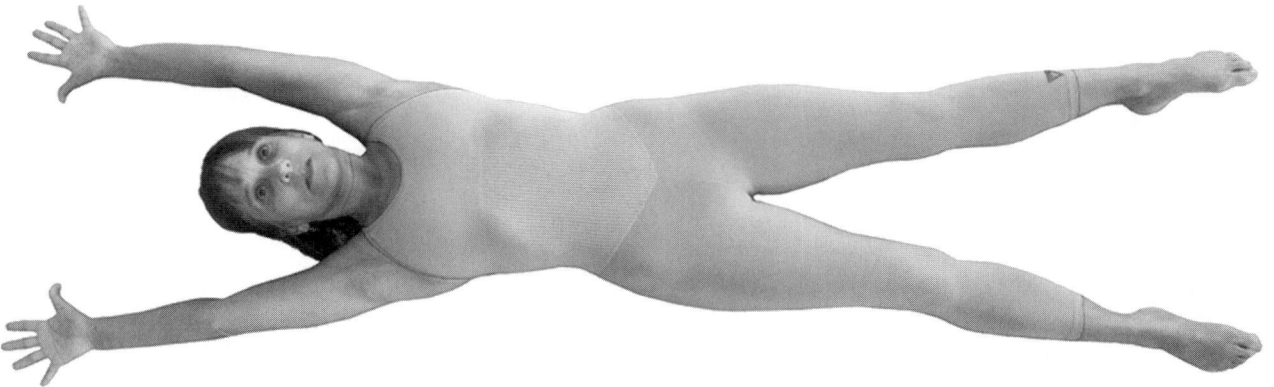

Fig. 51D – Full Body Stretch (Position #1)

Position #52 — Quad Recalibrator

This pose will get you dancing. "Quad Recalibrator" recodes chronic patterns of tightness in your front body, especially in the sensitive area from your femoral triangle (groin area) to the top of your feet. Balancing tensile forces in the superficial front line corrects the postural dysfunction of carrying the head too-far forward of the spine. This forward head carriage is prevalent in our culture, and is the main cause of upper back and neck aches. Years of forward head-carriage causes shoulder and arm pain, headaches, and eventually kyphosis (excessively rounded upper back). Deeply stretching the groin area will also help to take pressure off of the leg muscles and the hamstring area.

This pose is also excellent therapy for healing poor knee tracking resulting from tightness in the quadriceps, psoas, and groin. Hip imbalances, short-leg syndrome, low back pain, flat feet, plantar fasciitis, and shoulder pain are also alleviated when this pose is practiced with regularity.

Fig. 52A – Quad Recalibrator, forward

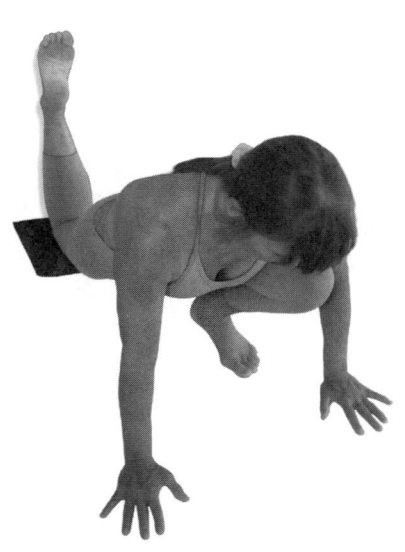

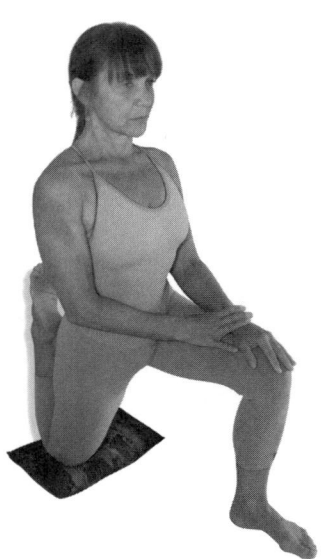

Fig. 52B – Quad Recalibrator, upright

CAUTION: If you have chronic knee pain or have had a knee replacement or surgery, you may need to skip this pose. If you are unable to point your foot well, this pose may be uncomfortable to your ankle joint. You may want to keep practicing the previous "Psoas Lunge" until your ankle becomes more flexible. We do not get comfortable by being uncomfortable and we do not get out of pain by being in pain.

Begin the pose in front of a wall, on your hands and knees with your palms down. The wall should be behind you. Place a pillow near the wall, and slide your right knee onto the pillow, with the top of your foot against the wall in a pointing position. Slide a small pillow or towel behind the foot going up the wall if there is pain in the top of your foot.

Use blocks under your hands if you cannot lean forward without rounding your upper back. Take a Core SIP Breath as you begin to lean forward while pressing your back thigh towards the floor and pushing into the top of your back foot, as in **Fig. 52A**. Keep your spine in natural alignment as you take a deep breath, holding and accentuating the action of your thigh muscles for a few seconds. Focus on feeling the pull of the entire superficial front line of fascia. Exhale and release tension as you deepen the stretch of your thighs. Practice contracting the muscles that feel tight several times, then bring your hands to your front knee and bring your trunk to an upright position as shown in **Fig. 52B**.

As you come up, make sure that your left shin is directly above your ankle and perpendicular to the floor. How close you put your right knee towards the wall is going to determine the intensity of the pose, so find an edge where you feel some intensity but nothing that you could label as pain or strain.

Bring your trunk upright, with your rib-cage aligned above your hips and your hands on your left thigh. Bring your left sit bone towards your inner left thigh, keeping your trunk elongated and your hips level. If you are feeling too much intensity or any pain, come down and slide your knee away from the wall a few inches. If you are not feeling much stretch, then slide your knee closer to the wall, creating more intensity.

Now take a breath, and hold it while tightening and engaging your thigh muscles. Practice tightening into what feels tight. As you exhale, release the extra tension but stay in the action of the pose. Keep the length of your trunk as you press down with your feet, and square and level your hips. Imagine you are drawing your front foot back, without actually moving it.

Usually you will feel your muscles lengthen with that first hold. At this time you can do two or three more PNF contraction exercises. After the first or second contract/release, if you want to feel more intensity, carefully slide your knee closer to the wall. After you finish with the right side, repeat the entire procedure on the other side.

Note: You may notice that one of your thighs feels tighter than the other. Because humans have a dominant hand, we are stronger and more contracted on that dominant side: right-handed = strong and tighter right thigh; left handed = strong and tighter left thigh. Tight thigh and psoas muscle-attachments pull your hips forward, putting tremendous strain on your pelvis, the lumbar spine, and the hamstring muscles. This leaves them chronically sore and tight. Practice the "Quad Recalibrator" and you will relieve chronic low back pain and restore fluid movement in your legs, feet, hips, and knees.

THE SPINE ALIGNER SERIES

POSITION #53 — SPINE ALIGNER

The "Spine Aligner" is a "green" pose that gives you the tools to by-pass unnecessary effort, creating sustainability within your body. This amazing pose gives you youthful posture, and teaches you to sit comfortably by activating your inner ring of support in the core fascia and muscle line. The "Spine Aligner" has fundamental principles of internal support that can be applied to everything that we do, particularly activities that require sitting (like driving a car and working at the computer). It is essential that the poses we do support functional movement, as this ensures that good posture becomes innate and that optimal alignment is maintained at all times, not just on the yoga mat. Sitting, after all, is where most poor postural and breathing habits become ingrained.

The "Spine Aligner" creates synergy between your psoas and quadratus lumborum (QL). These two muscles work in synergy to balance and stabilize your spine in all movements. Regular practice of this pose keeps you flexible, aligned, and fit, balancing the interactions between your inner and outer hip rotators and supporting the lumbar and sacral areas.

This pose also re-patterns the slouching alignment habits usually created by sitting in a chair. It wakes up our core spinal and breathing muscles, allowing them to support us with energy and efficiency.

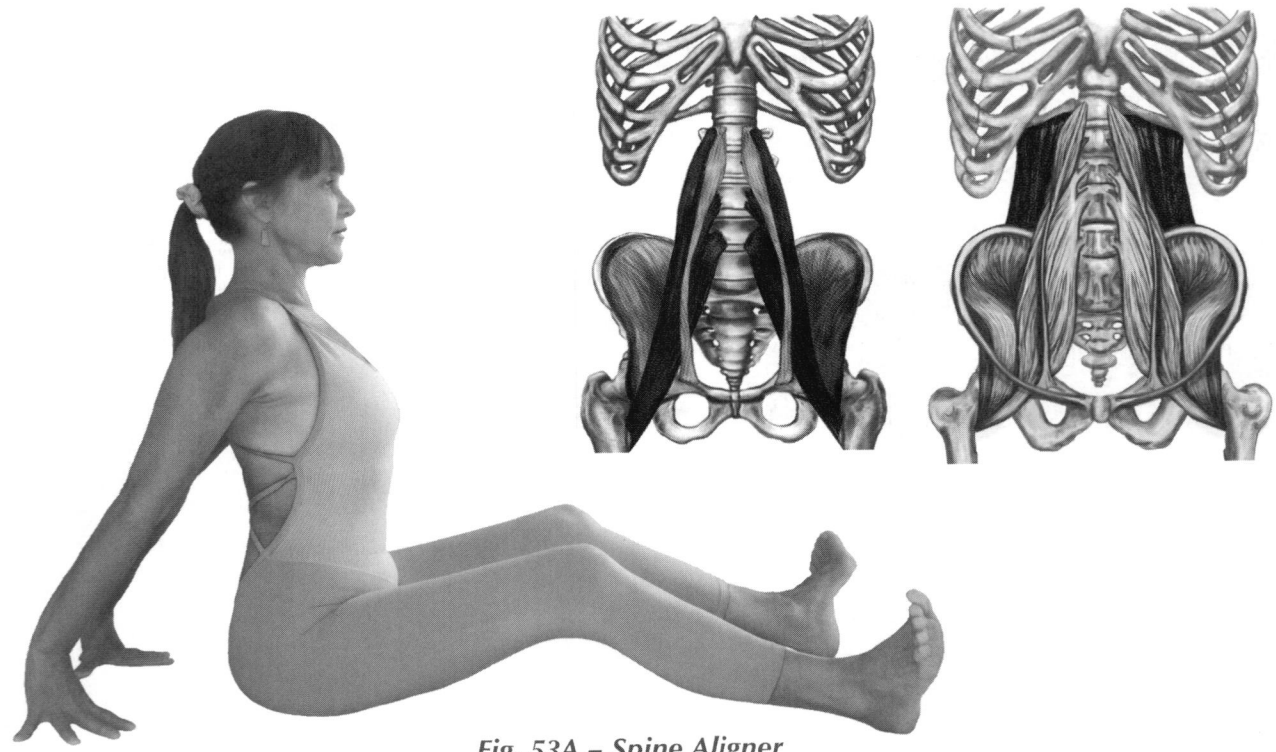

Fig. 53A – Spine Aligner

The "Spine Aligner" can be done with a chair (**Fig. 53B**) if you are not comfortable sitting on the floor. From a seated position, place your heels on the corners of your mat while pressing through the balls of your feet. Keep your knees slightly bent and your toes spread apart. Keep your knees apart as though you were sitting on a horse, and check that the level of your knees is even with the top of your hips. Initiate an action to bring your inner thighs together without actually letting your knees come closer to each other; maintain the wide-leg positioning shown in **Fig. 53A**. You may place a yoga block or Pilates ring between your knees to assist in this action. This action balances the dynamic between your inner hip rotators and your outer hip rotators, keeping the sacral platform lifted.

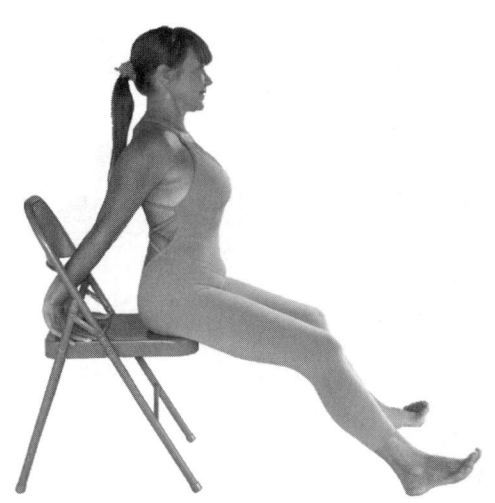

Fig. 53B – Seated Spine Aligner

Spread your buttocks apart so that you can balance on your sit bones. Place your hands on the mat behind you, fingers pointing towards your hips. If there is strain in your forearm, face your fingers outwards, with your thumb pointing towards your hips. Keep your arm muscles firm and contracted, with your shoulder blades pulled down away from your ears. (**Note:** If there is pain in your fingers or wrists, balance on fists with your palms facing away from your body. You may also use blocks.) Press through the balls of your feet while lifting and extending your toes back towards your shins. Keep your toes spread wide and actively extended as you press your heels into the mat. Your toes should be spread with your feet slightly turned out as though pressing on a gas pedal. Knees should be bent to reach the level of the top of your hips. Make sure the knees are not bent too much or too little. Keep your shoulder blades down and this balance of actions between your inner and outer hip rotator forces.

Begin to inhale using the SIP Breath while sensing how breath movement causes your spine to lengthen during inhalation. Keep the extension that comes into your spine even as you exhale. Stay in the pose and continue to breathe space into your spine and length into your waist. Breathe in and visualize your psoas muscle group. Think about your psoas connecting from your inner thigh bone to your lower spine and your diaphragm (**Fig. 53A**). Remember that as you breathe in, the psoas and QL muscles are activated to assist in spinal extension. In this pose, you activate the psoas for deep breathing and core stabilization, instead of having to rely upon the peripheral muscle engagement patterns typically acquired from sitting in chairs. Inhale and visualize the psoas acting as a rooting foundation for the downwards contraction of your diaphragm, and acting as a guide wire down through its attachment at the inner thigh bone.

Sometimes dysfunctional posture habits become so ingrained that we cannot sense when we are misaligned. You may even feel like you are leaning slightly back when you are actually naturally aligned. Position yourself sideways or laterally to a mirror so that you can see your spine alignment from the side. If you tend to have forward head carriage, it may feel unfamiliar to have your spine in alignment and the

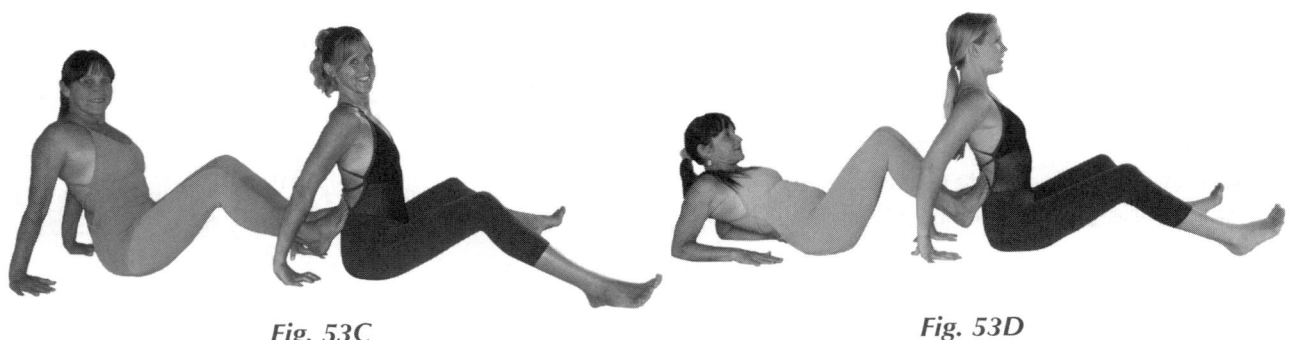

Fig. 53C   *Fig. 53D*

Michaelle uses her feet to help establish the natural 30 degree angle of the sacral platform at the same time Rayna and Kris turn on the inner movements of breathing to hold the adjustment.

weight of your head resting atop your spine. Holding your head up with extra effort from your throat or upper shoulder can become an ingrained habit that feels "normal." If you have become accustomed to working these muscles extra hard, then it may feel odd to let go of such habitual patterns.

Feel the lumbar curve in your lower back and the natural inward and upward tilt of your sacrum. Retain awareness in your feet throughout the exercise. Keep your feet slightly turned out as you balance on the middle of your heel. Breathe in and notice your arches. Don't let your feet fall open or lose activation of your inner thigh rotators, or your sacrum will flatten and you will lose the curve in your lower back. Straightening the knees will also cause you to lose your sacral tilt and lower back curve.

Continue core breathing, using the SIP Breath to draw air in through your mouth. As you inhale, feel the expansion generated in the upper chest muscles as you resist down with the shoulder blades. Breathe five to ten times, sensing your breath and your being. The weight of your head is resting atop your spine. Your face, neck, and jaw are relaxed. Turn your head side to side to bring awareness and to determine if you are holding tension in any of these areas. Such tension can transfer all the way to your pelvic floor and lower body, making the pose feel uncomfortable. Feeling compression in the SI joint is a sign that you are not engaging your upper psoas and transverse abdominal muscles enough to support an elongated spine and stabilized core. Inhale extension and core support into the spine. Maintain the lift as you exhale.

Teacher/partner adjustments as shown in **Fig. 53C** and **Fig. 53D** can help bring the curve into the lower back, enabling natural tilt in the sacrum. This adjustment combines with Core SIP Breathing to engage core muscles and initiate natural spine alignment patterning.

Every position in YogAlign is painless. There may be intensity when you engage muscles that have been inactive, but there should never be any pain. Pain leads to strain, not to gain.

Note: If you cannot engage the curves of your spine, make sure that you sit on a chair and use a strap around a post or doorknob to pull yourself up into alignment. Practice the SIP Breathing technique to maintain extension while holding onto the strap. Soon your core will become strong enough to maintain natural alignment without the strap.

POSITION #54 — TWISTING SPINE ALIGNER

Twist poses tone your abdominal organs while creating kid-like spinal flexibility in your spiral and lateral rotational movements. Balancing the tensile forces in the spiral line of fascia is the focus in this pose. "Twisting Spine Aligner" tunes the inner hip rotators, taking tensile stress off of the iliotibial (IT) band and lower back region. Strong inner hip-rotators and adductors help maintain the sacral lift by preventing the outer hip-rotators from dominating sacral tension forces. Over-engaging the outer rotators flattens the sacral platform and loads up tension in your low back muscles, vertebrae, and hip socket. The balance of forces between your rotator groups is strongly determined by the positions of your legs and feet. As with the "Spine Aligner," the "Twisting Spine Aligner" can be done sitting in a chair if that is more comfortable for your hips or knees. If you cannot sit on the floor with knees bent and retain your lumbar/sacral curve, sit up on a yoga block or chair (**Fig. 54B**).

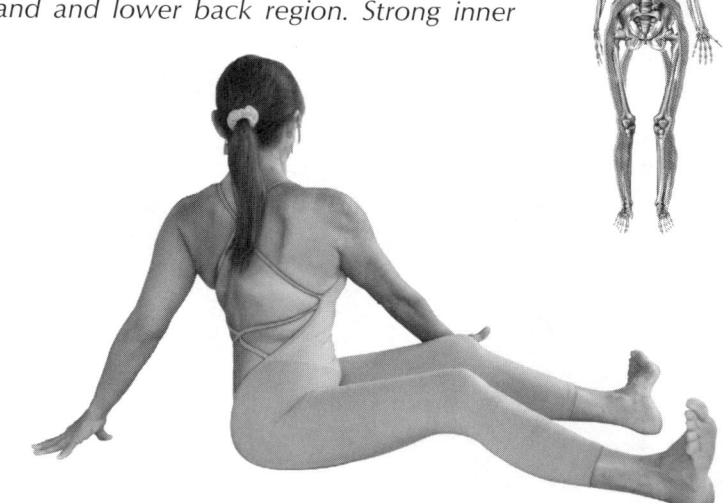

Fig. 54A – Twisting Spine Aligner

From the "Spine Aligner," continue breathing length and extension into the spine and waist. Position yourself in front of a mirror so that when you twist, you can see your spinal curves from the side. This cannot be emphasized enough: the sacrum should have a natural tilt that allows it to act a shock absorber; it should not be held flat. Squeeze in on your thighs without letting your knees move closer together. You may place a yoga block or Pilates ring between your knees to assist in this action.

If you are using a strap to hold proper alignment, hold both ends in your right hand. Inhale and twist to the left, placing your left hand behind you, fingers pointing away from the body, with your shoulders back and down. If you are not holding a strap, bring your right arm to the outside of your left thigh with your palm facing out and fingers spread wide. Keep the curve in your lower back and the lift in your sacrum. Exhale as you retain the length of your waist, powered by your inner ring of core support.

Stay in the twist, and inhale with a SIP Breath; this time gently hold in your breath. Make sure that when you hold your breath your shoulders are down and

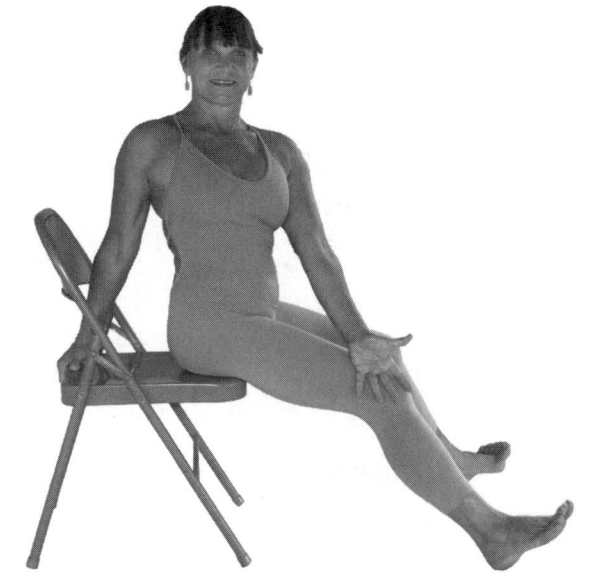

Fig. 54B – Seated Twisting Spine Aligner

you are not trying to hold too much air. Keep it comfortable. Add extra tightening to your trunk muscles as you twist from your abdominal area. Hold for 10-20 seconds and exhale with a lift of your waist, releasing the extra tightening of your trunk muscles. Notice the ease of the twist, and keep focusing on alignment and the body in its entirety. Inhale back to the center, noticing the difference between your right and left sides.

Repeat the twist, this time to the right. Stay awake and present in your entire body, noticing if you are straining any part of your body and creating tension. Turn off extra effort and let your breathing process align, tune, and support you from the inside out. When you are perfectly aligned, your body will feel as if you are floating. When this happens, visualize your brain developing new neural pathways to keep you aligned in this posture automatically, without ever having to think about it. You can create a new you!

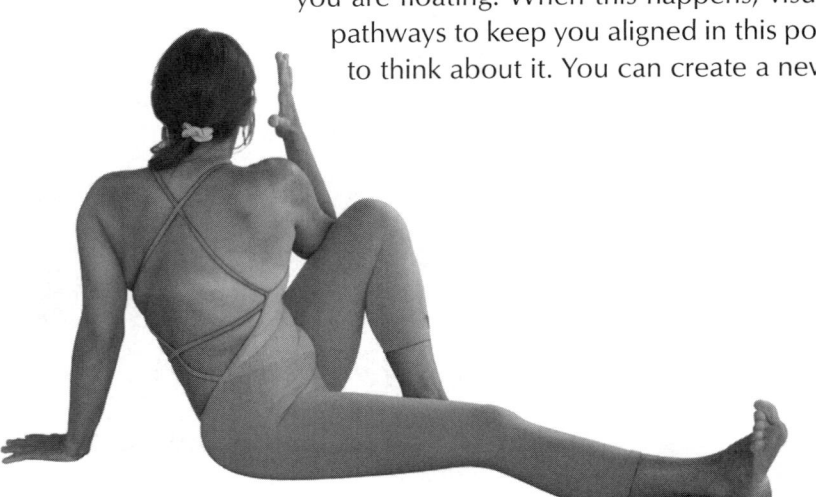

Note: Use extra caution when doing spinal twists. If you reverse your natural spinal curves while trying to actively twist your trunk, you are putting your spine in great danger.

Fig. 54C – INCORRECT: Spinal Twist

See **Fig. 54C**, and notice how there is no curve in my lower back spine. Notice the flattened lumbar curve. There is no correct way to do this type of spinal twist. The human body is simply not designed for this body position. Doing twists with either or both legs straight has greatly contributed to the epidemic of yoga and stretching injuries.

Lumbar discs are compressed and sacral ligaments get strained and overstretched when the body is not supported from the core and aligned in the natural curves that allow the flexible rod actions of your spine. Such body positioning is obviously a danger to your spine, but notice how it affects breathing, too. Do not do poses that prevent the downward piston-like movement of your diaphragm muscle. If in doubt, see if you can take a deep breath. If you cannot, the pose is not serving your body.

The best twist is basic and simple, and always keeps the sacral platform lifted and the spine aligned in its natural curves. If your spine is not in natural alignment while twisting, you are likely doing your body more harm than good, on a number of levels. Keep it simple and enjoy the benefits of non-compressive spinal twists. Avoid poses requiring you to straighten your legs or wrap your arms around your knees to bring your hands together. These movements in your periphery only serve to compress your internal body.

POSITION #55 — ADVANCED SPINE ALIGNER

Posture is tuned up to perfection and the core line of fascia is tuned into balance with regular practice of the "Advanced Spine Aligner." Through the practice of this pose you will learn to "turn off" the extra effort that leads to tension and thickened fascia in your upper neck, back, and shoulders. Gain strength, power, grace, and ease in movement with this super pose. Relieve lower back pain and soreness over your entire body. "Advanced Spine Aligner" also helps to heal knee injuries, sciatica, IT band inflammation, and even TMJ.

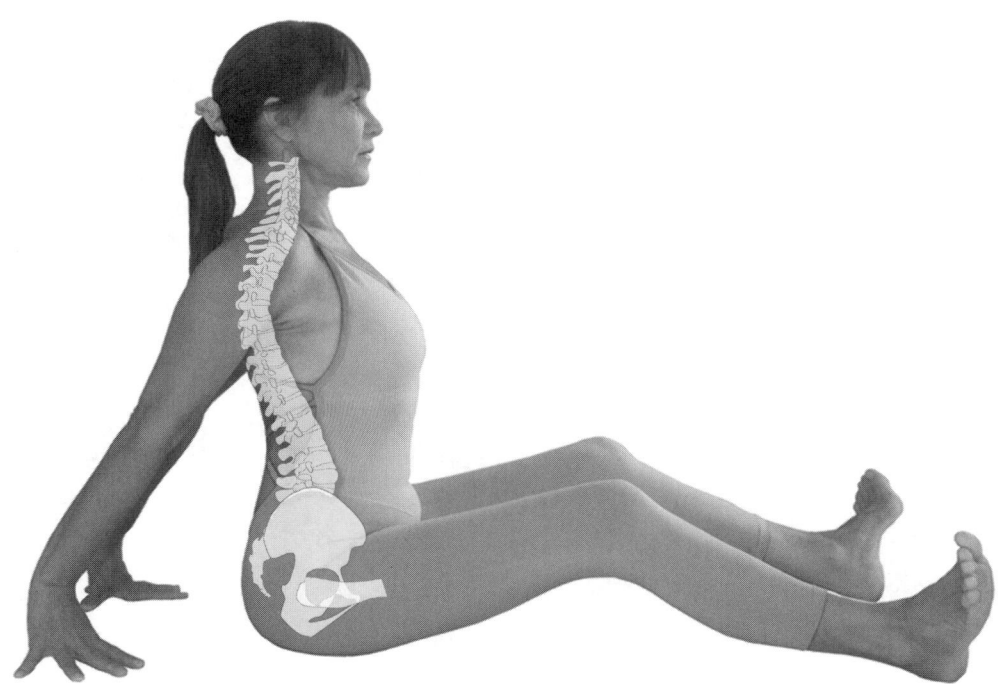

Fig. 55A – Spine Aligner

To begin the "Advanced Spine Aligner," make sure that you are sitting on the bottom of your sit bones with the curve maintained in your lower back and sacrum. Sit sideways to a mirror and check your alignment if possible. If you feel tightness in your hips, sit on the edge of a chair to do the pose. Place your hands behind you as shown in **Fig. 55A**. (**Note:** You can also put a strap around a post in front of you, and pull on the strap [with arms out in front] to bring yourself up into natural alignment.)

Resting on your fingertips with your palms facing away from your trunk, draw down with the tips of your shoulder blades. If you have wrist pain, you may balance on your fists. Keep the alignment in your feet, with your toes extended and spread apart. Pretend there is a block between your knees and squeeze into the imaginary block without moving your knees. (You can also place an actual block or fitness ring between your knees.) These squeezing actions will regulate the balance between your inner and outer hip rotators. Keep your feet active and the tops of your knees level with the top of your hips. Use a mirror and check your alignment from hips to head. Connect with the feeling of your sacrum. If you feel tension, you

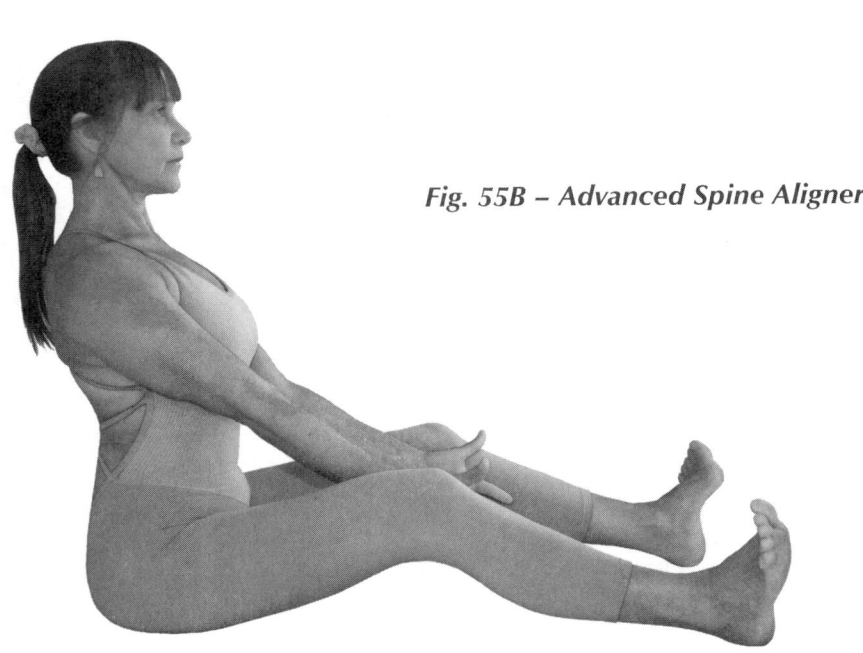

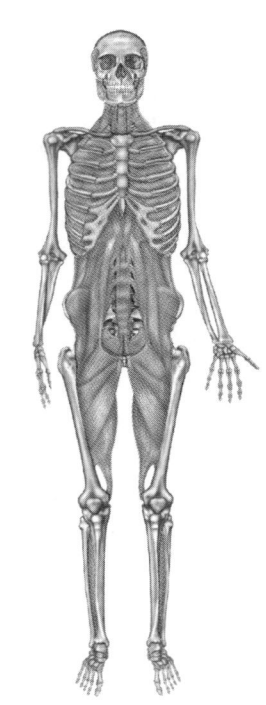

Fig. 55B – Advanced Spine Aligner

may need to use the strap or sit on a chair or yoga block to get your knees lower than your hips. Inhale with a Core SIP Breath and hold for a few seconds. As you exhale, open your mouth as widely as you can and extend your tongue, making sure that you are not jutting out your chin when you exhale. Keep relaxed. Your head should be light as it balances on top of your spine.

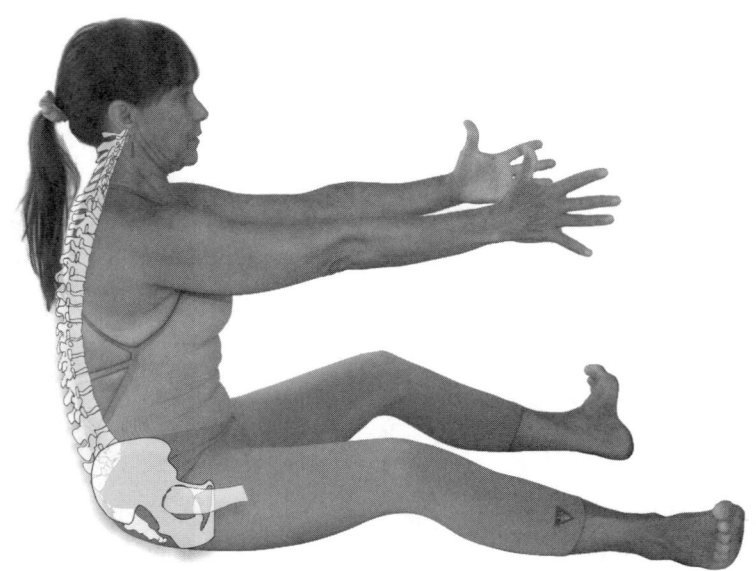

Fig. 55C — INCORRECT: Spine Aligner

The "Advanced Spine Aligner" **(Fig. 55B)** requires you to release your hands from behind you, bringing them to your front, and placing them between your knees. The palms face each other, and the fingers are spread, with thumbs pointed up and shoulder blades down. Use the SIP Breathing technique to engage the muscles and fascia of your deep front line and sense the connection to your core. Try to use your arms to spread your knees apart as you resist with your inner thighs. Your arm muscles are toned as you hold this resistance and focus upon your alignment.

Focus. Notice how the process of inhalation engages the muscular actions of your breathing tube and supports the lift of the front of your spine.

Mind your alignment. If your alignment looks like what is shown in **Fig. 55C**, you should practice the "Spine Aligner" with a strap, as explained above. Notice the reversed spinal curves and flattened sacral platform in this incorrect alignment. Sitting and exercising in this position results in bad posture, and causes damage to spinal discs and nerves.

There is serious long-term danger in performing straight-leg seated and forward bend poses as shown in **Fig. 55C**. In addition, what you cannot see is that my diaphragm is unable to engage for deep breathing— exactly what happens when I sit poorly in a chair.

In **Fig. 55D,** Zack is clearly uncomfortable, his spine is compressed and he has lost the natural curves in his back. This is not a measure of flexibility nor can you get flexible doing this. The most common yoga injury is lower back strain and the right angle, leg straight position is the reason why.

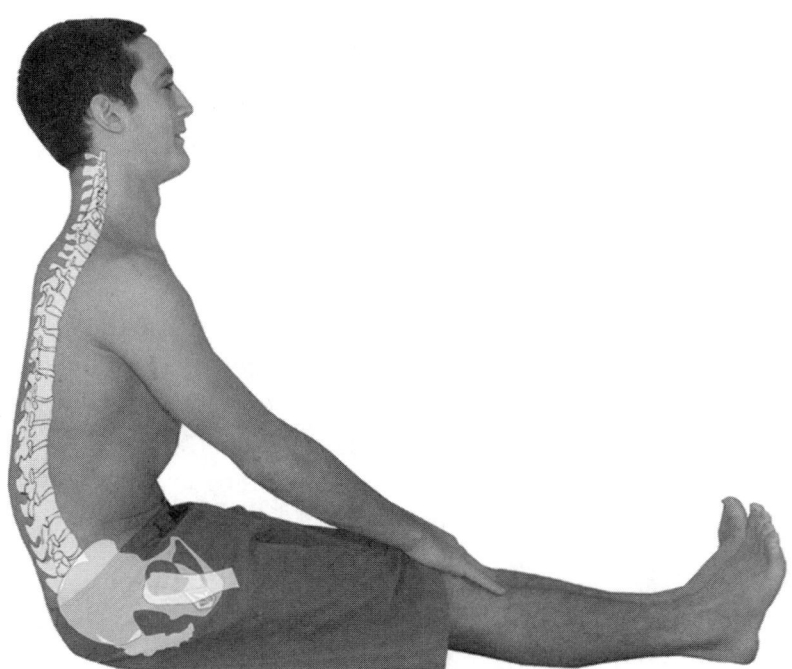

Fig. 55D – INCORRECT: Sitting with straight legs and extended toes reverses the natural shock absorbing curves of the spine and sacrum.

SOS: Save Our Sacrums!

POSITION #56 — ROCKING SPINE ALIGNER

Super-charge your core and create balanced muscle actions in your spine with the "Rocking Spine Aligner." This pose gets your trunk and breathing muscles engaging together as stabilizers. The brain establishes muscle patterning faster when you practice conscious breathing as you move. The benefits of the "Spine Aligner" (Position #53) are available in this pose too, but here you get to rock and roll!

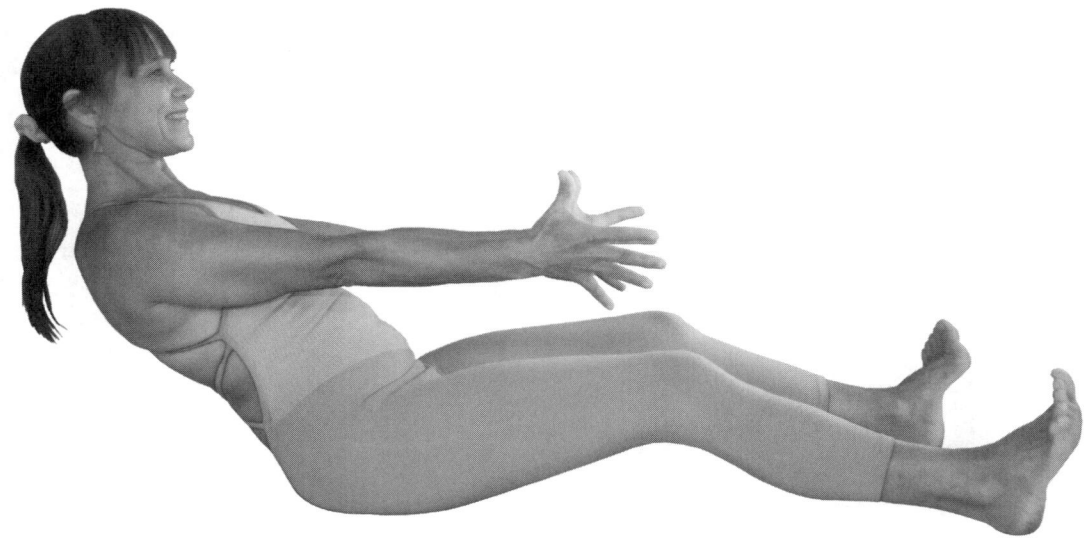

Fig. 56A – Rocking Spine Aligner

Position your body in the "Advanced Spine Aligner" (Position #55) and practice a Core SIP Breath. Feel the connections that engage your deep core line to bring you to center. Keep the resistance between your hands and thighs, and begin to exhale slowly, staying long in your waist. As you exhale, extend through your tongue, toes and fingers as you draw in with a strong belly action, keeping your waist area lengthened even as your exhalation muscles contract. Keep the knees pressing inwards without letting them open. Begin to lift your hands up so that your arms extend in front of your chest. Practice drawing your arms back to your core, keeping your fingers wide open.

Take another SIP Breath, rocking back as you use the movement of inhalation to bring you back up to sitting. Do not try to lead yourself back up by pulling from your head or neck. The roll-up should feel fluid and easy. If you cannot roll back up, go back to the seated "Spine Aligner" (Position #53), and practice rocking, going a little further back each time, without actually reclining on the floor.

Sit tall for the exhale while staying long in the waist. You may continue the wide open mouth exhale or make the "ssssss" sound through your teeth to extend the exhale. Keep your spine in its natural curves at all times. Repeat the entire exercise until you feel as though your core is alive and awake.

On your next Core SIP Breath, go to the floor into the "Full Body Stretch." Open your fingers wide and point your toes. Draw your arms deep into their sockets, and connect the foundation of your arms back into your core through the front, back, and lateral muscular fascia lines.

Stay reclined for the entire exhale, feeling your waistline pull in as the inner belly and rib cage contract, pressing air out of your lungs. To roll back up, use the SIP Breath to return to the seated "Spine Aligner." Stay in the "Spine Aligner" for your exhale, keeping your core muscles engaged and your spine extended, maintaining natural spine alignment and sacral integrity.

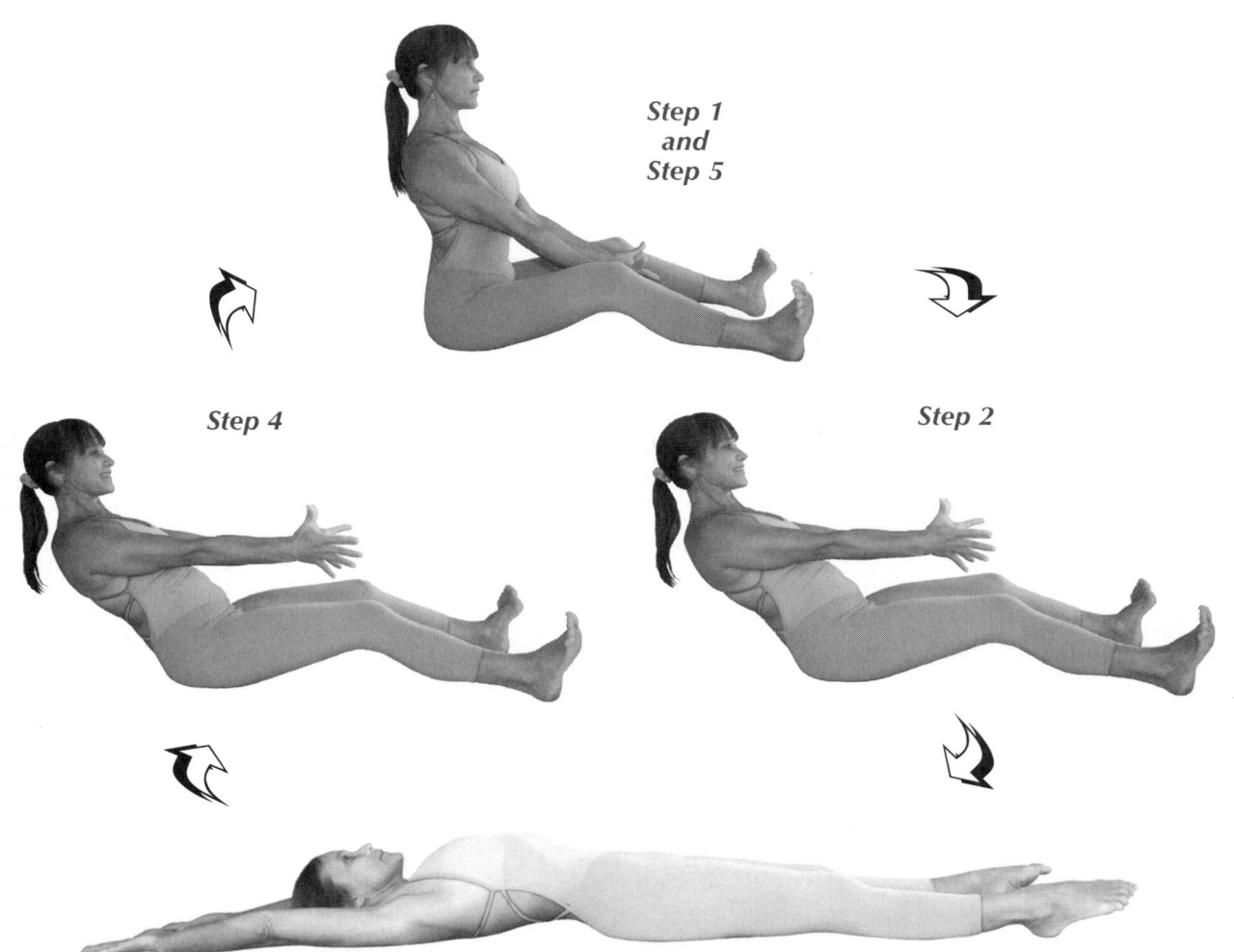

*Step 1
and
Step 5*

Step 4

Step 2

Step 3 – Full Body Stretch (Position#1)

Fig. 56B – Five Steps of the Rocking Spine Aligner

Note: You can hold your shins or support your trunk by placing your hands on the floor when you come up to the seated position, especially if you need help staying lifted in natural alignment. Keep the "gift of the lift" by lengthening the belly as you contract to exhale. This trains your core trunk muscles to eccentrically engage—lengthening as they contract.

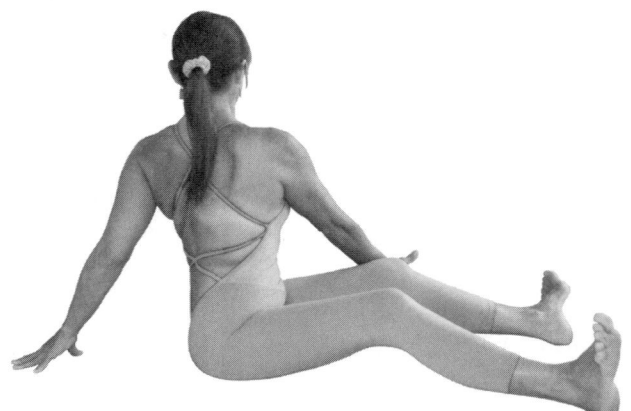

Fig. 56C – Twisting Spine Aligner (Position #54)

Stay in the "Full Body Stretch" noticing the energy in your center.

You can now add a twist to the rocking spine aligner each time you come back up to sitting. Use the same principle of alignment as in previous twists, keeping the spinal curves in neutral and moving from the abdomen. Keep engaging your knees inwards (without letting them actually move) to get the hip rotators balanced. Keep your waist long and your spine extended. Begin to experiment with PNF muscle exercises, holding breath and muscle actions for a moment in the "Twisting Spine Aligner" (Position #54), accentuating muscle engagement, and releasing on exhalation into a deeper supported twist. You can vary these movements and tone your core, align your spine, and massage your back in just a few moments.

After a few weeks of practicing, your core muscles will start to engage automatically with the actions of stabilization providing lift, support, and extension to your spinal area. This will serve you much better than having a tight "six-pack." Your waist will elongate, providing more space for your internal organs, and eliminating the "pot belly" look. Have fun and improvise different movements, but always keep your attention on sensing your whole body, staying in alignment and using conscious core breathing.

When you have completed the pose, "Spinal Roll" your way up to your hands and knees and roll your hips around in circles, feeling the undulation of your spine.

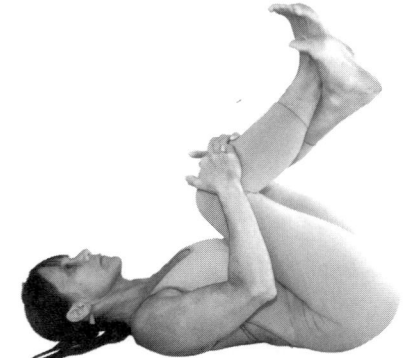

Fig. 56D – Exhale, rock knees held above hips.

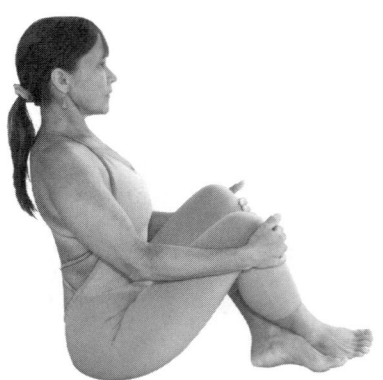

Fig. 56E – Inhale, roll up.

POSITION #57 — THE GLIDER

"The Glider" pose is great for swimmers, surfers, and paddlers. This pose establishes arm movement patterns that originate from your core and are synchronized with your breathing. Like all YogAlign poses, "The Glider" will improve your posture as well as core strength. You will get toned in the back body, flexible in the front, and balanced in the shoulder girdle and rotator cuff. "The Glider" also equalizes fascial forces between the connective tissues of the superficial front line and the superficial back line.

With regular practice, the forces of flexion and extension in the superficial front and back lines equalize, helping to relieve chronic neck and back pain. One can truly sense the fascia web in this pose, especially when there is restrictive tissue in the belly and front body.

Many athletes paddle with poor posture, pulling from the cap of their shoulders, with their chins leading the way. Poor alignment and lack of connection to the core is highly inefficient and leads to strain, pain, and injuries, sometimes requiring surgery. The movements in "The Glider" will train you to paddle efficiently, powered from your diaphragm and a strong but flexible belly, both of which enable you to move with grace and ease while in perfect natural alignment.

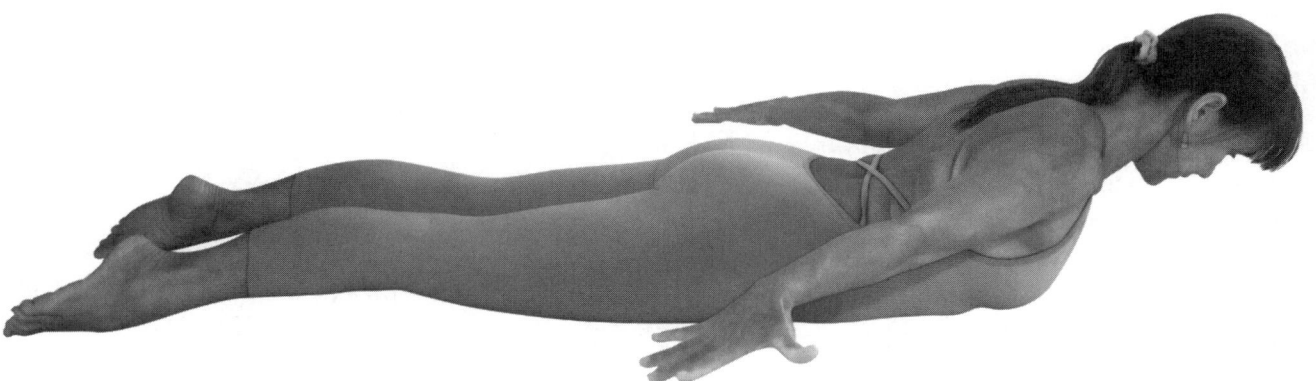

Fig. 57A – CORRECT: Glider

Lie on the floor, belly down, with your forehead on the mat. Bring your arms back like glider wings, keeping the palms pressed down to the mat and the arm muscles "turned on." Open your fingers wide and press your hands into the floor. Keep your arms deep in the socket and pull the tips of your shoulder blades towards your hips. Begin to use a SIP Breath to lift your chest and arms off of the floor. Return to the floor as you exhale and than again begin to press your arms deeply into the floor with your forehead resting on the mat. Inhale and lift your head, arms and shoulder girdle off of the floor together. Keep your hands and chest off of the floor, fingers wide open and the tops of your feet pointing and pressing down on your mat. Avoid lifting with your chin or leading with your head. Keep your neck neutral. Inhale and lift your head, arms and shoulder girdle off of the floor together. While you are lifted, continue to fire your arm muscles as though you are trying to press your hand towards the floor. Lift from your core using your breathing muscles for support. Your collarbones should be wide and your shoulders should be pulled away from your ears.

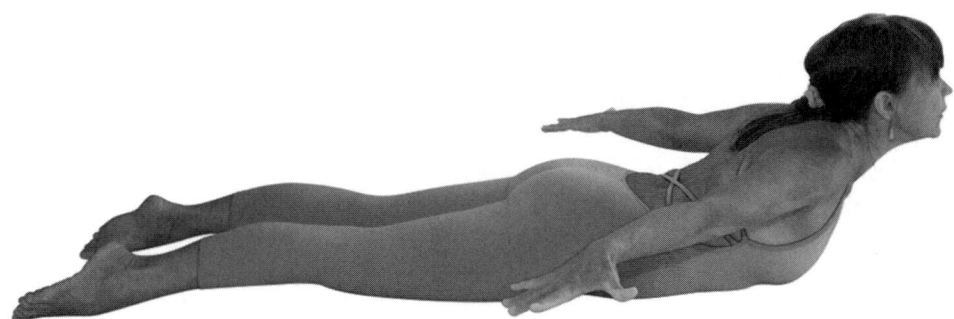

Fig. 57A – INCORRECT: Glider

Be aware of the sensations throughout your entire body. Imagine your body soaring like a glider or an eagle. Relax tension in the eyes and jaw. Focus on staying present in the moment. Avoid leading with your chin, which puts you at risk for neck compression. Use a mirror to check your alignment.

Try it with a Twist

With your fingers spread, lift your chest and turn to the side like a glider rotating from side to side. Be sure to keep in natural alignment, with your arms always pulling into your core center.

Repeat these movements, twisting from side to side, and then lie back down on the mat resting your head to one side, with your hands palms up at your side. Begin to press your ear toward the mat. Keep your shoulders drawn away from your ears and intensify the actions for a moment. Exhale and release the added neck tension and notice if your head now turns easier to that side. Turn your head to the other side and again press, tighten and release the muscle actions in your neck.

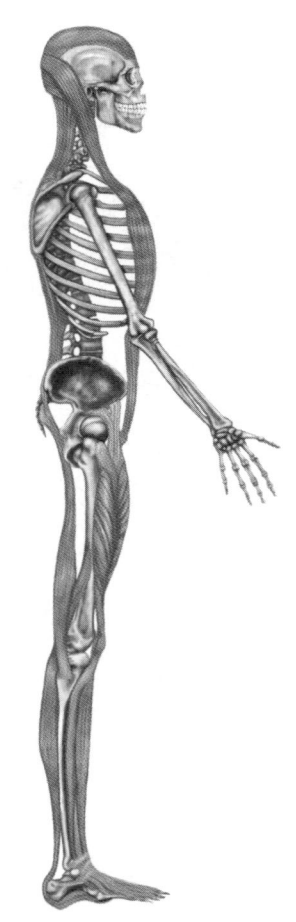

For variation, turn your head to one side while inhaling. Keep your head turned with your neck long when you exhale. Inhale and bring your head back to center. Repeat on the other side. Stay lifted and long when you exhale. Practice this movement with your hands in a fist, and then again with your fingers wide open. Release tension in the jaw and face by adding an open mouth exhale while lifted. Feel power in your tongue coming all the way from your abdomen as you press the air out. Extend your tongue as far out as you can, but avoid lifting your chin. Come down as you exhale and rest your head to one side of the mat and simply observe as your breathing process happens naturally. Take four or five breaths in that position and then then lift and turn your head to the other side, releasing any tension you feel in your neck. Bring your head back to center and prepare for the cobra pose.

POSITION #58 — THE COBRA

"The Cobra" is one of the most widely-practiced of all yoga poses. It massages and tones the extensor muscles in your back as it simultaneously tones your abdominal organs, stretches your belly, stimulates your thyroid gland, and keeps your spine strong and flexible. Like the "Glider," the "Cobra" will balance the fascial forces between the front and back body. The superficial front line is stretched from the top of your toes to your head, and the core line is strengthened in length and integrity.

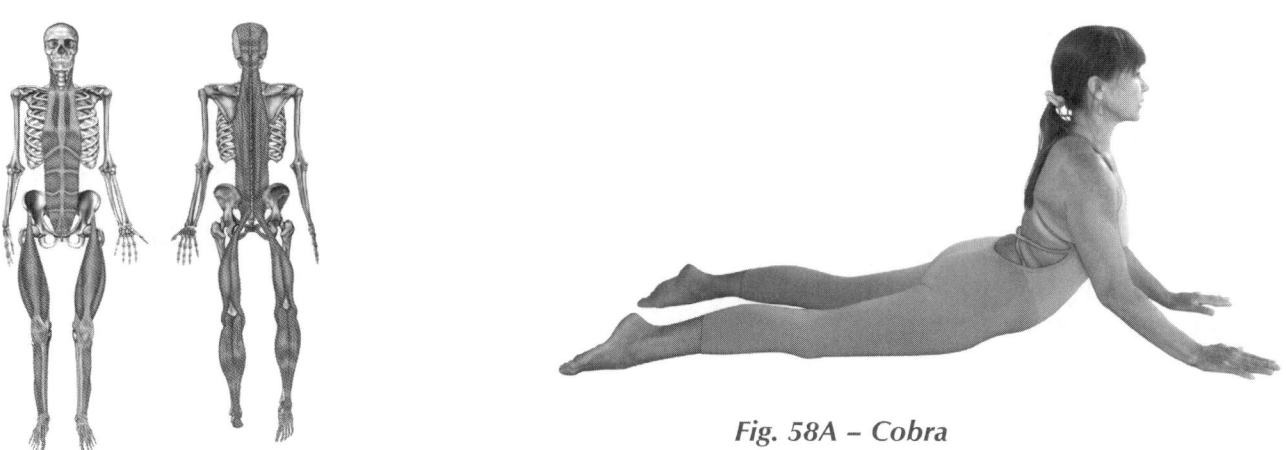

Fig. 58A – Cobra

You can flow from "The Glider" into "The Cobra." Set your palms on the floor underneath your shoulders, your forehead resting on the floor. If you feel any compression in your lower back, make sure to extend your hands further out in front of your chest or stay with the "Glider" pose. Keep your feet shoulder-width apart, toes spread, and press the tops of your feet into the mat. Draw your shoulder blades down and towards your heart, keeping your elbows at your sides.

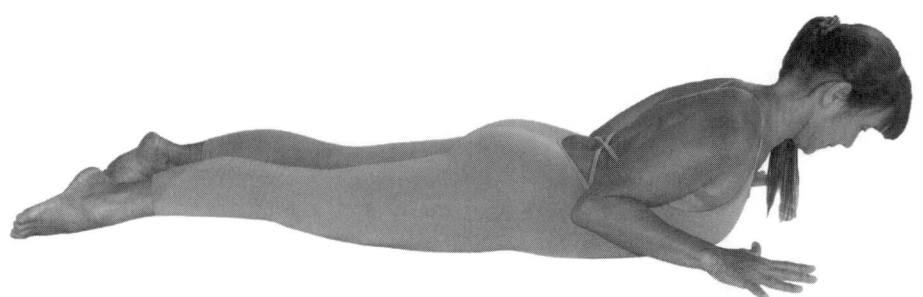

Fig. 58B – Cobra preparation pose

With your forehead resting on the mat, lift your hands a few inches above the floor with your elbows bent, shoulders down, and your fingers spread wide as shown in **Fig. 58B**. Inhale with a SIP Breath while lifting your chest from the floor without the use of your hands. When you cannot lift any higher, press your hands to the floor and continue lifting from your core. Keep your elbows slightly-bent, lengthening from the base of your spine to the crown of your head. When you need to exhale, slowly lower to the floor,

335

keeping your shoulders away from your ears while moving from your center. Inhale with your hands off of the floor and, with a SIP inhalation, lift your chest again. Slightly engage your buttock muscles to support your lower back, taking care to move slowly and avoid pushing hard, which will eliminate any lower-back compression.

After a moment of resting, bring your forehead to the center and begin to lift with your elbows bent to the side as you inhale. When you can no longer lift away from the floor, place your hands down and carefully come into the cobra keeping a bend in your elbows. As you exhale, stick out your tongue and feel your belly draw in. Think of the cobra snake hissing and extending its tongue. Hold the contracted muscles for a moment as you initiate the SIP Breath. Release the actions and notice how open and long your breathing process is now. You can also practice inhaling, holding the breath and tightening all of your muscles. As you exhale, go deeper and sense your entire body from your toes to your head.

When you first start practicing "The Cobra," begin by rising up on the inhale and lower with the exhale several times before you attempt to hold yourself up in the cobra position. Stay lifted and extended for a few breaths, using each inhale to lift yourself higher. Lower to the floor to rest, and then repeat the move from the beginning for each breath cycle.

As you do this pose, concentrate on using SIP Breathing to stabilize your rib cage and work your diaphragm. Over-lifting the front ribs with poor breathing habits can cause compression of your rib cage, shortening and compressing your back ribs, and the curve in your lower back. It's best to let your breathing process align your ribs from the inside out. If you still feel compression in your lower back, gently pull the bottom of your sternum (breastbone) towards your pubic bone. Do not lock out your elbows or lift your chin as in **Fig. 58D**. Stay neutral in the neck spine and keep your elbows bent, working and aligning from your core.

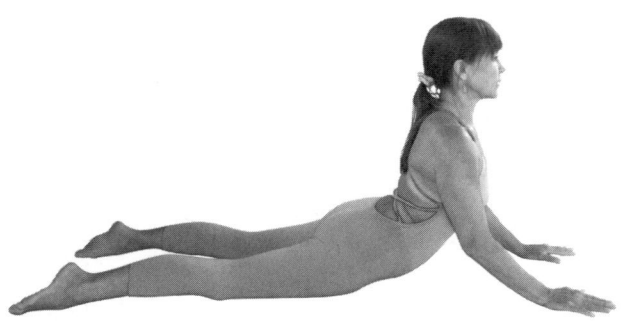

Fig. 58C – CORRECT:
Note neck and elbow position.

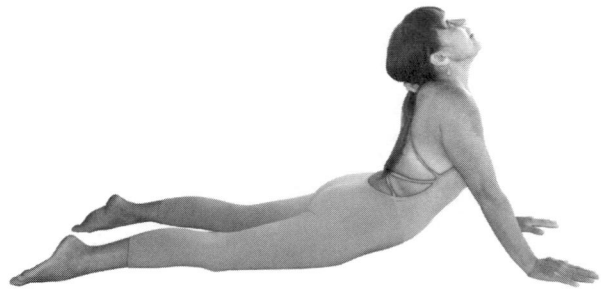

Fig. 58D – INCORRECT:
Compressed neck and locked out elbow position.

POSITION #59 — HIGH TO LOW PUSH-UPS AND HIGH DOG

Push-ups are a powerful way to stay strong and in-shape using your own body weight. By following YogAlign principles of core alignment, you can avoid injury or compression to your shoulder joint, wrists, or lower back spine while still enjoying the benefits of this exercise.

This exercise is broken up into a sequence of three positions, each of which is described below.

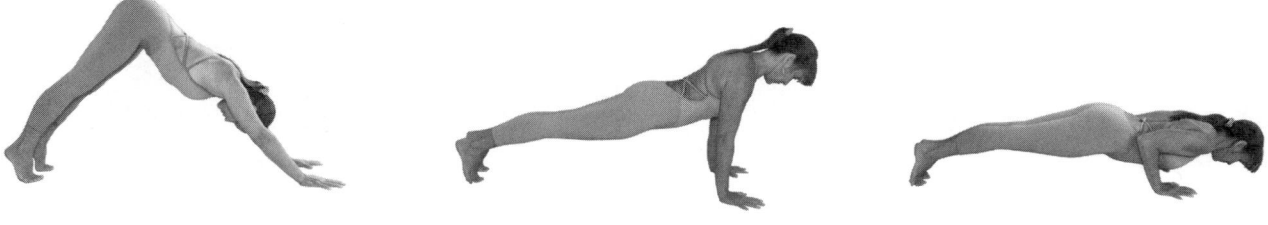

Fig. 59A – High to Low Push-ups

Start by lying on your belly with your hands palm-down on the floor by your shoulders. Inhale and press up into "High Dog" with your feet hip-width or wider **(Fig. 59B)**. Stay in natural spine alignment by keeping your heels lifted high and, if necessary, your knees bent. Press into your palms with your fingers spread wide.

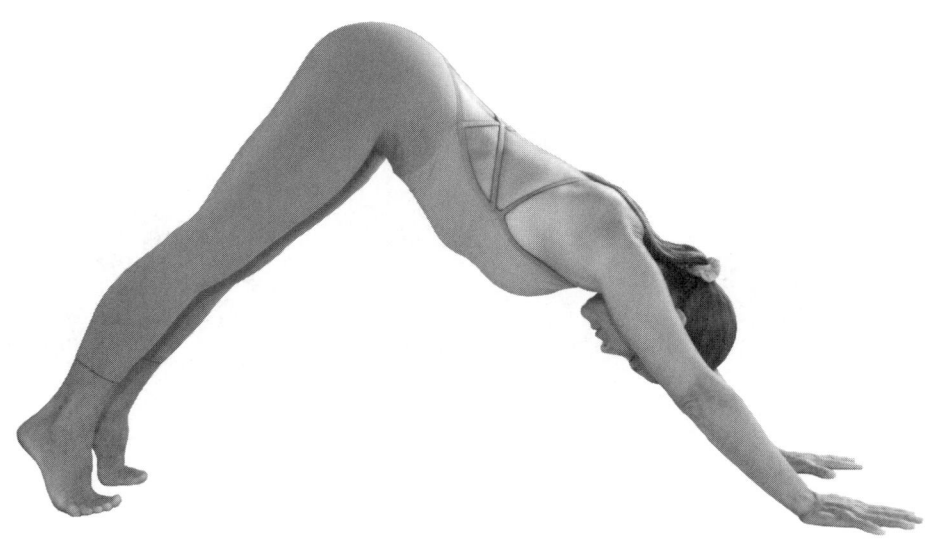

Fig. 59B – High Dog

Walk your feet and hands further apart. Inhale while bringing your shoulders above your wrists into the "High Push-Up" position. You may have to walk your feet back further in order to bring your shoulders above your wrists. Engage and stabilize the muscles in your arms, trunk, and legs. Exhale while staying in the "High Push-Up" pose as in **Fig. 59C**. Keep aligned and centered, with your shoulder blades down and your neck long. Retain these positions throughout the entire pose.

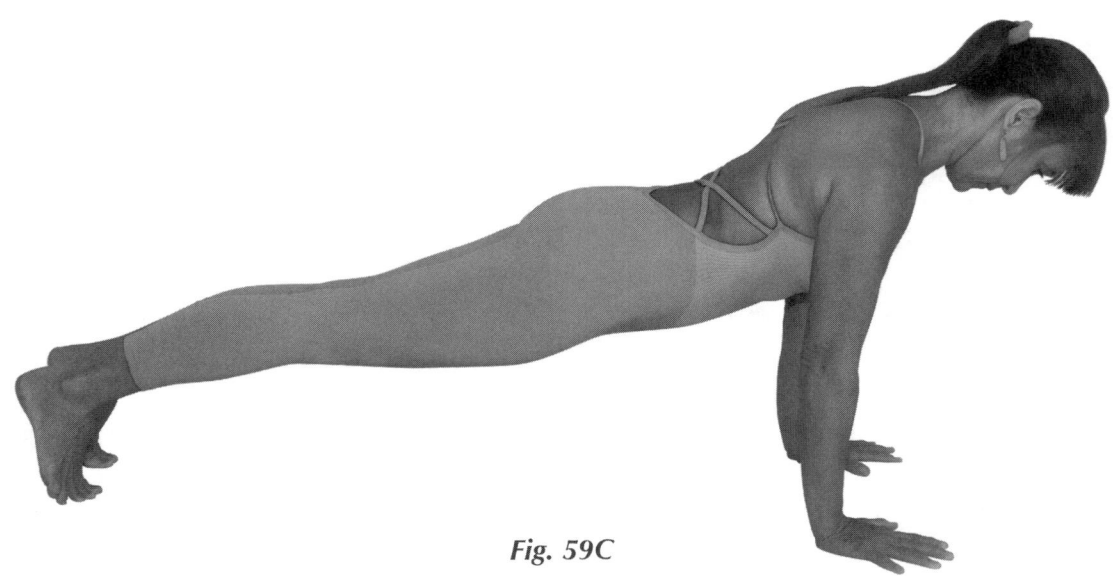

Fig. 59C

Use the SIP Breath and inhale your way down towards the floor. Keep your buttock muscles firm and make sure that you are inhaling as you slowly lower your body towards the floor. Stay balanced on your hands and on the balls of your feet for a few moments, then release to the floor and exhale. Inhale each time you push up or down. Do not lift from your throat; engage your breath from your core in order to balance your muscle actions.

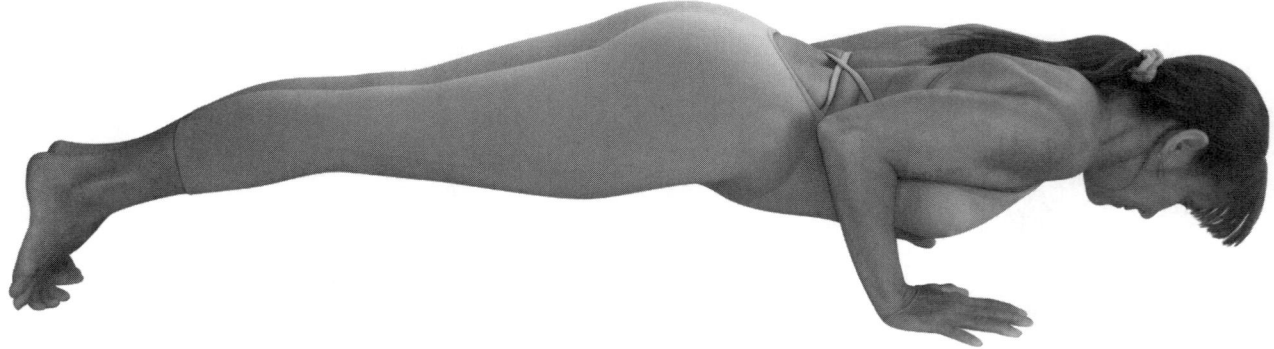

Fig. 59D – CORRECT: The low push-up position requires you to support yourself from your inner core, using the movements of breathing.

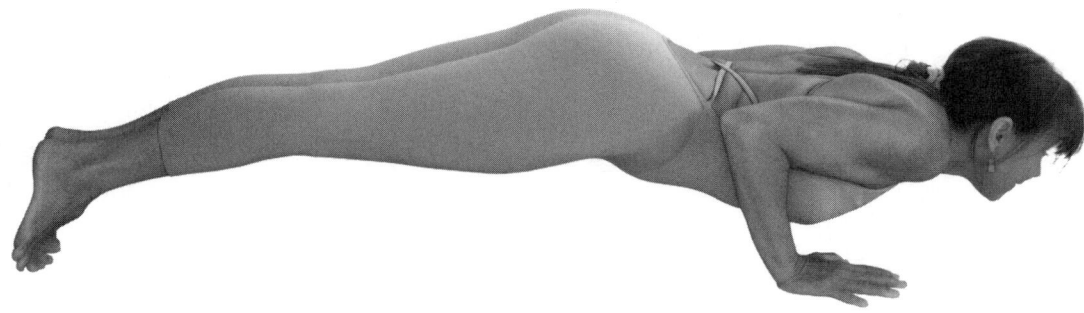

Fig. 59E – INCORRECT: Leading your push-up with your chin will get you nowhere fast, and will cause a lot of neck pain and arthritis in the long run.

The version of push-up shown in **Fig. 59E** will cause strain to the occiput (where the neck muscles attach to the base of skull). It is at this point that the neck muscles attach to the dura, or fascia sheath, that surrounds your brain.

These push-up poses should be done slowly and consciously using the movement of inhalation to push up or press down to the floor. People have been injured by moving too fast through this pose, engaging in poor spine and shoulder alignment. It is important throughout this exercise to use your core muscles to support you from the center. Lifting your head and leading with your chin reinforces forward head-carriage, upper shoulder tightness and muscle strain in the occiput. Practice feeling comfort throughout the neck region and never lift with your chin or lead with your throat as seen in **Fig. 59E**. If the pose hurts your wrist or shoulders, you can also balance on your forearms as show in **Fig. 59F**.

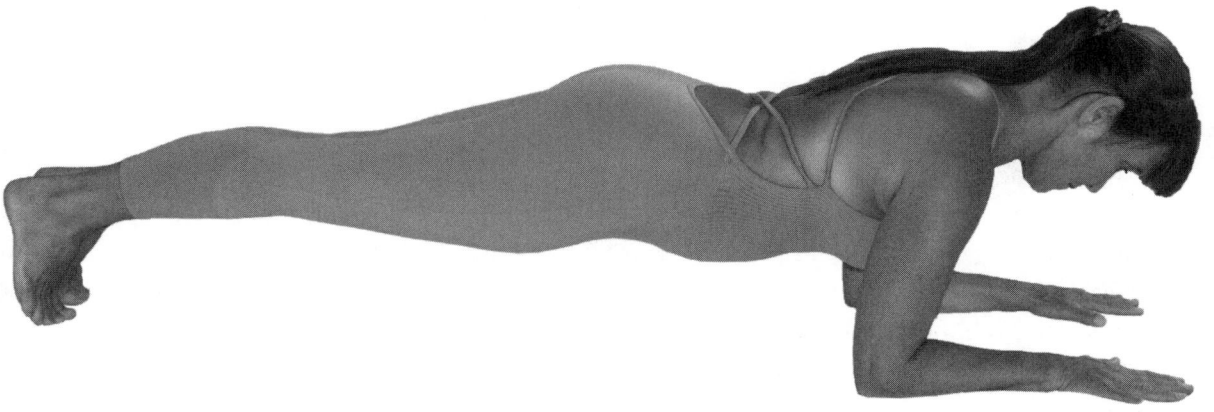

Fig. 59F – A Forearm Balance can be substituted for the traditional plank pose, which can be hard on the wrist joints.

Position #60 — Rocking Bow (Advanced)

"The Rocking Bow" is a prone back bend that opens your heart while strengthening the muscles of extension in your back. With this pose you can tone your arms, abdomen muscles and inner organs. Make sure to warm up for this pose and include self-massage of the arms and shoulders. "The Rocking Bow" helps you gain tremendous strength in your shoulders and back body. Your glutes and the backs of your legs gain tone as they work hard to extend your hip joint, and your stomach muscles (as well as your entire front body) get a huge stretch from your toes to your jaw. Do not do the Bow pose if you have a herniated disc, impinged nerves, or a history of lower back pain or surgeries.

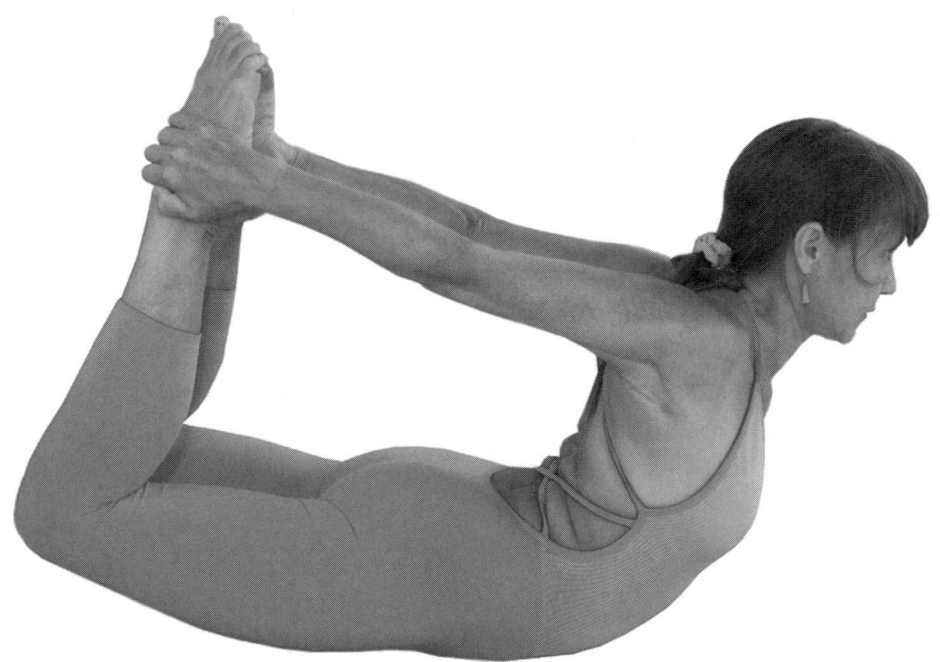

Fig. 60A – Rocking Bow

Lie on your belly, reach behind your back, and grab your ankles. Draw your shoulder blades down and back. Squeeze your inner thighs and do core breathing to stimulate active length in your psoas. Keep your feet active by pointing your toes and sense your entire body. If you feel any pain in your lower back, come out of the pose and practice "The Glider" (Position #57) instead. A deep SIP Breath activates the fascial connection from the diaphragm to the xyphoid process at the bottom of the sternum. This fascial pull created by the diaphragm contracting downwards keeps your front ribs "tethered," so that they don't pop out and rotate up along with the front rib cage, which causes the lower ribs to compress the lumbar spine area. Remember: the ribs are connected from front to back, so what comes up in the front goes down in the back. It is vitally important that you keep your lower back lengthened, keeping your rib cage level with your hips in order to avoid compressing the sacrum and lower back area.

Inhale as you slowly lift up into the bow, engaging your butt muscles from your core to your limbs. Exhale as you lower back to the floor and rest for a moment. Do four or five of these cycles with the breath, breathing up into "Rocking Bow" and exhaling back down to the floor. Focus on maintaining alignment in your spine and rib cage.

On your next inhale, stay up and hold the position, engaging your arms into the socket and lengthening internally from your body center. Avoid over-lifting from your chin and throat, as this will radiate compression throughout the entire spine. Still up, rock back and forth, using the breath and massaging your abdomen and organs as you roll.

Again, avoid reaching from your throat, which causes compression to the cervical and lumbar curves. Doing this over an extended period of time will eventually injure your discs and promote bone spurs. Engage using your core breathing muscles. Try to create and feel the balance in your spinal curves and in your fascial pathways.

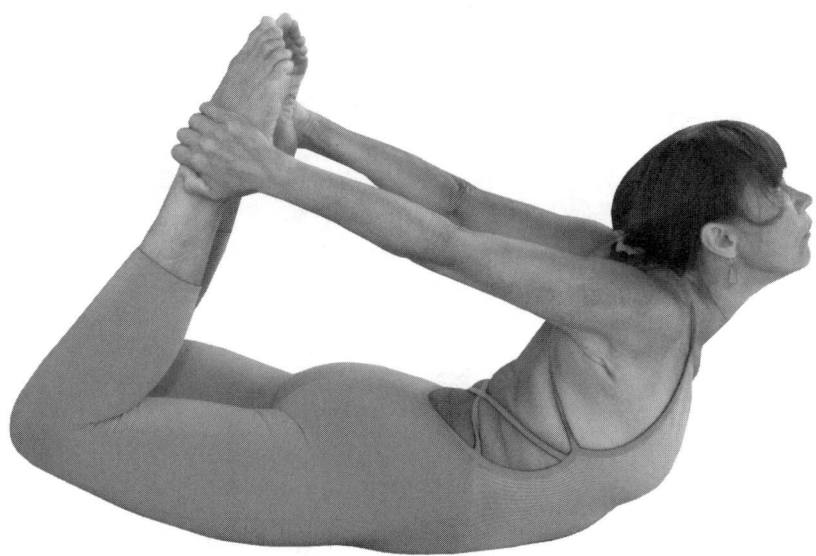

Fig. 60B – INCORRECT: Leading from the throat will compress your neck and lumbar spine.

POSITION #61 — BACKBEND ON A BALL

"Backbend on a Ball" opens and stretches the entire front of your body, enabling you to "let go," releasing both physical and emotional tensions. This pose is a super balancer for all of your fascia lines, but in particular for the core and superficial back and front lines. Having a ball enables you to do the back bend with either passive or active actions. To make this an active pose, you may press your hands against a wall to make your back stronger and your front longer. Like other backbends, this pose relieves compression on your interior spine, tones and massages your abdominal organs, and releases life inhibiting tensions in your belly area. (Remember that chronic tension in your belly engages fight-or-flight responses from your nervous system which inhibit blood flow to your abdominal organs, and slow metabolism, digestion, elimination, and sexual energy.)

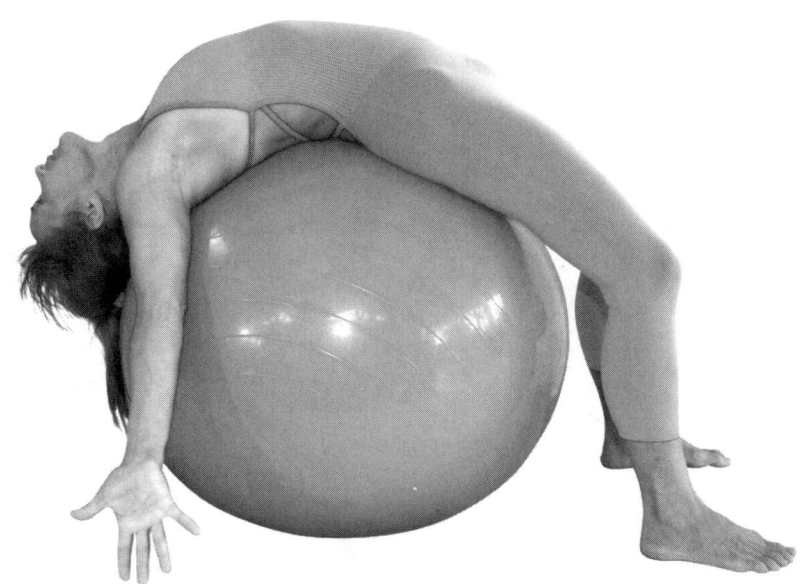

Fig. 61 – Backbend on a Ball

Start by sitting with your lower back and sacral area on the edge of the ball. Slowly lie back, resting your butt and mid-back on top of the ball. Continue to roll back until your neck and head are also resting on the ball, as in **Fig. 61**. It's best to position yourself near a wall so that you can use your hands to stabilize yourself, in case you start to roll sideways off of the ball. Open your arms out to the side with your palms up, your fingers wide open, and your arms pulled back into your trunk.

Ground through your feet and begin the SIP Breath, inhaling through

Caution: If you are not comfortable resting your neck and head on the ball, or you feel strain to the front of the throat, place a small pillow or towel underneath the back of your head.

your mouth and exhaling out of your nose. With the breath, and as you are comfortable, move your hands down the wall, keeping your arms deep in the socket. Keep your elbows from leaning out. Rotate your triceps under to protect your shoulder joints.

Take a deep breath, hold, and engage all of your muscles for a few seconds. Exhale and extend deep into the backbend. Release your jaw and neck muscles with an open mouth exhale. Let go of the unconscious fear that comes up in a deep backbend. When the body feels danger, the psoas and other muscles of the abdomen unconsciously contract, putting your trunk in a vice grip. Practice sensing your whole body and draw your limbs toward center as you radiate energy out through your fascia lines.

On your next exhalation push out all of the air and feel how your muscles contract. Hold the actions, keeping your stomach and rib muscles contracted as you begin to inhale with a SIP Breath. For a few seconds, continue to draw your navel towards your spine creating inner resistance. Release the exhaling muscles and feel the expansion of your ribs as the diaphragm moves down. Continue core breathing and note how much the outer belly stretches each time you inhale. By allowing the outer belly area to lengthen, the diaphragm is freed to move more deeply into your abdomen, toning your organs. As you exhale, the outer belly draws in and the diaphragm releases and moves back up towards the heart and lungs.

On your next inhalation, hold your breath, make fists, and squeeze all of your muscles tightly for several seconds. On the exhale, open your fingers and mouth wide, extend your tongue and draw your limbs into your center, going deeper into the backbend. Repeat several times.

To come out of the pose, slowly walk your hands up (and your feet away from) the wall, so that you roll up supported by the ball. Then slide down the ball until you are in a high squat, leaning against the ball to lengthen your lower back and traction your spine. Push the ball against the wall for more support. Stay here and enjoy the feeling of low back traction from this ball-supported squat.

Optional work while in the squat with the ball: Place a block between your thighs, resisting and squeezing your thighs together to further awaken the deep core line running from your diaphragm and psoas to your inner thigh adductor muscles, all the way down to the arches of your feet. Feel the core line as you inhale and sense the power of aligning from the center of your body.

NOTE: *To release back compression, or if you feel pain, it is ideal to lengthen internally using SIP breathing. However, you may draw the tips of your front ribs down externally to lessen compression in your back as well. Breathing from the core aligns your rib cage with your hips, and keeps pressure off of the lumbar and sacral areas. If you feel tension in the lower back, you need to work at releasing the psoas muscles through breathing. Do not push yourself too hard, but ease into a place of comfort and intensity.*

POSITION #62 — SUPPORTED BRIDGE POSE

The yoga "Bridge" pose is an excellent pose for opening the chest and arm lines of the superficial front line of the body. It has a stabilizing effect on the shoulders and strengthens the extensors along the back line. I recommend using a yoga block to support the sacral-lumbar area and to keep the extra weight off of the neck spine and cervical area. Avoid this pose if you have bulging or herniation of your cervical spine or lower back.

Avoid over-lifting your rib cage by practicing the SIP Breath and focusing on breathing with the side and back ribs.

Lie on the floor on your back, with a yoga block and strap within reach.

Bend your knees and with a light squeezing of your buttock muscles, begin to lift your hips off of the floor until you can rest on top of

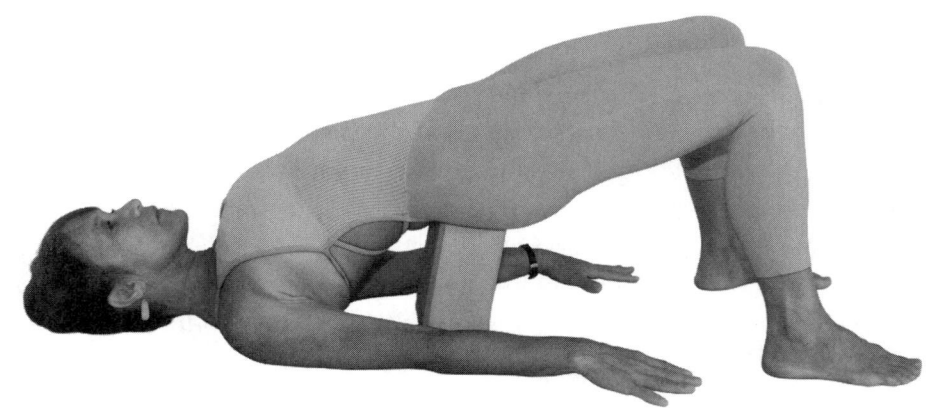

Fig. 62 – Supported Bridge

your shoulders. Put the block under your sacrum and then extend your arms, keeping them shoulder-width apart. Press your palms down into the floor, with your fingers wide open. If you cannot rotate your bones in the forearm comfortably to press the palms down, you can also turn your palms up.

Begin a SIP Breath to add length to your torso and to provide internal support. Feel the muscles and fascia in your heart and chest area expanding when you inhale and retain the feeling of length and openness when you exhale. Stay balanced on the top of your shoulders and press evenly into your feet with your toes spread. Keep a slight contraction in the lower part of your buttocks but do not squeeze too hard as you will add too much effort in your lower back region. Keep your inner thigh muscles gently contracted as though trying to bring your knees together without moving them.

If there is tension in your lower back, check that your front ribs are not popping out and leading to a compression in the back of the rib cage. You can use the SIP Breath to tether the ribcage to the pulling action of the diaphragm's descent, while guiding the tip of the breastbone into alignment with the hips. By doing this you get an internalized adjustment of posture that does not create tension in the extremities.

> **Note:** In YogAlign we recommend trying this pose with a strap and practicing neutral arm width to support functional body movements. Individuals who have very flexible shoulder ligaments may do this with ease; however, remember to balance the actions of flexibility and strength in all poses to avoid the dangers of ligament stretching and hypermobility in your shoulder.

POSITION# 63 — THE WHEEL (ADVANCED)

If you feel at ease doing the backbend on the ball and have no shoulder, low back or wrist injuries, you can proceed to do this more advanced pose: the "Free-Standing Backbend" or "Wheel" pose. "The Wheel" is a powerful stretch for the superficial front line and deep core line. It both strengthens your extensor muscles in the posterior of the back body and arm regions, and balances the muscle/fascial pathways of your functional lines. Ultimately, this pose stretches and tones your entire body. This pose also opens the heart and chest and can help alleviate insomnia and depression. Posture, too, is balanced, with the pose correcting forward head carriage and rounding of the shoulders.

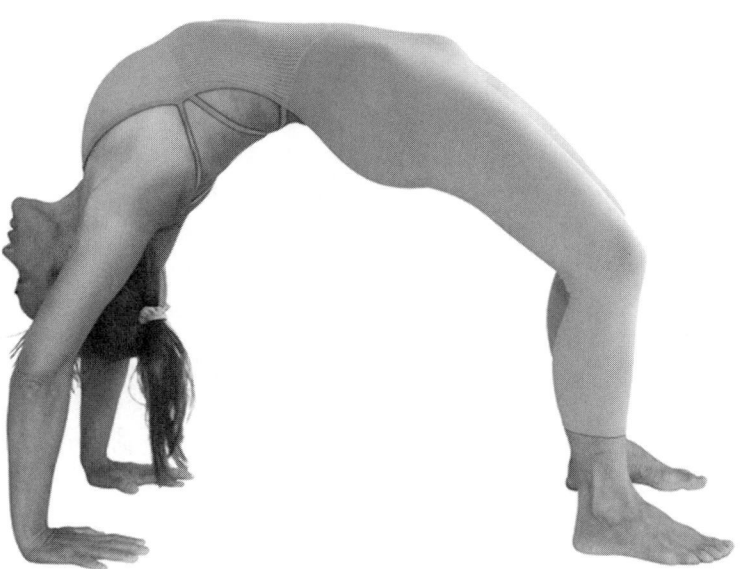

Fig. 63A – The Wheel

This pose will free your spine and relax your mind. Energetically, it opens your heart, helping you to release fear while building willpower and confidence. "The Wheel" is a finely-tuned balance between pushing and letting go. If you hold tension in your neck or try to lift from the top of your shoulders, you will not find a place of ease in this posture and you will possibly do more harm than good to your structure. Through this pose you can learn how to balance the actions of pushing and yielding at the same time.

For "The Wheel," begin by massaging your hands and wrists to bring blood flow and awareness to these delicate parts of your structure. If you have tension in your wrists or shoulders, you may use blocks placed against a wall to raise the level of your shoulders to your hips. Having your hands on the blocks will aid in releasing tension in your shoulders and wrists.

Do not attempt this pose if you have any serious wrist or shoulder pain. Instead, use the ball for your backbends rather than putting undue stress on your wrist joints. Remember, no pain means no strain, and you will not get comfortable by being uncomfortable.

From the "Supported Bridge Pose," move the block away from your sacrum area and begin to extend your arms overhead and bend your elbows, placing your hands (palms down and shoulder-width apart) underneath the tops of your shoulder. Stay balanced on your entire hand, pressing into the floor with your fingers wide and active.

Note: Draw your elbows in line above your hands, your forearms drawn in, and your shoulder blades engaged deeply, keeping them away from the tops of your shoulders. Feel the actions of your latissimus dorsi muscles as well as the muscles that stabilize your scapula.

Breathe in as you press with your hands and feet, keeping them evenly engaged. Lift your hips off of the floor and bring the top of your head to the mat, being careful not to compress your neck. Activate your muscles to pull your arms deep into their sockets, and connect with your lateral, or latissimus, muscles for extra support from your back. Your entire arm should be one long line of energy, beginning at your rib cage and hips. In the front, feel your arms connecting into your chest. In the side and back body, draw your muscle actions toward center and feel how your arms are like wings that extend from your core. Stay grounded in your legs with equal weight, and focus on feeling the effort of the posture being distributed throughout your whole body. Come down on an exhale and rest for a moment. Come up again, and press up into the arch, feeling your body extending and shining like a ray of light energy.

Relax your neck. Lift your heels off of the floor and gently contract your gluteals. Sense the alignment in your spine. Stay lifted in the front-body and rooted into your legs and feet. Take a deep Core SIP Breath and hold, tightening all of your muscles for five seconds. As you exhale and release, press up higher into "The Wheel." Engage your hands and feet firmly and pull your limbs into the center of your body. If you are practicing with others, ask them to check your alignment to ensure that the tips of your ribs are level with the tops of your hips as shown in **Fig. 63A**.

Press on the inner edges of your feet and, if you feel tension in the knees or lower back, let your feet turn out slightly. Lumbar compression in this pose can occur due to shortened psoas muscles, or over-lifting your chest using your front ribs. Breathing deeply will help to activate your diaphragm, creating a fascial pull that aligns your ribs to your hips. If you still feel compression, tip your lower ribs towards your pubic bone to bring your back ribs away from your hips. If you continue to have pain in your lower back, practice the "Free-Standing Backbend" on a ball. Wait until you have the strength and awareness in your deep psoas muscles to push up into this backbend without a struggle. Come down slowly to the mat and rest with your knees bent for a moment, letting your back muscles relax and soften. Slowly rotate your knees from side to side and then end with a full body stretch.

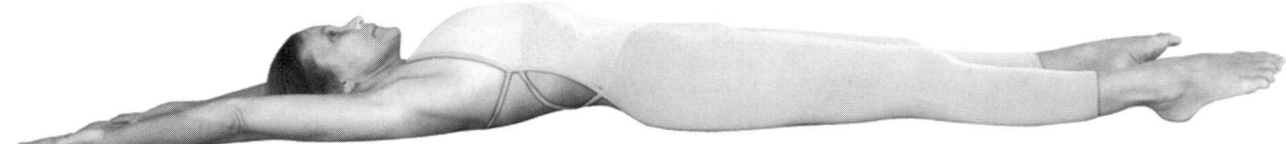

Fig. 63B – The Full Body Stretch (Position #1)

POSITION #64 — HANDSTAND (ADVANCED)

The "Handstand" is a fun pose that invokes the sense of being a kid. This pose creates energy and is an effective mood elevator, calling upon the strength and flexibility of your entire body. "Handstand" also tones your entire body and is a great pose for developing balance and inner core strength. The pose fine tunes your vestibular system, which affects balance, eyesight, hearing, and kinesthetic awareness—the sense of where you are in space. In particular, the muscles affecting your scapula are balanced and made flexible in order to support the weight of your lower body. Practice "Down Dog" and "Traction Dog" before attempting to do the handstand. If you learn the building blocks of YogAlign, which strengthen the lower trapezius, rhomboids, lats, serratus anterior, and the pec minor in synergy, you will be tuned and ready to try this pose without any risk of joint injury, pain, or strain to your wrists or shoulders.

Always make sure your poses look like you are standing well with aligned posture, no matter in which direction your body is going. Make sure that the surface you are practicing on is level and firm. Do not use an extra thick, soft yoga mat as it could lead to overstretching of your wrist ligaments.

You can do this pose safely against a wall to give you the opportunity to fine tune your balance without worrying about falling over. Start by massaging your hands and wrists to bring blood flow and awareness to your wrist joints. Position yourself on your hands and knees, shoulder-width apart, about a foot from the wall. Consciously place your hands on your mat or the floor with your fingers wide and your arms connected into your shoulder sockets. Free your neck, keeping it lengthened and aligned with the rest of your spine. Feel your arms connecting to your lats and back extensors at their foundation in your core.

Traction Dog: Preparation for a Safe Handstand

From your hands and knees, lift up into "Traction Dog," keeping your shoulders away from your ears, your forearms aligned and your upper arm bones lifted to prevent hyperextension of your shoulder joint. Try to retain these muscle actions. Position your legs as though you're about to start running, with one leg forward. Inhale and kick your back leg up to the wall, followed by the other leg.

Note: *You will likely be more comfortable kicking up with one leg more than the other; however, once you are proficient in "Handstand," it is recommended that you also practice kicking up with your less dominant leg, to balance the back and leg muscles.*

Once in the inverted position, let your head drop to neutral and balance on your hands, pressing evenly with your palms and fingertips. Keep your shoulders pulled away from your ears to maintain the connection to your core. Inhale

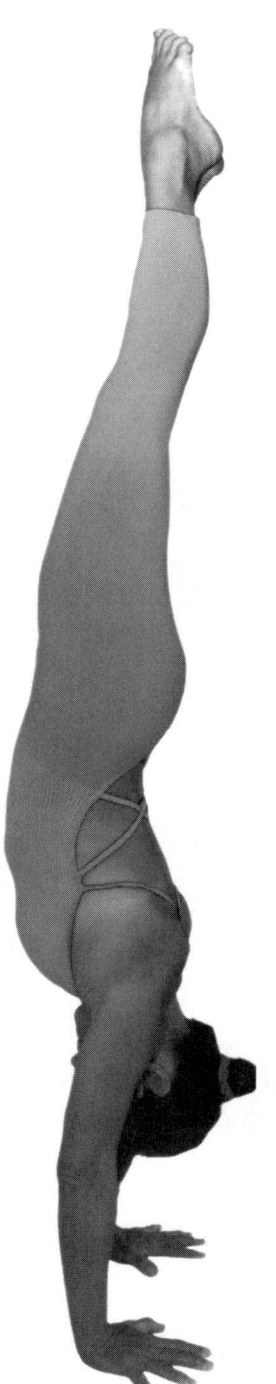

Fig. 64A – CORRECT: Handstand

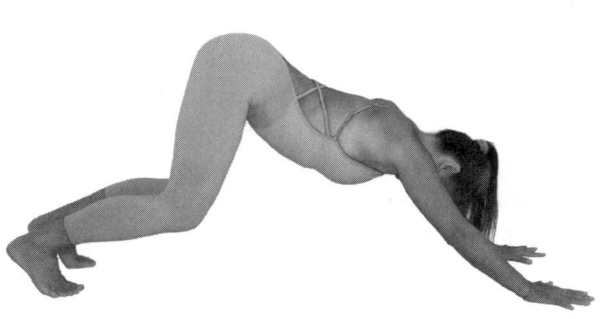

Traction Dog (Position #29)

with a SIP Breath and feel yourself lifted and steadied by a strong internal ring of support. Keep one foot balanced on the wall and extend up with your opposite leg while keeping both of your feet pointed or flointed.

If you feel balanced, bring your other foot away from the wall, bringing both legs together. Squeeze your inner thighs and glutes, staying active in your feet while practicing core breathing to generate support from your center. Sense your entire body and listen to the sounds around you. Avoid thinking. Practice being in the now, and balance the efforts of your eyes by consciously looking with both eyes.

Equalize your vision for balance. To perfect your balance you must equalize the amount of effort between both of your eyes. All modern humans have a tendency to be side-dominant. The over-engagement of one side of your eye muscles can create just enough muscle tension to pull you to one side and prevent you from finding perfect balance. If you are right-handed, practice gazing predominately through your left eye. If you are left handed, emphasize your gaze through your right eye. Alternatively, you can also wear a patch on your dominant eye. In all poses, you should strive to have a gaze that is balanced in both of your eyes. When doing inverted poses, it becomes particularly crucial that your eyesight is balanced.

YogAlign principles recommend keeping your head in neutral rather than lifting your chin to support yourself. When you lift your chin, the neck spine compresses and shortens, as shown in **Fig. 64B**.

Come down slowly with control, bringing down one leg at a time while keeping your hands engaged. Come to standing or kneel down with your hips on a block and massage your hands and wrists again. Notice how you feel and whether your energy has shifted or increased. Do your hips feel level? Do you feel as though you are more aligned, with more freedom in your breathing process?

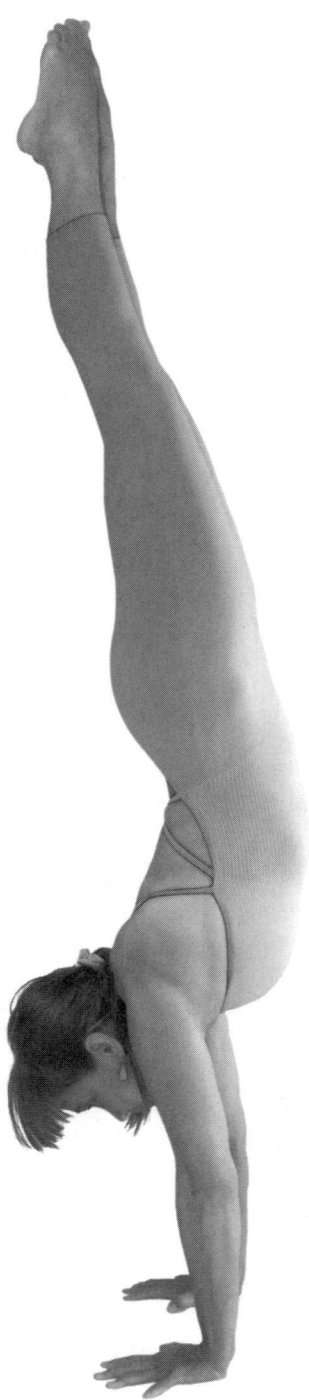

Fig. 64B – INCORRECT: Handstand

Position #65 — Forearm Stand (Advanced)

"Forearm Stand" is a powerful inversion calling upon the strength and flexibility of your entire body. Like the "Handstand," the "Forearm Stand" requires balanced actions in the muscles that stabilize the position of your scapulae. You must have a very strong, stable, and aligned shoulder joint to attempt this pose.

Inverting your body in "Forearm Stand" massages and tones your abdominal organs. One gains a sense of power, the will is sharpened, and fears and anxiety are alleviated with regular practice. The muscles and fascia of the core line, the spinal muscles, and the diaphragm are enlisted to stabilize your spine with eccentric contractions. The legs and gluteals become strong and toned, with the ring of support that occurs when you do the YogAlign SIP Breath.

In the YogAlign version of the "Forearm Stand," the pose is done with the head in line with the spine rather than letting the chin lift upwards. Lifting the chin shrugs your shoulders, causing a loss of core spinal integrity, which can in turn lead to hyperextension of your lower back and compression of the lumbar sacral area.

Using inhalation to find your inner ring of support is especially important in this pose, as the weight of your legs and torso is above non-weight bearing joints in the shoulder and neck spine, putting them at risk for injury. Strength and synergy in the lower trapezius, rhomboids, lats, serratus anterior, and the pec minor will give you the balance and tuning you need to do this pose without risk.

When you come down from the handstand, keep your legs active and bring them down one at a time. Always use a wall or a partner to spot you, to avoid injury.

Come onto your hands and knees about a foot away from a wall, positioning yourself sideways to a mirror in order to monitor your spine alignment. Come up into the "Traction Dog" pose (Position #29) by first turning your palms up towards the ceiling and pressing the tops of your hands into the floor. Keep your elbows in line with your shoulders and

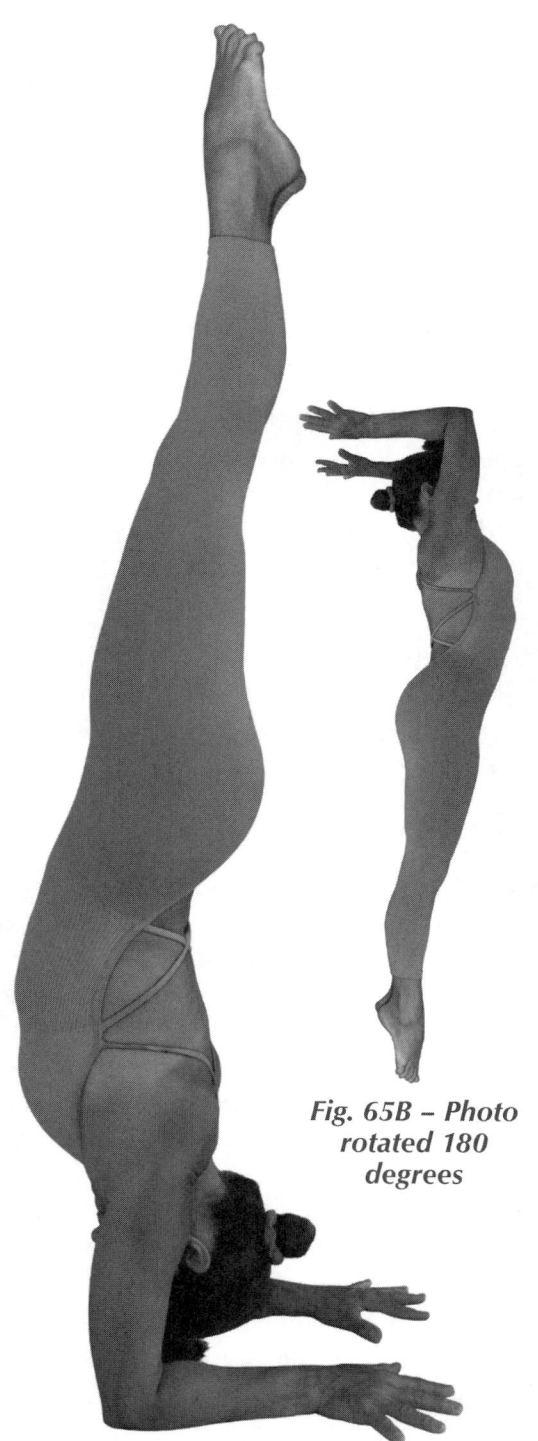

Fig. 65B – Photo rotated 180 degrees

Fig. 65A – CORRECT: Forearm Stand

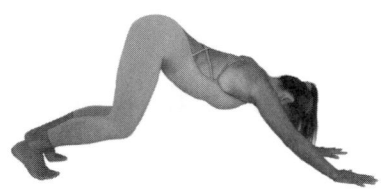

Traction Dog (Position #29)

your arms engaged into their sockets. As you press your hands into the floor, notice that your arm bones engage back to the core through the fascial connections of your arm lines. Retain these actions and next, slowly turn your palms to the floor, keeping the integration of the muscles in your back and especially rooting down with your scapula.

From "Traction Dog," bring your forearms to the mat, keeping your shoulders well away from your ears. Press your hands and the balls of your feet strongly into the mat. Keep your fingers and toes spread. Inhale, lift your hips and kick your legs, one at a time, up to the wall. Your arms should stay in the same position while you keep the back of your neck long, without lifting your chin. Avoid strain in the shoulder and don't let your elbows wing out to the sides.

Practice Core Breathing to find your inner ring of support. Squeeze your inner legs and buttock muscles as you press on the inner edges of your forearms. Concentrate on keeping your scapulae moving towards your hips and heart. Point or floint your feet up to the ceiling while actively spreading and extending your toes and letting your neck hang loose. Hold the pose from the very center of your body by enlisting the power of your breath. Stay here for several breaths, until you feel yourself unable to hold the core alignment. Come down from the pose carefully, one leg at a time.

Avoid lifting your head in this pose as it will reinforce forward head carriage. Do not practice the inverted shrugging pose (a.k.a. "The Nixon Version"). It looks bad, feels bad, and worse, it may damage discs in your cervical spine or cause injury in your rotator cuff. Always ask yourself: Can I breathe deeply? Do I have the spinal curves in natural alignment?

Mind Your Alignment

When doing inverted poses, strive to keep optimal alignment as though you were in a natural standing position. Looking at **Fig. 65A**, notice that my head is not touching the mat; when this same photo is rotated 180 degrees (**Fig. 65B**), I look as though I am standing with good posture, because the effort of the pose is engaged from my inner core muscles rather than from my neck and upper trapezius muscles. Many people do the forearm stand with their head lifted up and their neck and back spine hyper-extended and overarched, as shown in **Fig. 65C**. There is danger when you burden your neck spine and shoulder joints with the weight of the lower body, especially when you are not in natural alignment. Many people have incurred injuries in the neck and shoulders doing inversions with poor alignment that exert unnatural force and weight on delicate joints. Do not do a pose if you feel unnecessary pressure or force in any part of your body. When you are aligned in breath and spine, you will feel connected to your core with an equalized effort throughout your entire body—as though you are floating in the pose.

Fig. 65C – INCORRECT: The shrugging forearm stand puts intense pressure forces on the shoulder joint, neck spine and the dura matter.

POSITION # 66 — ACTIVE CHILD'S POSE WITH NECK ROLLS

"Active Child's Pose with Neck Rolls" releases chronic neck, jaw, and back tension. Headaches, TMJ, vertigo, and poor posture can be healed with regular practice of this pose. Your knees are kept at least shoulder-width apart to allow you to lean forward without overly rounding your upper back or compressing your anterior spine. The superficial back line is stretched, and tenseness and soreness in your neck muscles is re-patterned and alleviated. Circulation in the lymph glands in your armpits is increased, enhancing your immune functions. The neck rolls use PNF exercises to release tense facial muscle patterning from the neck muscles of the occiput region, where the muscles of the neck spine join to the base of your skull. Do not attempt this pose if you have severe bone spurs, whiplash, or disc herniation in your cervical spine.

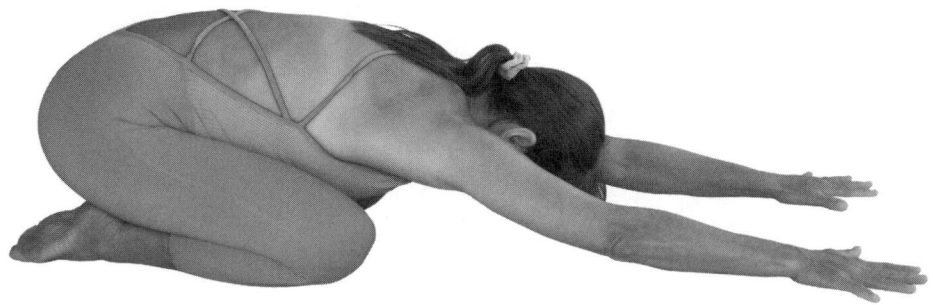

Fig. 66A – Active Child's Pose

Begin on your hands and knees with your fingers spread wide and palms pressing into the floor, as in **Fig. 66A**. Keeping your front spine lengthened, shift your hips back over your heels moving your knees further apart, allowing space for your belly to rest between your thighs. Press your hands down, keeping your elbows lifted as you draw your shoulders away from your ears, lengthening your neck. Use the movements from your breath to stretch your rib cage from the inside out. If you feel discomfort in your knees or the tops of your feet, place a block under your hips.

Neck Rolls

Inhale and drop your elbows and forehead to the floor. Lift your hips and begin to roll forward as in **Fig. 66B**. Keep the weight of your head and shoulders on your forearms with no pressure on your neck spine. Exhale back to "Active Child's Pose" (**Fig. 66A**), lifting your elbows off of the mat and pressing down with your hands to actively stretch your shoulder girdle. On your next inhale, roll forward and do the "Neck Roll" as above keeping the weight of your head and shoulders on your forearms, with no pressure on your neck spine (**Fig. 66B**). Stay in this position and practice PNF by further tightening the areas that feel contracted. As you exhale, release that tension and roll in deeper. Keep weight off of your neck and spine at all times. For extra health benefits, massage your neck-to-skull attachments in this position while keeping weight on the elbows and off of your neck.

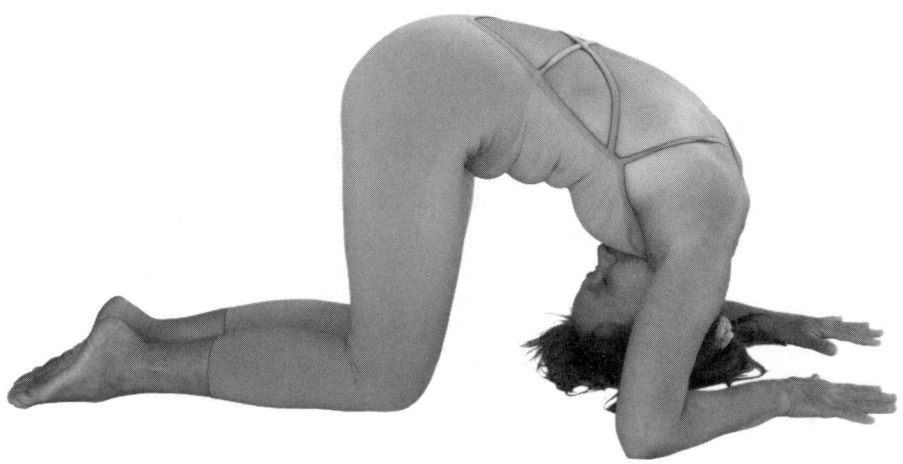

Fig. 66B – Neck Rolls

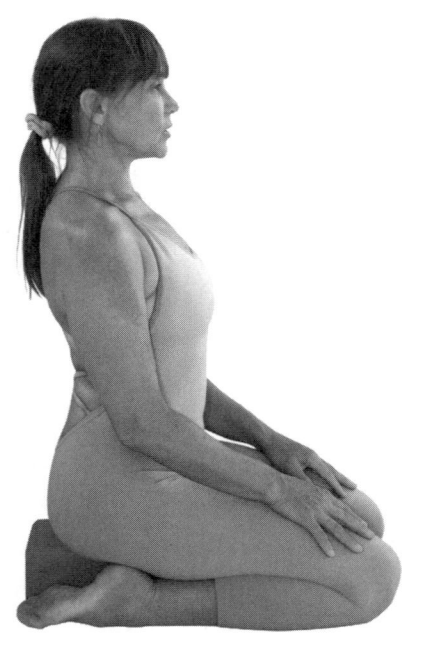

Fig. 66C – Drink in the effects of the neck rolls and feel your head "floating atop your spine."

Roll back to the "Active Child's Pose," straightening your arms and lengthening your spine. Turn your head to the right, lift your hips, and complete a neck roll with your head looking right. Repeat the PNF exercise three times by tightening the areas that are contracted and feel tight. Release, and begin the "Neck Roll" returning to "Active Child's Pose" on the exhale. Alternate the "Active Child's Pose" and the "Neck Roll" going back and forth a few times, until you feel a release of tension.

Turn your head all the way to the left now and repeat the PNF exercise on this side. Stay here as long as you are comfortable and massage the side of your neck. Roll back to the "Active Child's Pose" and notice what you are feeling. Is there more mobility as you turn your head? Come into a kneeling position, placing your hips on a block, and focus on how your neck feels, noticing the effects of the pose (**Fig. 66C**). Feel the weight of your head balanced atop your spine as though it is floating there effortlessly.

Position #67 — Monkey Squat

Before the invention of the chair, squatting was part of everyone's daily life. Today, few people can squat without pain or injury. The "Monkey Squat" helps release tension in your hip and legs. This is a pose that will tone your pelvic floor and abdominal organs and, in particular, your bladder. In cultures where squatting is done every day, people stay flexible and aligned well into advanced age. Prostate and colon cancer, knee and hip replacements, and osteoarthritis are rare in cultures that still squat. This pose also aids the digestive and elimination processes and brings a feeling of lightness to your body.

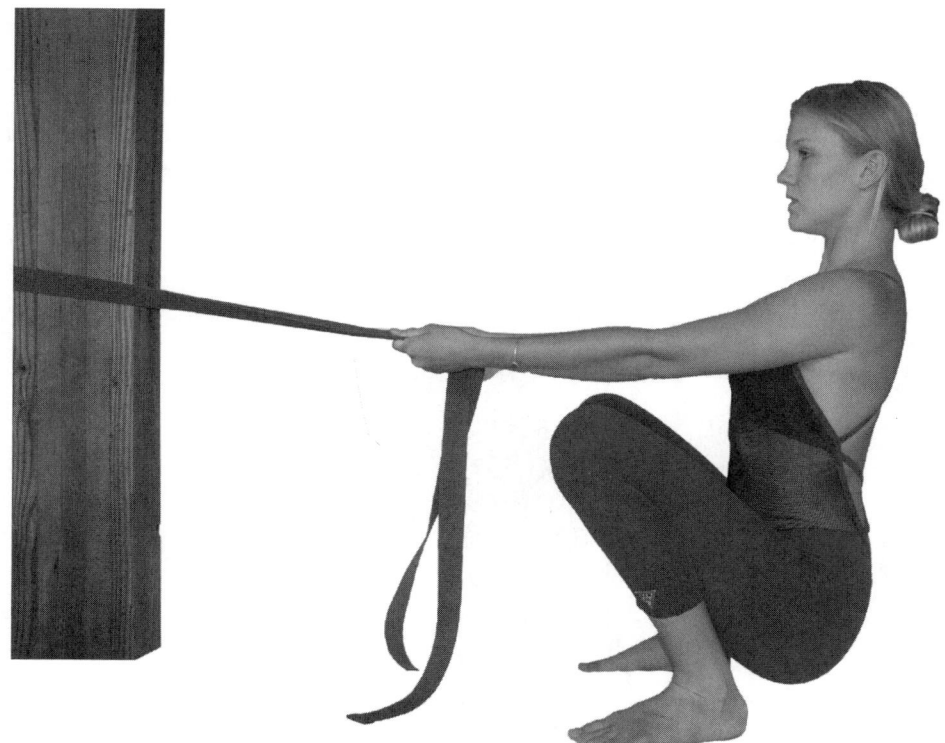

Fig. 67A – Using a strap enables you to pull back, lengthen and traction your spine.

Unless you are a seasoned squatter with excellent knees, it is best to use a strap for support in this pose, to keep compression off of your knees. Place a strap around a post, doorknob or tree, holding one end in each hand. Slowly drop into a squatting position, with arms straight and engaged strongly through your lats to your hips and into your trunk. Activate your shoulder blade muscles to keep the blades stabilized and your neck elongated. Position the strap just below shoulder level, and keep your feet slightly turned out. Stay up on the balls of your feet as you slide back, pulling on the straps while you squat with a lift in your waist, curve in your lower back and your entire spine and skull in natural alignment.

Continue in a squatting position with your feet slightly turned out and your hands on the floor in front of you. Move from one foot to the other like a monkey, balancing on the balls of your feet. Practice core breathing and elongate from your center. If you can squat without a strap, place your elbows between your thighs and press your hands together into "Namaste," as in **Fig. 67B**. Begin to practice Core Breathing and notice how your pelvic floor widens, allowing your sit bones to engage towards the floor on the inhale.

If possible, use a mirror to observe your spine from the side. Look for proper tilt in the sacrum and natural curvature in your lower back. Use Core Breathing to awaken the psoas and achieve more elongation in your spine. Don't let the upper back round or the lower back flatten. Keep extension in your spine and elasticity in the movement of your diaphragm. Lower your heels towards the floor only if you can do so without compressing and shortening the front of your body.

Don't stay in a squat if your knees are tight or sore.

Practice PNF techniques by holding your breath for a few seconds and tightening your muscles. As you exhale and release, lengthen your front spine and keep your head aligned, resting atop your spine. Keep a tilt in your sacrum with your shoulder blades engaged. Your neck feels free and your head is floating.

Practice squatting to stay young forever. You can squat on many occasions, even in daily tasks such as gardening or using the toilet.

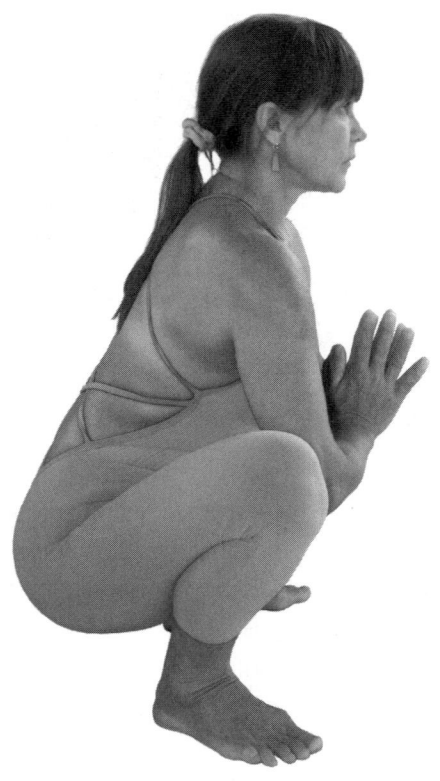

Fig. 67B – Monkey Squat

POSITION #68 — WIDE-LEG FORWARD BEND

This pose balances the muscle/fascia lines in your legs, keeps your hips flexible, and tones your pelvic floor. Hip rotators are strengthened and balanced while your inner thighs tone and relax. You can practice PNF in this pose to make fast progress in becoming flexible without strain.

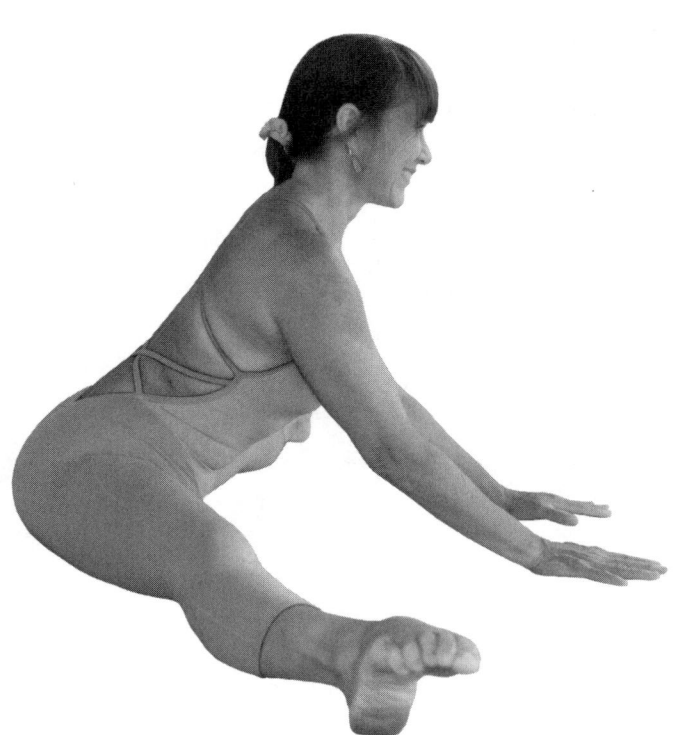

Fig. 68A – Wide-Leg Forward Bend

To do a "Wide-Leg Forward Bend" from a seated position, first open your legs as widely as possible with your toes pointing or flointing. If you lose the curve in your lower back, bend your knees until the curve reappears. Place a small pillow under your sit bones if you cannot get your hips level or if you cannot get your sacrum and lower back into the curves of natural spine alignment. Position yourself on the bottom of your sit bones by pulling the flesh of your buttocks back up and out of the way. Point or floint your feet being careful not to extend through your heel in the braking position. If your upper back rounds or you lose the curve in your spine, bend your knees even more.

Place your hands on the floor behind your trunk with your fingertips pointing in towards your hips. Lean back on your hands and breathe deeply, opening your chest and front spine. Practice tightening and releasing your engaged muscles using PNF exercises to recode your neuromuscular patterning and reset the resting muscle lengths for more flexibility.

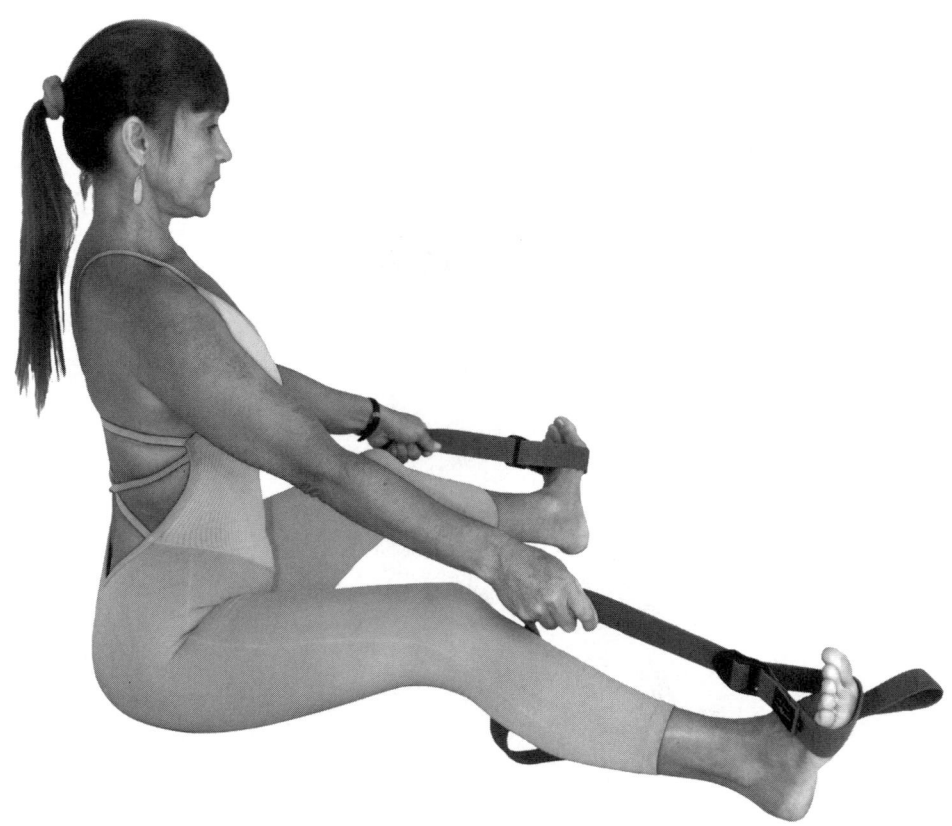

Fig. 68B – Spine traction to forward bend, with strap.

From here, if you feel that you can't even begin to lean forward, put yoga straps around the balls of your feet as in **Fig. 68B**. Bend your knees, if necessary, to get your spine into natural alignment. Keep the shoulders down and your spine aligned, lifted and active.

Notice the feeling of your breathing tube or trachea as you inhale. Feel how it extends with inhalation and keep the lift as you exhale and progress in the pose. Use a mirror to check for natural spine alignment, making sure that your ear is in line with the middle of your shoulder and your head is in line with your spinal column. Look for a 30-degree tilt of your sacrum and an inward curve of the lumbar spine. Your rib cage should be aligned above your hips. The SIP Breath can assist you in finding alignment and extension from your inner core. If this pose feels intense and your upper back wants to round excessively, stay here; otherwise, you may begin to lean forward.

If you are quite flexible and can lean forward without the use of the straps, bring your hands in front of you while keeping the length and lift of your front spine as in **Fig. 68A**. Practice breathing and keeping extension from your center. Your sacrum (sacroiliac) joints should feel stable and supported before you attempt to lean forward. Stay lifted in your front spine as you begin to lean forward. Place your palms on

Essential YogAlign Poses

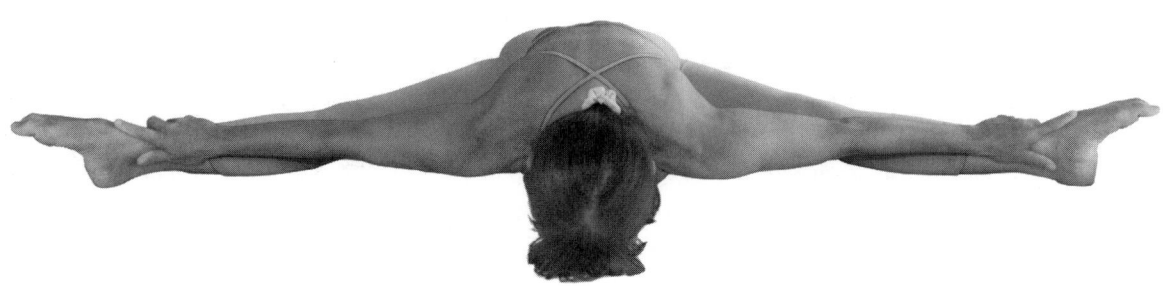

Fig. 68C – If you lean over, keep your toes pointed!

the floor in front of your trunk. Stay on the base of your sit bones, and avoid rounding your upper back or flattening your sacral lumbar area in order to lean further forward.

Inhale with the SIP Breath technique and hold the pose, pointing your toes, activating your entire body, and extra-tightening your muscles. Exaggerate the muscle tightening, focusing on your pelvic floor muscles. When you exhale, relax the pelvic floor muscles and continue engaging your feet in a point or floint. Stay lifted, keeping the core extension that comes from the inhalation process. You may be able to go towards the floor as in **Fig. 68C**, but do not attempt this if you have to round your upper back in order to get there.

Inhale and hold your breath, squeezing what feels tight while you keep extending and lengthening. Exhale, holding your extension and length as you lean farther forward. Don't let the body shorten when you exhale, but keep the "gift of the lift." Open your mouth wide when you exhale and feel tension running out of your body like water.

When you come up, softly shake out your legs and prepare for meditation by doing a "Full Body Stretch."

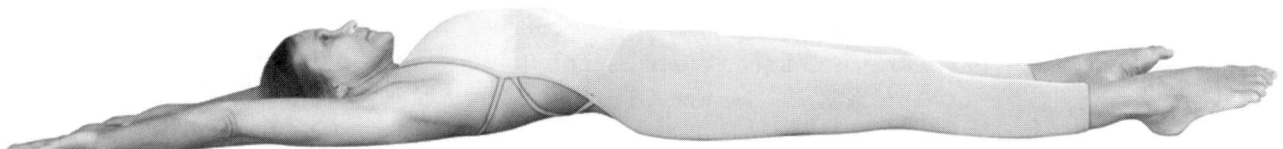

Fig. 68D – Full Body Stretch (Position#1)

Position #69 — Meditation

In the ancient Yoga Sutras, the path of yoga is meant to prepare you for meditation and God (or source) realization. Yoga is a tool that helps us remove the obstacles that keep us from feeling connected to our true source. It is only our thoughts that keep us suffering and the demands of our ego that keep us believing that we are separate. By the regular practice of meditation we can clear our mind of the thoughts that keep us suffering in the past and projecting into the future. In meditation, we learn that we are the awareness behind our thoughts. We are intrinsically connected to all that is. Through the practice of meditation, our mind chatter drops away and we can then experience the truth of who we are. Beyond thoughts and concepts is our true nature—the force of life itself.

Come into a seated position with a block or bolster under your hips. Use as many blocks as you need in order to sit in ease with no pressure on your knees, hips or ankles. The position in **Fig. 69** is a great way to meditate because it is very natural, and it allows for easy maintenance of good posture and spine alignment.

Mediation is a practice in witnessing the present moment. Be aware of the antics of your mind. The mind is much like a theater in that you can use it to watch movies about the past and the future, or you can use it to watch the programming of the present time. When you start to over-identify with the mind and go into the future or the past, you miss what is occurring in the present. When you do this, you miss your life because you are not fully experiencing it. This is why so many of us feel like our lives are speeding by. When your mind is racing to the past and future, it is similar to driving too fast in a car. The scenery is going by so fast that you miss the beautiful details and subtlety of living.

Make sure that your higher awareness is running the projector and that you are actually experiencing the present moment. If you have a lot of thoughts arising from the past or future, observe them in the same way that you are listening to the birds, and then bring your awareness back to the present moment.

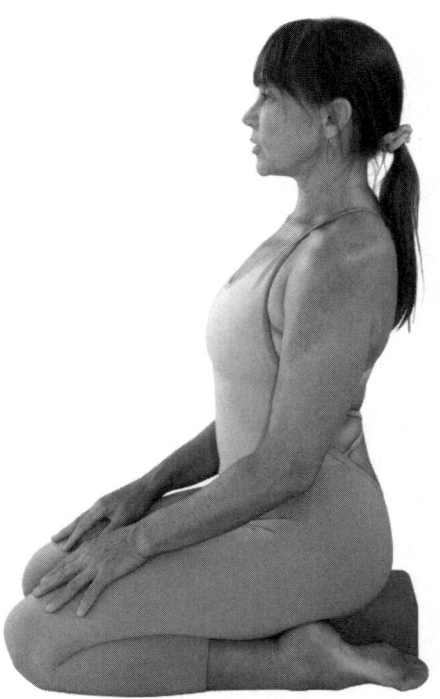

Fig. 69 – Meditation is ideal when sitting in a natural spine position supported by your inner core.

Much of the suffering we feel in our lives comes from identifying ourselves with our mind. Our mind is a great tool, but who we are is not just the thoughts coming from our mind. With over-identification on the past and future programming of our minds, we become trapped by a poverty of thought that keeps us frozen in fears or biases, preventing us from seeing things as they really are. We can use our mind to make decisions and process information when needed, but it is wise to learn meditation techniques that reduce the excess thoughts leading to worry, fears and expectations.

There is much wisdom in the simple saying that "tomorrow never comes but today is always here." We are never the same in any given moment and even our perception of who we are is limited by our linear thinking processes. In Meditation, we simply allow ourselves to reside in the moment without trying to label or judge the experience. We begin to shift to a place of "being." When you practice sensing your body, watching the breathing process and noticing the sounds around you all at the same time, there is a huge shift in awareness. This shift takes you to the eternal present, which is where life happens.

Many of us are on a quest to find meaning and to figure out the deep mysteries of life. We want to grab on to something and define our life. Sometimes when we try too hard to define life, these thoughts can keep us bound up in the future and prevent us from enjoying life in the now; consequently, we feel as though life is speeding up and passing us by. The truth is that there is no need to define life, because you are life. Simply witness the feeling of the forces in your being, take a breath and know in every moment that you are life itself. Life is here within us and it is only our thoughts about the past, future, and what we have or don't have, that keep us in a state of suffering and unacceptance.

To liberate one's self from the tyranny of our own minds, meditation is the yogic path to understanding, training, and transcending our mind to serve our highest good. We can direct our body to do poses or to exercise, but calming and training our mind is the most important work that we do both in yoga and in our life. The question becomes: how do we train our mind to be peaceful? For many, meditation is very difficult and we feel the chaos of our thoughts. The harder we try to turn off the mind, the more we are engaging the mind. This action is much like the monkey chasing his own tail. The best way to calm the mind is simply to practice feeling your body and breath, and to sense the world around you.

One of the tools to help you stay with the present is to sense "The Five B's"—Body, Breath, Birds, Breeze, and Being.

1st B
Sensing your BODY in its entirety.

2nd B
Sensing the feeling of your BREATH happening naturally.

3rd B
Sensing the BIRDS singing nearby or any sounds occurring in your environment.

4th B
Sensing the feeling of the BREEZE and the air around your body.

5th B
Sensing the Now of all of these B's or BEING at once, without judging, naming or labeling them.
Just sense and witness what is happening now, in this moment.

As you sit in meditation, practice simultaneously sensing these five B's. You can shift to a higher awareness and natural state of being in the moment by simply shifting to a feeling state. You can meditate all throughout your day and be aligned, present, and in the Now.

POSITION #70 — REST POSE AND FACE MASSAGE

The "Rest Pose" is called Shavasana *or "Corpse Pose" in the yoga tradition. Here, you relax and let go of the effort to move your body and focus instead on just being and feeling. We add a self-massage of the face to the "Rest Pose" in the YogAlign practice. It takes only a few minutes and does so much for your body and spirit.*

Here you can become a human being and not a "human doing." It is very important to give your body a chance to unwind and also to learn to calm the mind when your body is still. By being the witness to your body in its entirety, the movement of breath and the sounds occurring, you can shift to your higher awareness and connection to source, where you can experience a sense of inner peace.

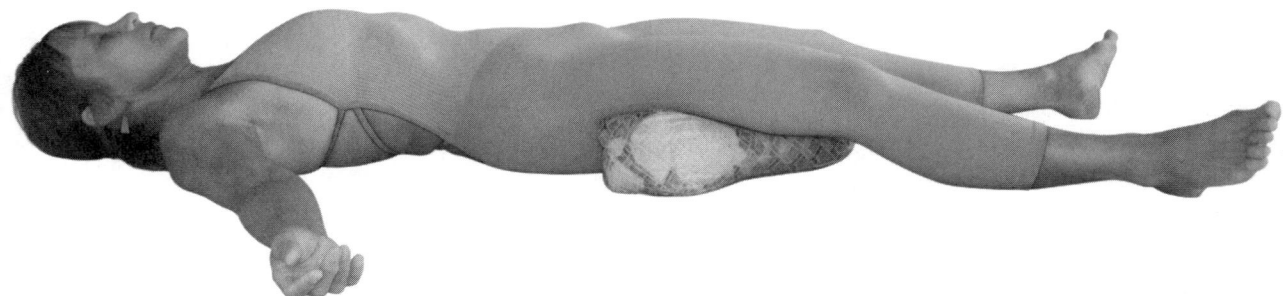

Fig. 70A – Rest Pose

Lie on your back with bolsters under your thighs to support the natural curves in your spine. It is important that you not lie in "Rest Pose" without some kind of support under your knees or thighs; this is essential for proper back support when reclining. The organs are heavy and can press weight into the vertebrae of your lower back. **Caution:** If you have serious lower back pain or injuries, do the pose while lying on your side with a small pillow supporting your neck and another one between your knees.

Begin to massage your face, starting with your scalp muscles (**Fig. 70B**). Stay present with your natural breathing process as you massage deeply around your skull, sensing the thin layer of scalp muscles, and massaging gently into any tenderness that you feel. Massage your ears on the inside and outside, paying attention to where the ear muscles connect to the jaw. Deeply massage your ear-to-jaw connection. As you go deeper into relaxation, let your body breathe on its own. Simply be present and observe its rhythm without attempting to control or direct.

Move down to the temples and massage in slow circles. Listen to your body and allow it to inform you of where it needs to be massaged and with what kind of pressure. Move from the temples to the jaw, starting at the hinge point. Massage the entire length of your jaw all the way to your chin. Use your thumbs to massage the muscles under your chin. Use your fingertips to massage the outside of your gums in your lower jaw. Move from the center of your jaw towards the molars. Switch to your upper gums and work your way back to the upper molars and then out to the hinge of your jaw, completing a circle.

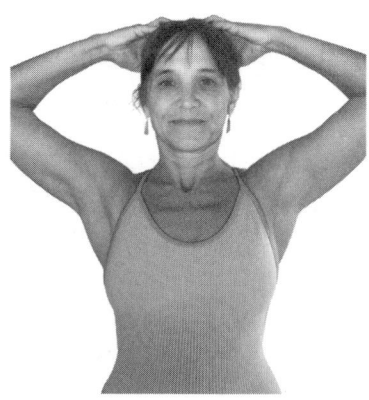 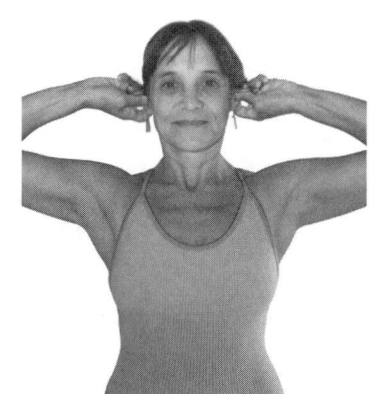 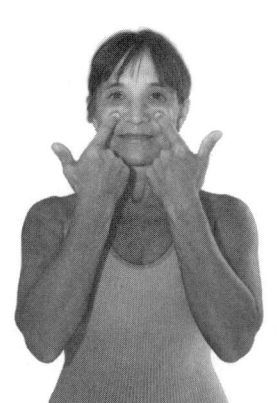

Fig. 70B – Face Massage

Press your index fingers into your sinus points at the base of each of your nostrils. Massage gently in circles, tracing the cheekbone all the way back to the jaw. Gently press into your upper and lower eye sockets, massaging softly. Move back up to the forehead and use your fingertips to massage from the scalp to the outside of your eyebrows. Hold your thumbs into the depression at the start of your eyebrows and your fingertips into the middle of your forehead for a few seconds. Go back to your scalp and press gently into the very top of your head, looking for soreness and massaging those areas gently but firmly.

Rub your hands together very quickly, feeling pranic heat start to build up. To get even more heat into your hands, take a Core SIP Breath while rubbing the hands together. Hold the breath and pull up on your pelvic floor as though you are trying not to pee and continue to rub your hands. Exhale and release the pelvic floor, quickly placing your heated hands on closed eyes. Let the heat melt tension from your face and skull. When the heat subsides, brush your hands down the front of your body, finishing with your arms out to your sides on the floor, with your palms facing up (**Fig. 70A**).

Slide your shoulder blades down your back so that your shoulders are level as you rest. Check that your chin is not lifted. It should be at the same level as your forehead. Place a small pillow under the back of your head if your chin is higher than your forehead. Your neck is long and your shoulders are drawn away from your ears as in (**Fig. 70A**).

As you lie on the floor, feel as though your skin is softening. Allow the boundaries of your body to disappear as though you are turning into a liquid pool of energy. As you sense your whole body, let the involuntary breathing process take over. Let the breath just happen, as you simply observe your body in its entirety. Keep observing your breathing process. Feel your entire body and be aware of any sounds or sensations outside your body. Witness whatever is happening in the present without labeling or judging whatever it is.

As you hear the sounds of birds or wind in nature, remember that the same force that is singing through the birds and powering the wind is making your body perform countless complex organ and cellular functions to give you this life. You are not in control of the running of your body, the life or god force is. You do not have to tell your heart to beat or your liver to function. The body works 24/7, and you get to experience the joy of living in the sacred space of your body, without handling all of the millions of details that your body takes care of automatically.

Listen again to the birds or any music or sounds around you without labeling or judging them. Observe the feeling of the breath moving in and out of you. Feel the connection to the forces of life and cultivate a sense of gratitude for the wonderful gift that is your life. Life flows like a river and we are all part of the flow. Continue to focus on the experience of feeling and being. When thoughts come that distract you back to the past or forward into the future, simply observe the thoughts as you would your breath, then return to the 5 B's. Be aware of the consciousness in the space between your thoughts. Observe yourself observing your thoughts and do nothing but the practice of being aware without judgement or opinion. Simply watch and observe your entire being in the moment, as you listen to the sounds of nature. Stay in the "Rest Pose" for 10 to 20 minutes and soak up the deep inner peace that comes to you when you reside in the present moment.

The five B's: body, breath, birds, breeze, and being.

Do not forget to hear the bees buzzing too.

"Namaste" and aloha,

Michaelle

YogAlign Postures

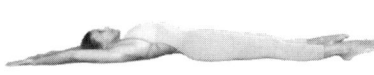

#1 Full Body Stretch

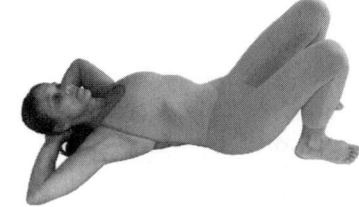

#2 Reclining Breath Tuning

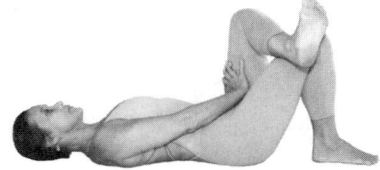

#3 PNF Hip Recalibrator

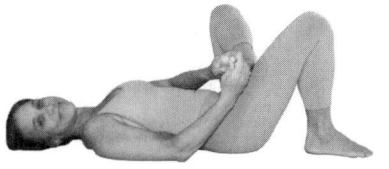

#4 Reclining Foot Massage

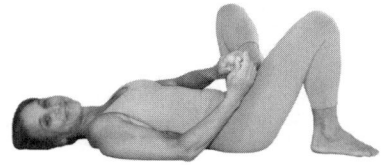

#5 Toe Weave and Foot Shake

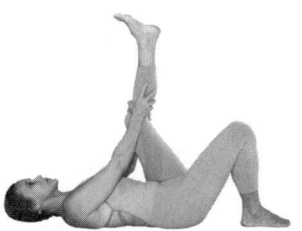

#6 Leg Massage

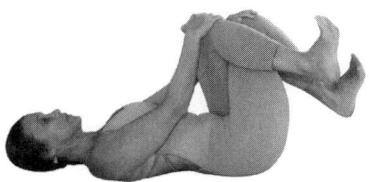

#7 Thigh Squeeze

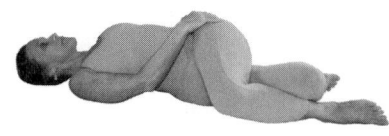

#8 Twist Massage

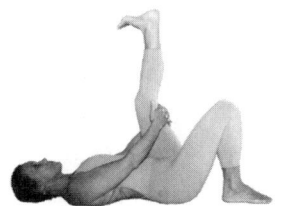

#9 Leg and Foot Recalibrator

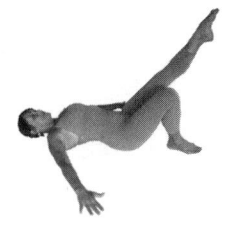

#10 Core Connector

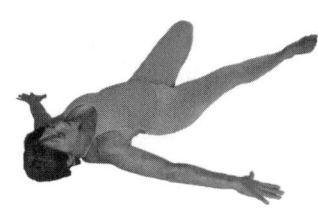

#11 Leg Circles/Hip Lubricator

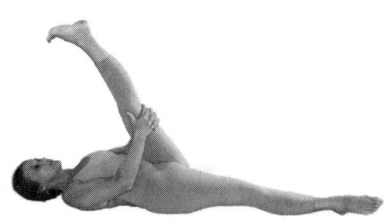

#12 Leg Wrestle

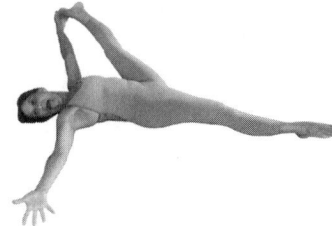

#13 Star

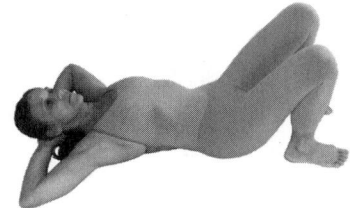

#14 SIP-Ups

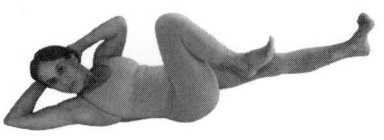

#15 Bicycle SIP-Ups

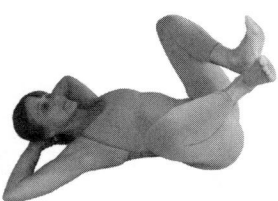

#16 Core Synergizer

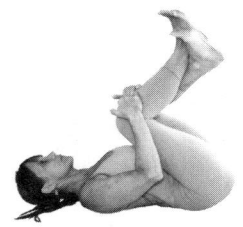

#17 Spinal Rolls

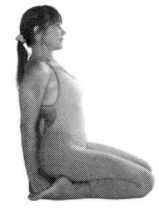

#18 Arch Tuner and Ankle Roller

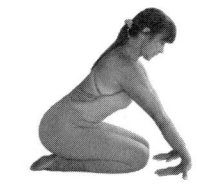

*#19 Wrist Opener &
Arm Massage*

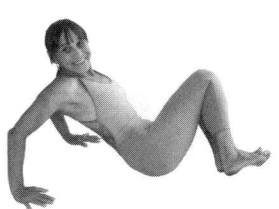

#20 Rotator Rolls

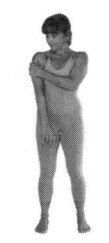

#21A Self-Massage Tune-Up

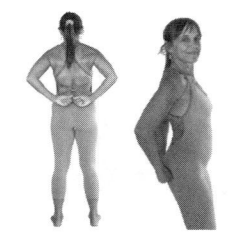

#21B The Poi Pounder

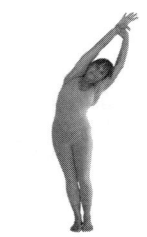

#22 Swaying Tree

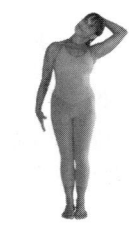

#23 Neck Elongator

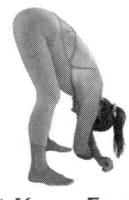

#24A Bent Knee Forward Bend

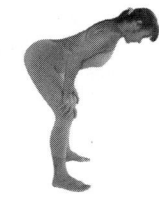

#24B Half Forward Bend

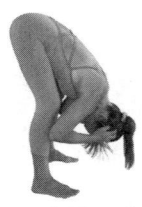

#25 Inverted Head Massage

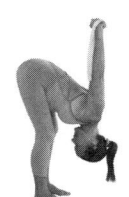

*#26 Inverted Shoulder
Balancer*

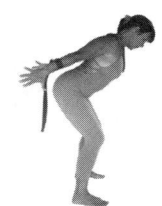

*#26B Half Inverted Shoulder
Balancer*

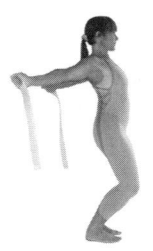

#27 The Rainbow

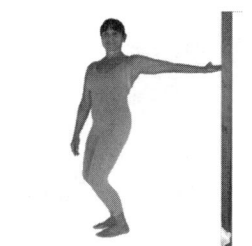

#27C Shoulder Arm Tune-Up

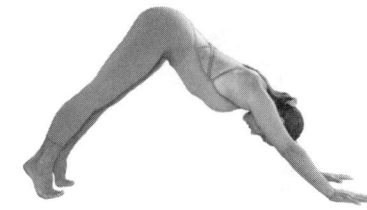

#28 High Dog

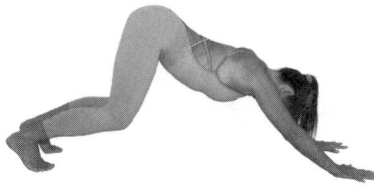

#29 Traction Dog

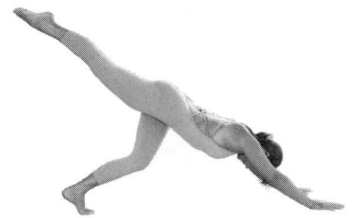

#30 Core Dog

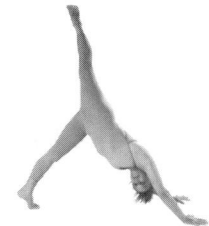

#31 Psoas Dog

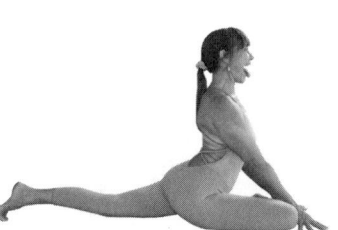

#32A Cobra Pigeon

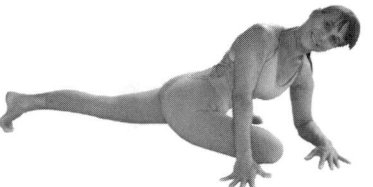

#33 Twisting Pigeon

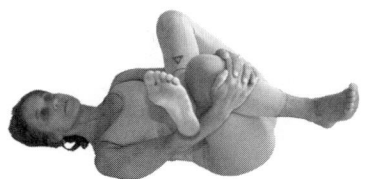

#34 Reclining Pigeon

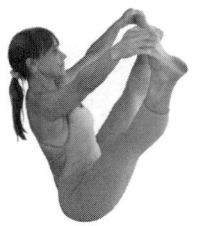

#35 Open Boat

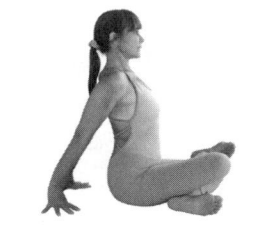

#36A PNF Hip-Balancer

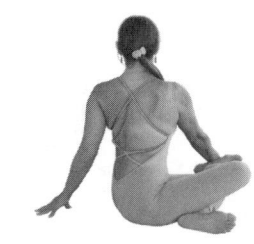

#36B Twisting Hip-Balancer

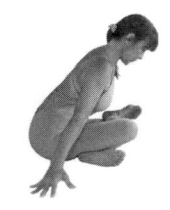

*#36C Forward Bend
Hip-Balancer*

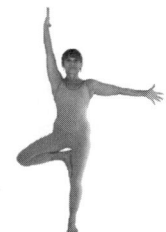

#37 Tree

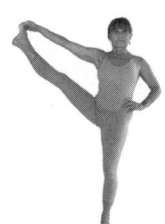

#38 Tree Star

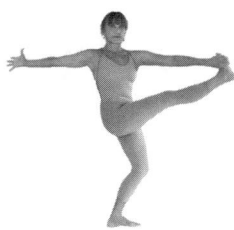

#39 Twisting Tree

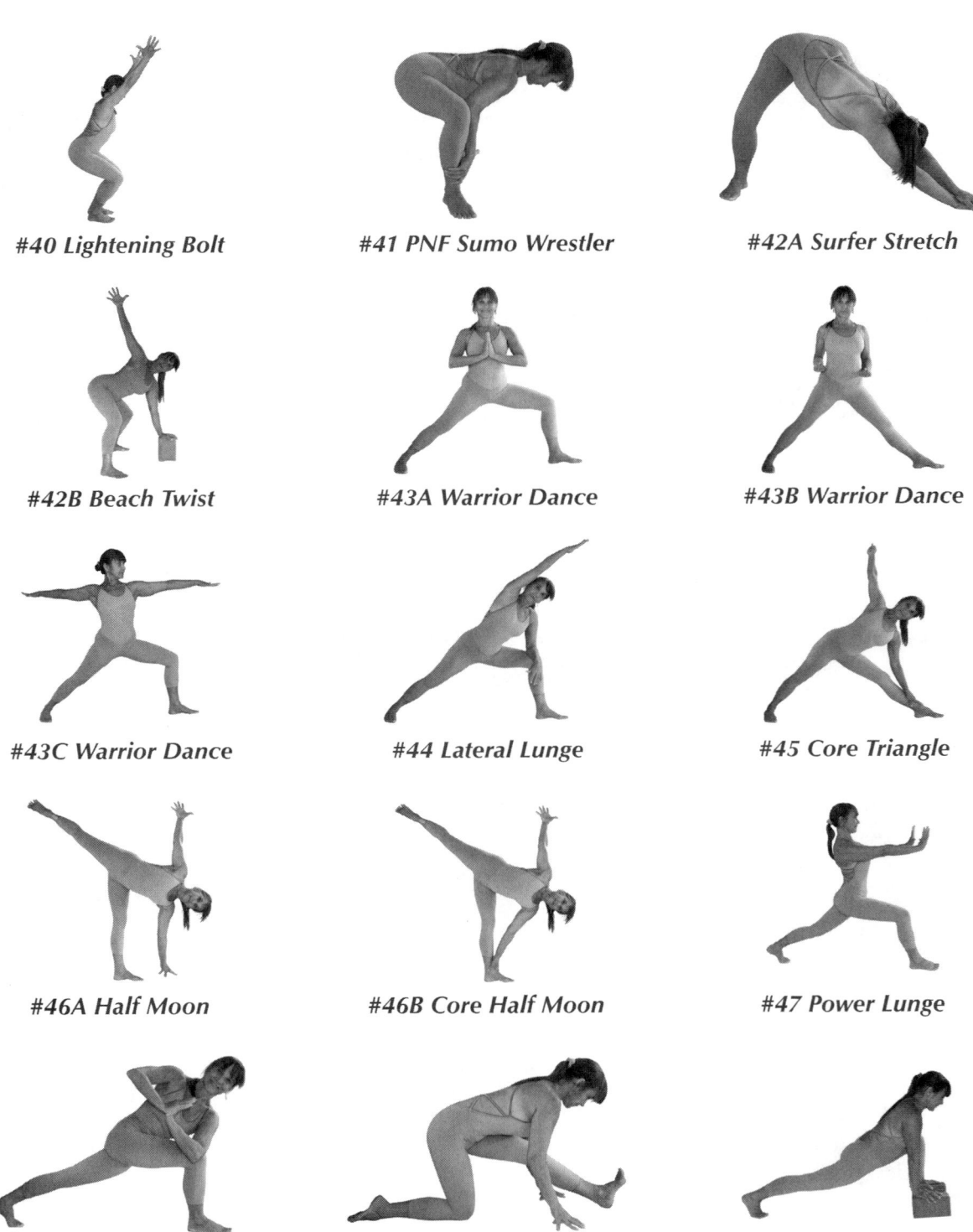

#40 Lightening Bolt

#41 PNF Sumo Wrestler

#42A Surfer Stretch

#42B Beach Twist

#43A Warrior Dance

#43B Warrior Dance

#43C Warrior Dance

#44 Lateral Lunge

#45 Core Triangle

#46A Half Moon

#46B Core Half Moon

#47 Power Lunge

#48 Twisting Lunge

#49 Half Split

#50A Runner's Lunge

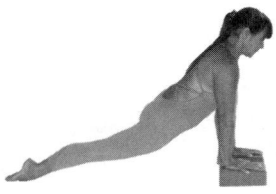

#50B Psoas Lunge

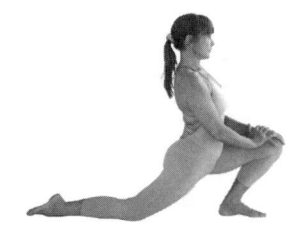

#50C Upright Psoas Lunge

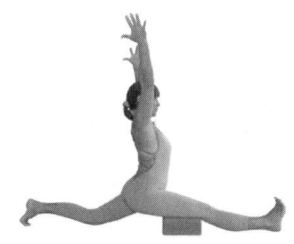

#51A Whole Body Recalibrator

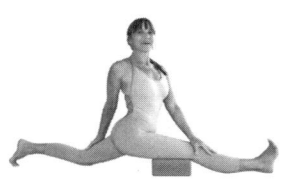

#51B Twister

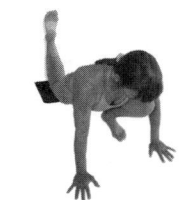

*#52A Quad Recalibrator,
forward*

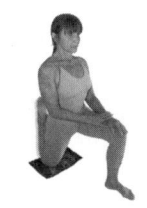

*#52B Quad Recalibrator,
upright*

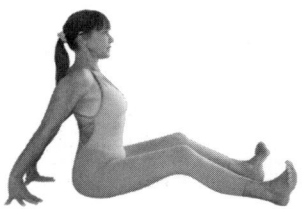

#53A Spine Aligner

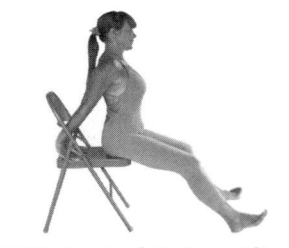

#53B Seated Spine Aligner

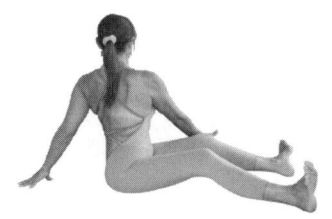

#54A Twisting Spine Aligner

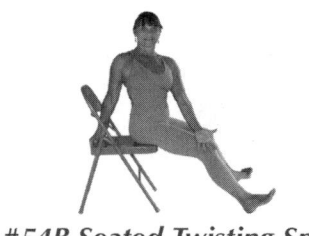

*#54B Seated Twisting Spine
Aligner*

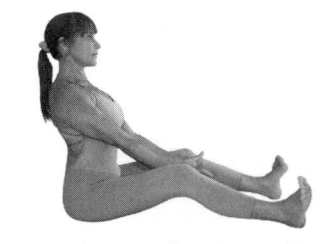

#55 Advanced Spine Aligner

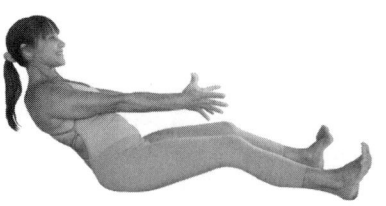

#56 Rocking Spine Aligner

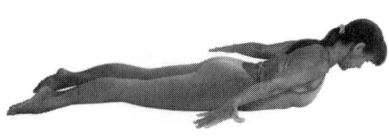

#57 The Glider

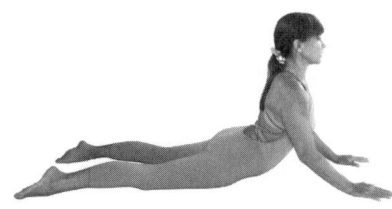

#58 Cobra

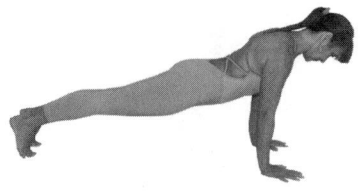

*#59 High to Low
Push-Ups*

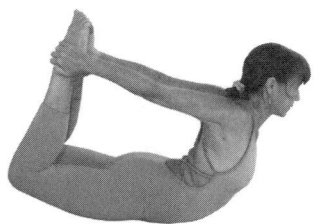

#60 Rocking Bow

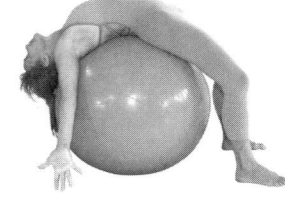

#61 Backbend on a Ball

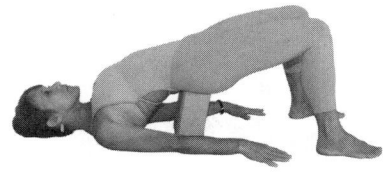

#62 Supported Bridge

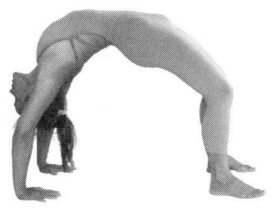

#63 Wheel

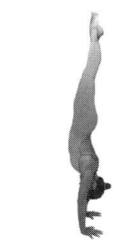

#64 Handstand

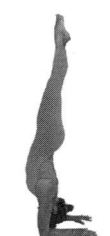

#65 Forearm Stand

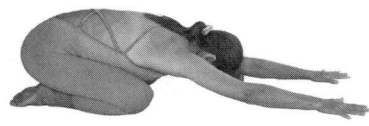

#66A Active Child's Pose

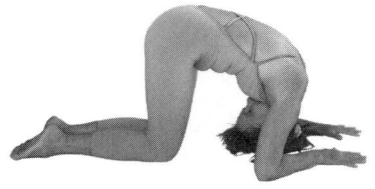

#66B Neck Rolls

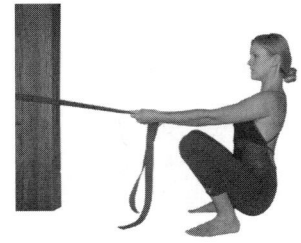

#67A Monkey Squat with Strap

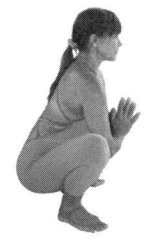

#67B Monkey Squat

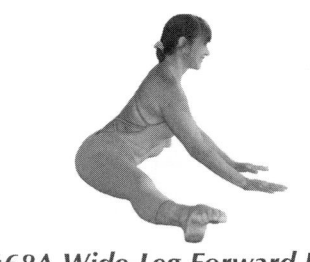

#68A Wide-Leg Forward Bend

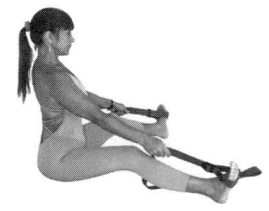

#68B Spine Traction to Forward Bend w/Strap

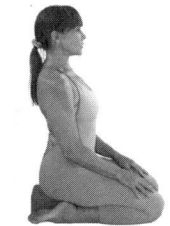

#69 Meditation

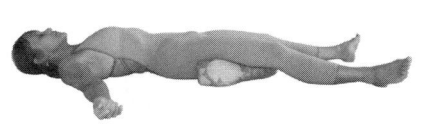

#70A Rest Pose

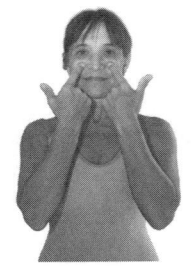

#70B Face Massage

POSTURES NOT RECOMMENDED FOR SAFETY REASONS

Incorrect Positions and Reasons Why You Should Avoid Doing Them

The following images are for viewing only and are not recommended as part of a yoga practice.

Down Dogs Can Be Bad Dogs

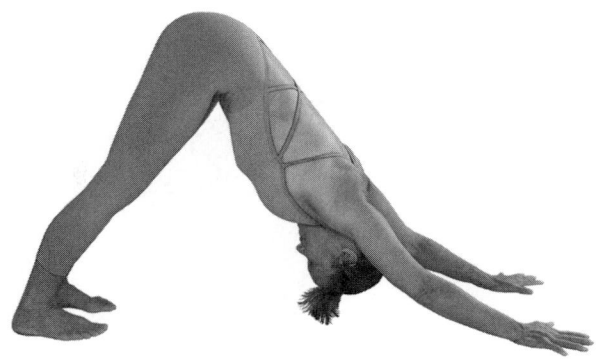

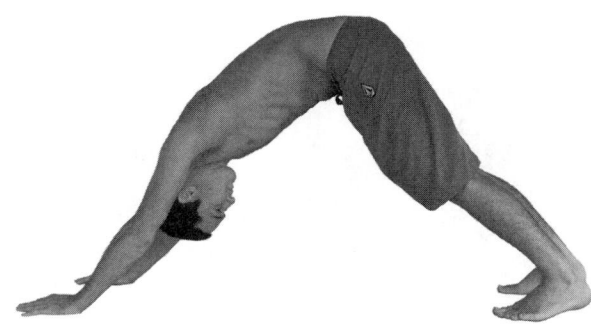

Hanging in the ligaments

Pushing the chest too far forward hanging from the shoulder and knee ligaments causes excessive overstretching of the support structures of the shoulder, lower back spine and knees. In the long term, joints are destabilized and weakened.

Spine compression in the right angle

Pushing down the heels puts excessive pressure upon the discs, compressing the spine. This will not lengthen the hamstrings.

The Spine Compressors

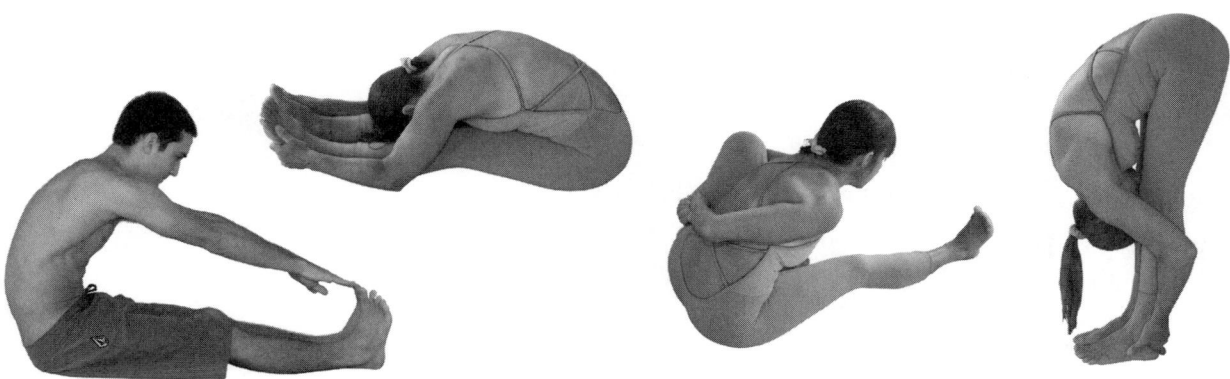

Contracting (shortening) the front to stretch your sore back makes no anatomical sense as the cause for the sore back is a short or weak front body. This contraction trades a short-term, false sense of stretching for long-term instability in the spine. Whether you engage in this straight-kneed, forward-bent posture while standing or sitting, the discs in the anterior spine are being compressed, and the spinal and sacral ligaments along the entire back line of the body are being overstretched.

The Neck Crunchers

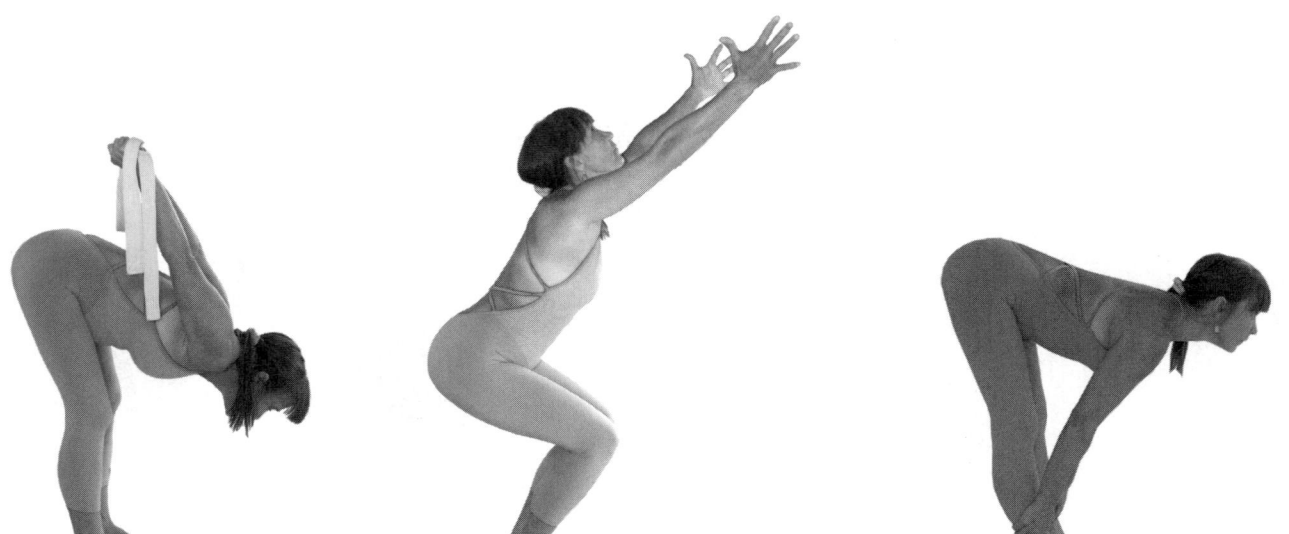

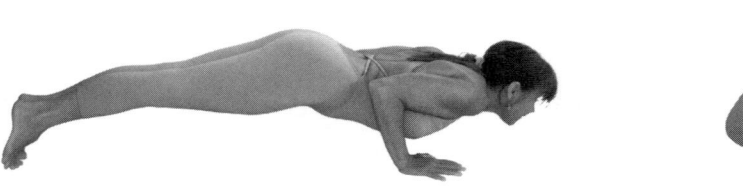

Leading with the chin reinforces forward head carriage while destabilizing the neck and shoulder girdle. Thrusting-forward and leading with the chin in a yoga pose takes you away from centered integrated movement patterns.

Repeated practice of these positions can cause neck spurs and chronic tension in the occipital region at the base of the skull, where your vision and balance centers intersect. Note the alignment in the photos and you will see me leading with my chin, compressing my neck, and shrugging my shoulders around my ears. With repeat practice, these movements reinforce muscle tones that actually inhibit breathing and enforce poor postural habits. These pose versions are multi-tasking at its worst.

Namaste Overhead—
A "Looks-Harmless-But-Isn't" Pose

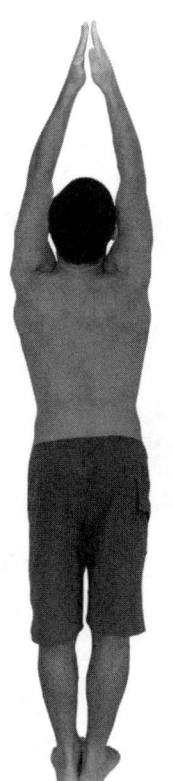

Many hatha yoga classes encourage practice of the sun salutation with a lifted chin, and the hands touching above the head. Although it does not look especially dangerous, hands pressed together overhead is one of the least functional of all body movements. When you try and touch your hands together, your shoulder blades must lift which causes a collapse of your upper chest. This pose cultivates bad posture habits that lead you to move from your extremities instead of from your core center. Avoid this arm movement to prevent poor posture and movement patterns such as forward head carriage, neck tension, hard upper traps, and shoulder joint destabilization. Lifting your chin in this pose habituates leading with the chin, which, as we have seen, is harmful in itself.

The Disc Damage Pose

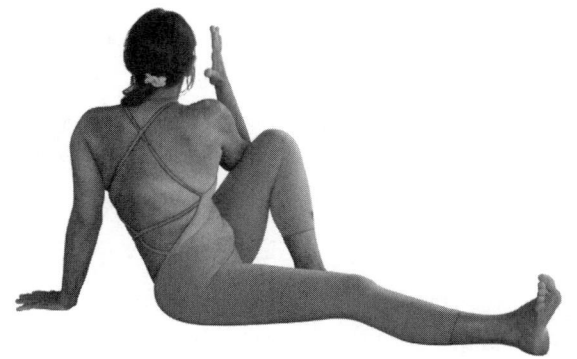

Doing a spinal twist with one or both legs straightened drags the sacrum down and leads to compression of your lumbar vertebrae and overstretching of the sacram-to-hip ligament structures. All four curves of your spine must be in neutral in order for spinal twisting to be beneficial.

Poses That Quickly Age Your Spine

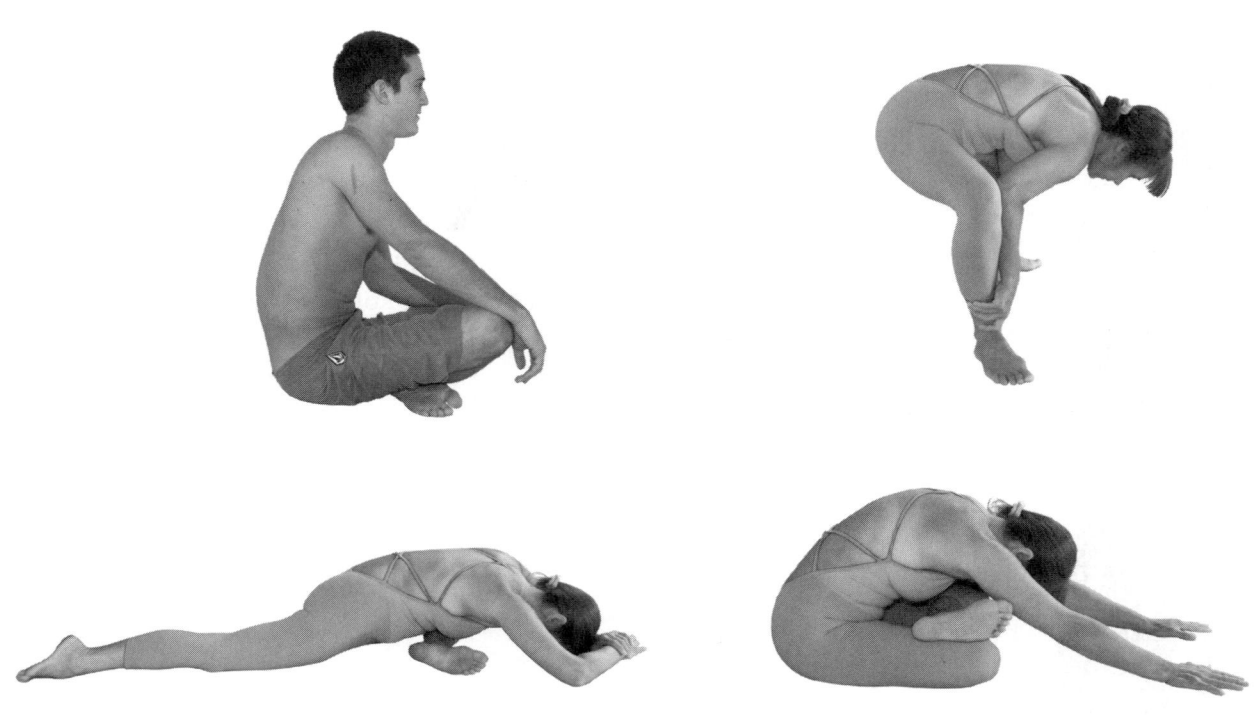

Leaning over your knees with the upper back rounded puts enormous stress on the knee joint and entire spinal column. The biggest danger is that the damage is slow and insidious. Ligament stuctures don't have a lot of pain receptors , so you don't feel your sacral ligaments stretching out until your sacrum sags and you've lost its vital function as a shock-absorber for the spine. You don't notice that your heart and diaphragm are compressed, nor do you sense the constant pressure and overstretching in your knee ligaments. The fact is that bending over with your spine rounded in the upper-back area will actually reinforce many of the poor posture habits that you are using yoga to try and change. In every pose, notice if you can easily take a deep breath, and always retain awareness of whether or not your body is in good standing posture.

Poses Most People Hate To Do For A Good Reason

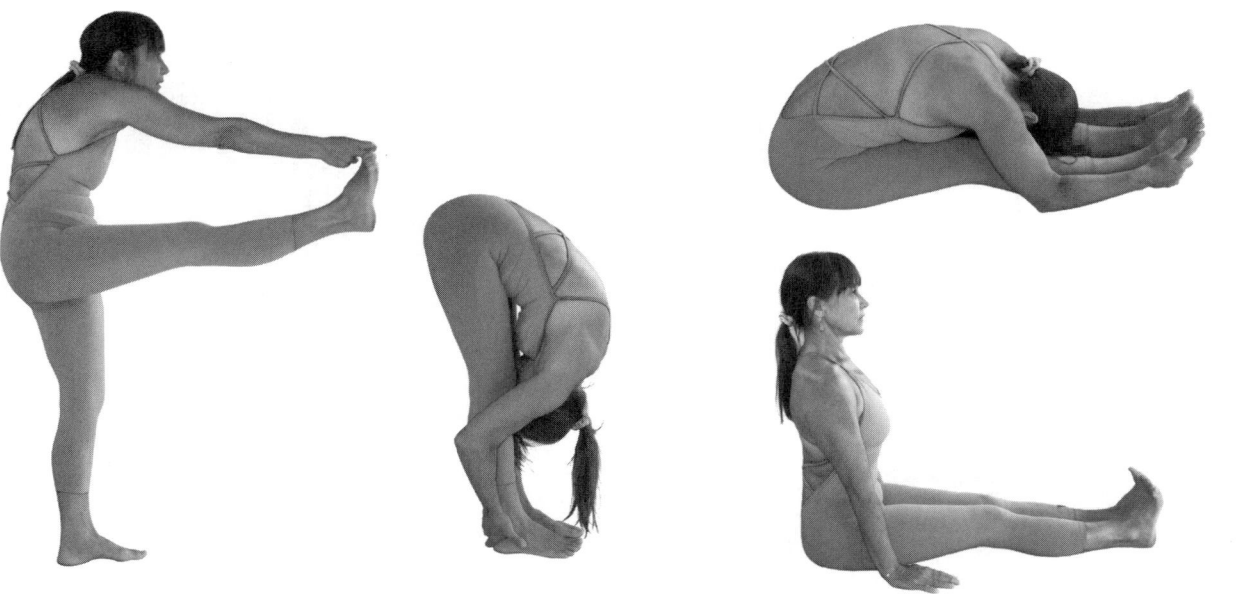

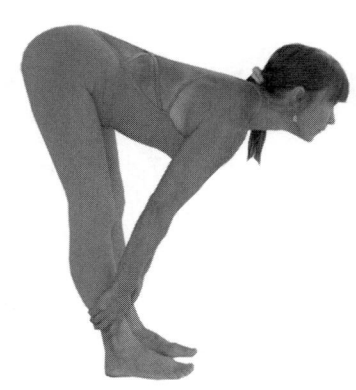

Poses in which you keep both knees straight at once are not natural for the human body and have no biomechanical value. Remember that keeping both knees straight engages fascial pulleys that send strain and tension to the lower back, leading to destabilization of the sacral platform. Keeping our knees straight also encourages us to rely upon our extremities (and not our core) for balance. The oft-repeated (and misinformed) direction to keep our knees straight in these poses only leads to compression and rounding in the spine. Engaging the body in this position weakens the ligaments of the spine, hips, and knees while compressing the anterior portions of the spinal discs.

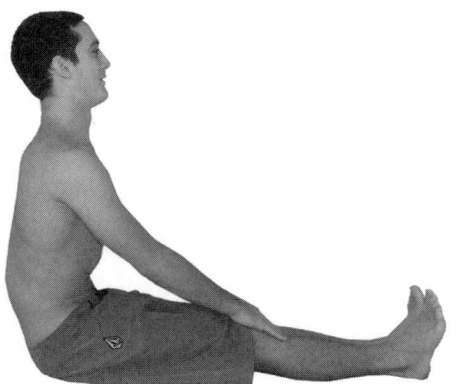

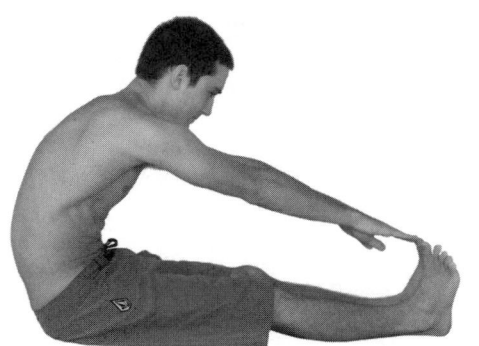

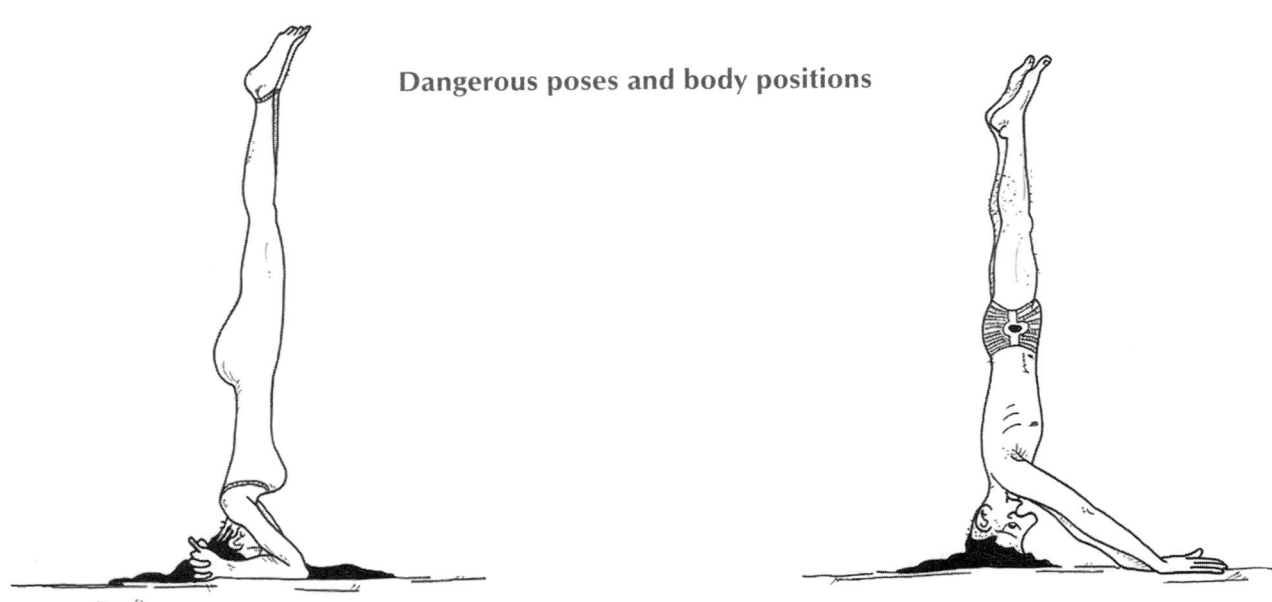

Dangerous poses and body positions

The headstand is a very risky pose that I do not recommend in the YogAlign method, as the risks definitely outweigh the benefits. Carrying the entire weight load of the lower body on the fragile neck spine is playing Russian Roulette with your spinal health. There are safer ways to create inversions and tractions of the neck and upper body that do not carry the dangers associated with these positions.

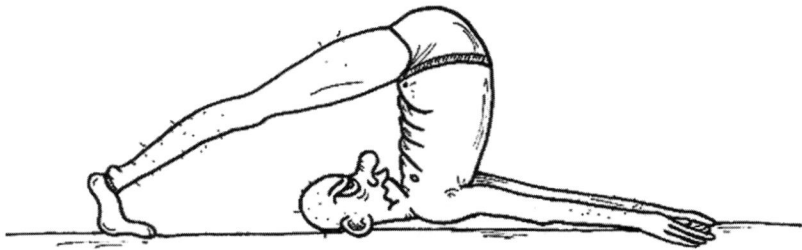

In these drawings are examples of poses so highly dangerous that I won't even demonstrate them. Plow, head, and shoulder stands have caused many yoga injuries including disc herniation, bone spurs, nerve impingement, compression fractures, and overstretching of the important neck and back ligaments that stabilize your spine. These poses and can even cause a stroke from the constriction of the carotid artery. Leave the plow in the field.

If you have ever suffered a yoga injury or you know someone who has, please go to
www.yogainjuries.com and take a survey about your yoga injury.
The goal is to create a data bank of information for yogis to get the facts on what poses are causing
injuries, as well as the circumstances surrounding (and severity of) these injuries.
In the future we hope to publish the results and establish a baseline of information about yoga injuries.

BIBLIOGRAPHY

Adler, Susan S., Beckers, D., Buck, M. <u>PNF in Practice</u>. Wurzburg, Germany: Springer Medizin Verlag, 2008.

Bernard, A., Steinmüller, W., Stricker, U. <u>Ideokinesis: A Creative Approach to Human Movement and Body Alignment</u>. Berkeley, CA: North Atlantic Books, 2006.

Biel, Andrew R. <u>Trail Guide to the Body: How to Locate Muscles, Bones and More,</u> 3rd ed. Boulder, CO: Books of Discovery, 2005.

Bond, Mary. <u>The New Rules of Posture</u>. Rochester, VT: Healing Arts Press, 2007.

Calais-Germain, Blandine. <u>Anatomy of Breathing</u>. Seattle, WA: Eastland Press, Inc., 2006.

Calais-Germain, Blandine. <u>Anatomy of Movement</u>. Seattle, WA: Eastland Press, Inc., 1993.

Couch, Jean. <u>The Runner's Yoga Book.</u> Berkeley, CA: Rodmell Press, 1990.

Cranz, Galen. <u>The Chair: Rethinking Culture, Body, and Design</u>. New York, NY: W.W. Norton & Company, 1998.

Desikachar, T.K.V. <u>The Heart of Yoga</u>. Rochester, VT: Inner Traditions International, 1995.

Dominguez, Richard H., M.D. and Gajda, Robert, PhD. <u>Total Body Training</u>. East Dundee, IL: Moving Force Systems, 1982.

Halpern,Brian, M.D. <u>The Knee Crisis Handbook</u>. Rodale Press, 2003.

Hanna, Thomas. <u>Somatics: Reawakening the Mind's Control of Movement, Flexibility, and Health</u>. Da Capo Press (Perseus Books Group), 1988.

Farhi, Donna. <u>The Breathing Book: Vitality & Good Health through Essential Breath Work</u>. New York, NY: Henry Holt and Co., 1996.

Franklin, Eric. <u>Pelvic Power: Mind/Body Exercises for Strength, Flexibility, Posture, and Balance</u>. Hightstown, NJ: Princeton Book Company, 2003.

Iyengar, B.K.S. <u>Light On Yoga</u>. New York, NY: Schocken Books, 1996.

Keller, Doug. <u>Yoga As Therapy</u>. DoYoga Productions, 2006.

Koch, Liz. <u>The Psoas Book</u>. Felton, CA: Guinea Pig Publications, 1997.

Lasater, Judith. <u>Yogabody: Anatomy, Kinesiology, and Asana</u>. Berkeley, CA: Rodmell Press, 2009.

Lasater, Judith. <u>What We Say Matters</u>. Berkeley, CA: Rodmell Press, 2009.

Lasater, Judith. <u>Yoga Abs: Moving from Your Core</u>. Berkeley, CA: Rodmell Press, 2005.

Menezes, Allan. <u>The Complete Guide to Joseph H. Pilates' Techniques of Physical Conditioning</u>. Alameda, CA: Hunter House Inc., 2004.

Miller, Elise Browning. <u>Yoga for Scoliosis</u>. Shanti Productions, 2003.

Myers, Thomas W. <u>Anatomy Trains</u>, 2nd ed. Edinburgh; New York: Churchill Livingstone Elsevier, 2009.

Neihardt, J.G. <u>Black Elk Speaks</u>. Lincoln, NE: University of Nebraska Press, 1979.

Novak, Janice, M.S. <u>Posture, Get it Straight!</u>, 2 ed. Andover, MN: Expert Publishing, Inc., 2006.

Porter, Kathleen. <u>Ageless Spine, Lasting Health</u>. Austin, TX: Synergy Books, 2006.

Long, Raymond, M.D., FRCSC. <u>Scientific Keys Volume I: The Key Muscles of Hatha Yoga</u>. Bandha Yoga, 2006.

Schatz, Mary Pullig, M.D. <u>Back Care Basics: A Doctor's Gentle Yoga Program for Back and Neck Pain Relief</u>. Berkeley, CA: Rodmell Press, 1992.

Schiffman, Erich. <u>Yoga: The Spirit and Practice of Moving into Stillness</u>. New York, NY:, Pocket Books, 1996.

Schultz, R. L., PhD, Feitis, Rosemary, D.O. <u>The Endless Web: Fascial Anatomy and Physical Reality</u>. Berkeley, CA: North Atlantic Books, 1996.

Selby, John. <u>Seven Masters, One Path: Meditation Secrets from the World's Greatest Teachers</u>. New York, NY: Harper Collins, 2003.

Singleton, Mark. <u>Yoga Body: The Origins of Modern Posture Practice</u>. New York, NY; Oxford: Oxford University Press, 2010.

Todd, M.E. <u>The Thinking Body</u>. Hightstown, NJ: Princeton Book Company, 1937.

RECOMMENDED PRODUCTS

Sitting in chairs is, in general, not promotive of good posture. It is recommended that you try to create a working environment that allows you to move around regularly. If you are desk-bound, consider creating an elevated workspace that allows you to perch at a half-standing/barstool height. Sitting on large exercise balls is an economical alternative to sitting in a traditional chair. You can still slouch in any chair so make sure to use the tools from the Spine Aligner poses to align using the movements of breathing. Best to avoid sitting in general but if you have to sit for long periods, here are some of the best chair alternatives availalble.

POSTERS OF THE FASCIAL LINES AND THE *ANATOMY TRAINS* BOOK

I highly recommend purchasing the book *Anatomy Trains* by Rolfer and educator, Thomas Myers. Available to buy from the website are large posters of the Fascial trains, books, DVDS, podcasts and articles. His website is a wealth of information on Fascial Tensegrity, Spacial Medicine, KQ (Kinesthetic Intelligence) and Physical Education for the 21st Century. Workshops, certification, and podcasts are available to anyone seeking to learn more about anatomy from a global perspective from Myers, the leading expert in fascial anatomy. Anatomy Trains is an important tool and reference center for body workers, movement educators, fitness trainers, yogis, and anyone interested in the function and structure of the human body.

www.anatomytrains.com
Kinesis Inc.
318 Clarks Cove Rd
Walpole, Maine 04573
888-546-3747

CHAIRS FOR OFFICE WORK

The Swopper chair: http://www.swopper.com/
HAG Capisco chair: http://www.ergodepot.com/HAG_Capisco_p/8106.htm
Salli Multi-Adjuster: http://salli.com/en/Products/Chairs/Salli+MultiAdjuster
Aeron chair by Hermann Miller: http://www.hermanmiller.com/Products/Aeron-Chairs

CAR AND TRAVEL

LumbAir back support products for driving: www.colonialmedical.com

EXERCISE, SPORTS AND YOGA

Expand-A-Lung breath-inhibition tool: http://www.expand-a-lung.com/

INDEX

[Index created with TExtract / www.Texyz.com]